Drug Discovery for
Nervous System Diseases

Drug Discovery for Nervous System Diseases

Franz F. Hefti, Ph.D.
Rinat Neuroscience Corporation
Palo Alto, California
and
Department of Neurobiology
University of California, San Diego
La Jolla, California

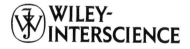
WILEY-INTERSCIENCE

A John Wiley & Sons, Inc., Publication

For general information on our other products and services please contact our Customer Care Department
within the U.S. at 877-762-2974, outside the U.S. at 317-572-3993 or fax 317-572-4002.

Wiley also publishes its books in a variety of electronic formats. Some content that appears in print, however,
may not be available in electronic format.

Library of Congress Cataloging-in-Publication Data is available.

ISBN 0-471-46563-1

10 9 8 7 6 5 4 3 2 1

Contents

Preface

Drug discovery has evolved to a complex, distinct process that engages many thousands of scientists, physicians, legal experts, and business specialists. The start of the first review journal *Nature Reviews Drug Discovery* in 2001 illustrates that the discipline has only recently gained adequate recognition as a unique effort that is separate from basic science. There are very few academic courses or textbooks that prepare for this activity. This volume attempts to fill part of this need, by providing the first introductory textbook to the drug discovery in the neurosciences. It is written for individuals who seek or have professional engagement in biotech and pharmaceutical companies, or in academic research groups involved in drug discovery research. It assumes that the readers have the basis of undergraduate education in general biology or physiology.

The neurosciences are a particularly difficult field for drug discovery, because of the complexity of the nervous system and the poor understanding of most psychiatric and neurological diseases. The currently available drugs were, in their majority, found by chance observations. A radical revolution is under way that reflects the enormous progress in molecular biology and several breakthrough discoveries of genes that cause nervous system diseases. Reflecting this progress, the book is organized by diseases and not by classes of existing drugs or molecular drug targets, as are most traditional books of pharmacology. While providing a historical perspective as necessary and useful, the chapters of this book emphasize the present and the future. It reflects the radical changes in drug discovery over the recent years and is written in the optimistic anticipation of rapid further progress.

Drug discovery and investigational science are community efforts. This book reflects thoughts and contributions of many colleagues for which I am very grateful. I wish to thank, in particular, those individuals with whom I have interacted closely over prolonged periods of time and who have profoundly influenced my thinking: Tajrena Alexi, Raymond Baker, Yves Barde, John Barrett, Michael Baum, Klaus Beck, Gene Burton, Jose Luis Castro, Charles Cohen, Alun Davies, Ariel Deutch, Millicent Dugich, Albert Enz, Caleb Finch, Beat Gähwiler, Bruce Glaeser, Hannes Gnahn, Menek Goldstein, John Growdon, Sarah Harper, Jukka Hartikka, Rolf Heumann, Ray Hill, Leslie Iversen, Beat Knusel, Vassilis Koliatsos, Heinrich Langemann, Paul Lapchak, Walter Lichtensteiger, Jeffrey McKelvy, Thomas McNeill, Eldad Melamed, Patrick Michel, William Mobley, Michael Moskowitz, Karoly Nikolics, Fukuichi Ohsawa, Doug Pettibone, Heidi Phillips, Scott Pollack, Donald Price, Ian Ragan, Cynthia Rask, Scott Reines, Arnon Rosenthal, Michael Rosenthal, David Shelton, Tracey Shors, Eric Shooter, Elliott Spindell, Hans Thoenen, Mark Varney, Jean-Marie Vigouret, Patricia Walicke, William Weiner, Hans-Rudolf Widmer, Bruno Will, and Richard Wurtman.

Thanks belong to my wife, Zena, for her understanding and support over many years of a life in science and drug discovery. I wish to acknowledge the National Parkinson Foundation and its president, Nathan Slewett, who have provided support for my academic research and been a source of motivation during many years. Drug discovery in the neurosciences is the professional passion of my life, because of scientific curiosity about our brains and the desire to help people suffering from nervous system diseases. Writing this book has been a very pleasurable experience. I am grateful to Luna Han, the editorial manager, for making it possible and for guiding me through the process.

Chapter 1

Introduction

Searching for drugs to influence the brain and nervous system is a fascinating and rewarding human activity. Many devastating and disruptive ailments that afflict humanity are diseases of the nervous system. Effective drugs are needed to relieve the often extreme human suffering. The brain is the seat of the human self, identity, and consciousness. Drugs that influence specific aspects of brain function will help us understand ourselves and conjecture the potential of humankind in this universe. Recreational drugs, street drugs, and drugs of abuse are part of modern society. Understanding how they work will shape the discussion concerning which ones to tolerate and how to prevent the use of the unacceptable ones. Hardly any conceivable human activity can compete with the broad spectrum of medical, philosophical, and societal topics touched by drug discovery for diseases of the brain.

Nervous system diseases have beleaguered humanity throughout history. In modern times most, if not all, of them continue to represent major unmet medical needs. Psychiatric diseases have been documented in antiquity and continue to disrupt the lives of the victims, their families, and whole communities. Schizophrenia impairs the ability to think coherently and distinguish between imagination and reality. Depression causes patients to become a burden to themselves and the people around them. Neurological diseases have become even greater problems in modern societies because of the increased human life span. Alzheimer's disease gradually destroys the brain physically and reduces active, elderly men and women to a primitive stage of cerebral function. Ischemic stroke in the brain brings severe disability and is one of the major causes of death. Drugs are needed to prevent, treat, and cure these diseases.

The human brain defines our place in the universe. What we are able to perceive, comprehend, and influence is determined by the brain and its ability to enhance its own function with devices. The quest to understand our brain, the research field "Neuroscience" bridges science and philosophy. Drugs affecting brain function will thus help us to understand our thought processes and our place in this universe. Drugs that modify specific mechanisms or specific subsystems of the brain are powerful experimental tools for neuroscience research. Drugs that alleviate pain such as morphine, aid in understanding the sensory nervous system. Drugs effective in depression help to identify the neuronal pathways that regulate emotional functions. We expect to find drugs that cure schizophrenia. They will assist in the quest to understand our thought and decision-making processes. We hope to find drugs that improve memory function. They will help in understanding memory mechanisms and in defining the cognitive potential of the human brain. New drugs and

Drug Discovery for Nervous System Diseases, by Franz F. Hefti
ISBN 0-471-46563-1 Copyright © 2005 by John Wiley & Sons, Inc.

information on their mechanisms of action will further accelerate the rapid progress of neuroscience.

Coffee and tea represent the most widely accepted examples of recreational drug use. Many societies tolerate, even encourage, the consumption of alcohol. In these societies problems are discussed and resolved "over a glass of wine." In some societies the consumption of cannabis is discouraged and punished by law, while others, for example earlier Islamic societies, found benefits in cannabis while discouraging the consumption of alcohol. Highly addictive drugs, such as morphine, heroine, and cocaine, destroy human lives and cause armed conflicts and war. We can help prevent these tragedies by understanding the mechanisms of action of the drugs. Research will be able to distinguish between beneficial and detrimental effects of recreational drugs and help society decide which ones to tolerate or to discourage.

1.1   ORIGINS OF NEUROPHARMACOLOGY

Nature has long provided a number of plant products that change nervous system function and behavior. Ethanol was most likely the first "neuroactive" drug utilized by early peoples. Through controlled fermentation it could be produced in reproducible ways and used for recreational and medical purposes. In Greek mythology, Dionysus, the son of the supreme god Zeus, conferred the art of winemaking to humans expressly as a gift of the gods to bring more joy to their lives. In many cultures, ethanol in beer, wine, and other fermented beverages has facilitated social contacts and interactions. Alcoholic beverages have been used to increase courage in battles and war. Besides ethanol, caffeine must have been one of the earliest known neuroactive drugs. Historical documents of China suggest the use of tea several thousand years before the current time. Caffeine-containing plants were probably discovered during prehistoric times and have found widespread use because of the pleasant stimulatory effects and success in fighting fatigue.

The oldest writings from China, Egypt, and Greece contain descriptions of hashish and other products of the cannabis plant, *Cannabis sativa*. They praise the perceived medical benefits for rheumatism, inflammation, and constipation. A wonderful description of recreational use has been ascribed to a poorly known female poet, Mahsati, who lived during the twelfth century in the geographical area of modern Azerbaijan (Gelpe, 1975).

Hashish enlightens the human mind,
An ass becomes who devours it like food.
Eating a little fights sadness,
In stupidity disintegrates who eats too much.

In a remarkably liberal way the poet uses an extended conversation among cognoscenti to portray and proclaim the various cognitive, sensory, and sexual effects of hashish. The precise understanding of the relationship between dose and effect, expressed in the cited segment above, implies that the participants were intimately familiar with the drug and were able to use it in a highly enlightened way.

The first known descriptions of opium, prepared from the seed capsules of *Papaver somniverum*, trace back to at least the fourth century BC. The statue of a poppy goddess (Fig. 1.1) from the Minoan culture on Crete in the Mediterranean is the oldest archeological artifact of human drug use. The euphoric effects of opium, probably also the resulting addiction, must have driven the widespread acceptance as recreational drug. Demand for pleasure and medical uses in the treatment of pain and other ailments has made opium an object for politics and war until recent times. Many other natural products served

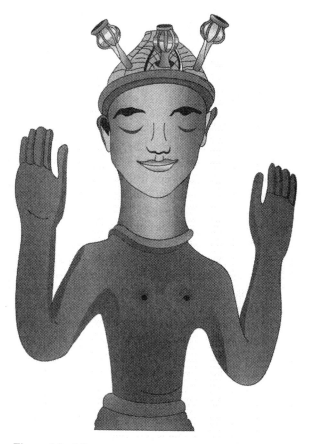

Figure 1.1 Minoan poppy goddess. Opium derived from the seed capsules of the opium poppy was one of the first medically useful drugs. The active ingredient, morphine, and its derivates are widely used for the treatment of severe pain up to this day. The statue is believed to originate from the late Minoan period in Crete, around 1500 to 1400 BC. (Archeological Museum of Heraklion, Greece)

medical and societal purposes. The native people of South America knew well before the times of written history about the beneficial effects of chewing the leaves of the cocoa plant, *Erythroxylon coca*. Hallucinogenic properties of the active ingredient, cocaine, served spiritual and religious purposes. The drug found use to combat hunger and fatigue during journeys or times of starvation. Belladonna, the extract of the fruit of *Atropa belladonna* with the active ingredient atropine, was known in antique times and used as sedative for medical purposes. Its effects on the pupil gave the drug its name "beautiful woman." Belladonna also has the dubious attribute of having been the most frequently used agent to poison people before modern times.

Hallucinogenic drugs were sometimes used on purpose, but often influenced humans and their history inavertedly. Peyote, derived from the cactus *Lophophora williamsii*, that grows in the North American desert, has been used by native Indians as far back as historical knowledge goes. Its stimulatory and hallucinogenic effects are caused by the active ingredient mescaline. In medieval Europe there were several periods when groups of people exhibited strange trance-like behaviors that included burning sensations and hallucinations, sometimes referred to as St. Anthony's fire. Already in the eighteenth century it was speculated that fungus contaminations of rye caused the disease. In modern times it has been discovered that such behaviors are elicited by the active ingredients of the fungus *Claviceps purpurea*, an occasional parasite growing on rye and contaminating the bread of its ignorant victims.

Progress from the naïve use of medicinal plant extracts to scientific understanding occurred only in the nineteenth century. In 1805 Friedrich Serturner, a young pharmacist in Germany, isolated morphine, the active ingredient of opium. Atropine was isolated in 1831, cocaine in 1860, and mescaline in 1897. These substances acting on the nervous system, together with biologically active compounds influencing other organs, helped to establish the new science of pharmacology in Germany, England, and France. Paul Ehrlich, who held academic positions in Berlin and Frankfurt and is often considered the intellectual father of pharmacology, formulated the concept that biologically active chemicals engage in a specific relationship with natural compounds of the body, similar to the relationship of key and lock. Ehrlich and John Langley, Professor at the University of Cambridge, England, used the term receptive molecule, or receptor. The concept that drugs specifically interact with receptor molecules has been the backbone of pharmacological theories since then. The model has been beautifully validated by modern molecular biology. Drugs have been shown to bind to receptors, thereby acting as receptor ligands in a selective way. Drugs bind to receptors with a measurable affinity. They stimulate receptors as agonists or block receptors as antagonists. Modern pharmacology has isolated and characterized the receptors and defined the interactions between drugs and receptors at the atomic level. It remains astonishing that researchers were able to conceive such a fertile theory and accurate predictions more than a hundred years ago.

The receptor concept and the availability of natural neuroactive drugs played an influential role during the formative years of modern neuroscience. A seamless link between neuroscience and neuropharmacology has existed throughout the twentieth century. Most modern textbooks of neuroscience describe the beautiful discoveries of neurons as cellular entities and the mechanisms of synaptic communication. From the point of view of drug discovery, it seems important to point out that Otto Loewi and Henry Dale, the two scientists credited with the discovery of chemical neurotransmission, were pharmacologists. Loewi was Professor of Pharmacology at the University of Graz in Austria, and Dale held the position of Director of the Department of Biochemistry and Pharmacology at the National Institute for Medical Research in London. Neuroactive molecules played a major role in their discovery of the first neurotransmitters, epinephrine, and acetylcholine. The modern concepts of chemical neurotransmission formulated by Loewi and Dale stood on the concepts of ligand—receptor interactions built by the early pharmacologists.

1.2 EXISTING DRUGS FOR NERVOUS SYSTEM DISEASES

Many of the drugs currently used in clinical practice and approved by regulatory agencies continue to reflect the early discoveries of neuropharmacology. While there are a large number of individual chemical entities, they fall into a relatively modest number of categories or drug classes. One or just a few such drug classes treat most diseases. Table 1.1 gives an overview. The table lists the broad psychiatric and neurologic indication areas typically used in textbooks of medicine and the available classes of drugs approved for treatment. The table and the following paragraphs serve as background and introduction for the detailed discussions in the subsequent chapters.

Pain medications are the most widely used and prescribed drugs. Every person has multiple experiences of the unpleasant feelings of pain during a lifetime. Pain sensations

Table 1.1   Major classes of drugs currently approved for the treatment of the most prevalent nervous system diseases

Schizophrenia	Dopamine D$_2$ receptor antagonists
	Clozapine
	Dopamine D$_2$/serotonin receptor antagonists
Depression	Serotonin/norepinephrine uptake inhibitors
	Monoamine oxidase inhibitors
	Lithium
Anxiety disorders	Benzodiazepine drugs
	Serotonin/norepinephrine uptake inhibitors
Alzheimer's disease	Acetylcholinesterase inhibitors
	NMDA glutamate receptor antagonist
Parkinson's disease	L-DOPA/DOPA decarboxylase inhibitors
	Dopamine receptor agonists
Acute brain/spinal cord injury and ischemic stroke	—
Sleep disorders	Benzodiazepine drugs
	Subtype selective GABA receptor ligands
Epilepsy	Benzodiazepine drugs
	GABA uptake inhibitor
	Drugs with unclear mechanism of action (valproate, lamotrigine, gabapentin, and others)
Pain	Nonsteroidal anti-inflammatory drugs (NSAIDs)
	Morphine and opiates
	Gabapentin
Migraine	Ergots alkaloids
	Serotonin receptor agonists

can be transient and irrelevant, when caused by minor injury to the skin, so that treatment of the wound itself is sufficient. More significant injuries that create pain for several days, such as burn injuries, are normally treated with nonsteroidal anti-inflammatory drugs (NSAIDs), compounds with a similar mechanism of action as aspirin. Many different variants of NSAIDs have been introduced into clinical practice over the decades. They differ in efficacy, duration of action, and their propensity to induce adverse effects. NSAIDs cause toxicity to the gastrointestinal system, resulting in gastric bleeding and intestinal injuries, when used over long period of times. Newer drugs with a higher degree of molecular selectivity have been developed to overcome this problem. In some products the older less selective drugs have been combined with molecules offering protection to the gastrointestinal surface tissues. NSAIDs are not sufficiently effective for treating highly intense pain. Morphine and its derivatives have thus remained the stronghold for treatment of conditions like severe burns, severe external and internal injuries, and intense pain associated with major surgery. While NSAIDs and morphine derivatives take care of many pain conditions, there evidently is room for improvement. None of the NSAIDs are without adverse effects and morphine derivatives are addictive.

Chronic pain, following neuralgias, nerve injuries, amputations, represents a particularly significant medical need. Besides NSAIDs, and morphine derivatives in extreme situations, gabapentin is prescribed for these conditions. Gabapentin is a remarkable drug that mirrors the difficult waters of neuroscience drug discovery. It is a structural analogue of γ-amino butyric acid (GABA), the principal inhibitory neurotransmitter in the brain, and was initially developed for the treatment of seizures to dampen the neuronal hyperactivity of the seizures. Clinical observations later revealed that gabapentin is effective for the treatment of chronic pain. Research on the mechanism of action failed to confirm a direct link to the GABA transmitter system. For most patients gabapentin does not fully stop the pain, and very high doses have to be prescribed for the beneficial effects. Many research groups have tried to elucidate gabapentin's mechanism of action to improve on it and make the "perfect gabapentin." Success has remained elusive so far. Despite the availability of gabapentin, NSAIDs, and morphine derivatives, chronic pain remains a very significant unmet medical need and a wide-open field for future drug discovery.

Migraine headaches and migraine attacks are a form of pain that can be very disruptive for their victims. Many patients use NSAIDs to reduce pain as the migraine attacks are progressing. Ergotamines were introduced in the first half of the twentieth century for the treatment of acute migraine attacks, most likely based on incidental observations during the widespread use of these compounds for the stimulation of the birth process. They have remained the only effective migraine therapy until the discovery of sumatriptan in the 1990s. Ergotamines affect several neurotransmitter mechanisms, and their mechanism of action has not been fully elucidated. In contrast to the introduction of ergotamines based on chance clinical observations, the discovery of sumaptriptan is one of the very few examples of a currently used drug that emerged from hypothesis-driven, rational drug discovery program. Migraine attacks were linked to abnormal dilatation of blood vessels around the brain, and specific serotonin receptors were identified that regulate cerebral blood flow (Humphrey, 1988). As discussed in more detail in Chapter 15, sumatriptan activates selectively the serotonin receptors of cranial blood vessels. Sumatriptan and its related compounds effectively treat and abort many migraine attacks. Many patients do not respond, however, leaving ample room for improvement and for novel drugs. In addition migraine prevention remains a significant unmet medical need.

Chapters 9 to 14 will be devoted to detailed discussions of drug discovery for neurological diseases, such as Alzheimer's disease, ischemic stroke, Parkinson's disease, sleep disorders, and epilepsy. The current treatment of most neurological disease is very poor. There are no drugs to slow down or stop progressive degeneration of the brain in Alzheimer's disease. Drugs are available that provide very modest improvement of behavioral functions. They increase the function of the neurotransmitter acetylcholine by inhibiting the degrading enzyme acetylcholinesterase (AChE). These AChE inhibitors are extremely toxic at high doses and work through the same molecular mechanism as nerve gases developed before World War II. Better treatment is badly needed to counteract the memory loss and stop the irreversible progression of Alzheimer's disease.

There is no effective treatment to protect nervous system tissue from degeneration following ischemic stroke or acute mechanical injury of the brain or spinal cord. The outcome of a stroke is improved in a small fraction of patients through the use of enzymes that digest the obstructing blood clot. Anti-inflammatory compounds are used to prevent the acute tissue response following mechanical brain or spinal cord injury. Strategies are widely pursued with the goal to prevent the cascade of degenerative events that lead to neuron loss following these injuries, but no such drug has reached clinical practice as yet.

The current therapy of Parkinson's disease represents the outstanding example of rational drug discovery among the drugs for brain diseases. Morphological studies on the brains of Parkinson victims carried out during the middle of the last century revealed a selective loss of neurons in the substantia nigra of the mesencephalon. This was followed by the discovery of dopamine as a neurotransmitter and the realization that dopamine is the transmitter of the substantia nigra neurons. The investigators leading these research efforts realized that therapeutic benefits might be obtained by providing the missing dopamine to the brain (Cotzias et al., 1969; Hornykiewicz, 1973). They identified the precursor of dopamine, L-dihydroxy-phenylalanine (L-DOPA) as the most suitable source for brain dopamine, and this compound indeed spectacularly improved the behavior of Parkinson victims. To avoid adverse effects outside of the brain, it was found necessary to combine L-DOPA with an inhibitor of the enzyme the converts it to dopamine outside of the brain (DOPA decarboxylase). Up to this day L-DOPA/decarboxylase inhibitor combination drugs have remained the cornerstones of therapy for Parkinson's disease. Additional drugs introduced later more directly affect dopamine transmitter systems but, while useful, have not changed the fundamentals of the therapy. Dopamine therapy of Parkinson's disease very effectively alleviates the symptoms. Unfortunately, the efficacy declines over the years and adverse effects emerge, and dopamine replacement therapy does not prevent the underlying disease process. Even in the situation of Parkinson's disease, where effective symptomatic therapy is available, there is a strong need for better drugs without adverse effects and able to stop the progression of the disease.

Sleep disorders and epilepsy are two major neurological disorders for which, fortunately, fairly effective therapy is available at this time. Both the induction of sleep and the block of seizure activity can be achieved by generally lowering brain activity. This somewhat simplistic link explains why often the same drugs serve in the treatment of both conditions. The sedative properties of barbiturates, derivatives of uric acid, were discovered early in the twentieth century. This class of compounds served for many decades as anesthetics, sleep inducers, and anti-epileptic drugs. During the recent decades barbiturates have been gradually replaced by diazepam and related benzodiazepines, because they are safer and do not cause death at higher doses. The sedative properties of the early benzodiazepines were discovered in animal behavioral studies. Only several years later did it became clear that barbiturates and benzodiazepines facilitate the function of GABA receptors in the brain, thus globally increasing the influence of inhibitory neurons and reducing the general level of neuronal excitability. During the recent decade GABA receptors have been fully characterized, and their molecular composition and function are now understood in great detail. Subtypes have been characterized, some of which play a crucial role in the induction of sleep. These subtype selective benzodiazepine receptor ligands have become widely accepted for the treatment of sleep disorders. For the treatment of seizures several new compounds have been introduced, some mechanistically linked to the GABA receptors, others with unknown mechanism of action. While seizures can be treated very effectively with the battery of currently available drugs, they are not ideal. Adverse effects, including sedation and drowsiness, limit their use, particularly in children and patients with severe seizure disorders.

Chapters 6 to 8 address psychiatric diseases in detail. Many of the drugs currently approved for treating mental disorders are descendants of compounds and discoveries made during the middle of the twentieth century. During that time several observations converged to the new hypothesis that neurotransmitter malfunctions in the brain underlie the symptoms of psychiatric diseases. The neurotransmitter role of norepinephrine and serotonin was established in those years. Reserpine, an alkaloid isolated from a plant medically used in India (*Rauwolfia serpentina*) that causes behavioral depression, was found to lower norepinephrine and serotonin levels in the brain. An investigational drug for tuberculosis, iproniazid, unexpectedly elevated the mood of tuberculosis patients. Iproniazid was characterized as inhibitor of monoamine oxidase, an enzyme that degrades norepinephrine and serotonin. A broad search for compounds able to elevate mood generated imipramine, later shown to block the removal of norepinephrine and serotonin from the synapses. Norepinephrine and serotonin, together with related neurotransmitters such as dopamine, were called monoamines or biogenic amines. The described observations provided the basis for the "biogenic amine hypothesis of affective disorders." Imipramine became the first widely used antidepressant.

Following the discovery of imipramine, many other inhibitors of monoamine removal were identified and introduced into clinical practice. Early compounds did not distinguish among the various monoamines and inhibited the removal, or uptake of norepinephrine, serotonin, and the related amines. More specific molecules gradually replaced the nonselective monoamine uptake blockers. Prozac, the best-known antidepressant, selectively blocks the uptake of serotonin. More recently introduced drugs are selective inhibitors of norepinephrine uptake. The current antidepressant drugs, while effective, are not ideal. Their beneficial effects become apparent after several days of treatment only, they are not as effective as desired, and they have adverse effects. Depression is a widespread and sometimes fatal disease. More effective and safer drugs are desperately needed.

Antidepressant drugs are often used to treat the depressive phase of manic-depressive illness. The manic phase responds to benzodiazepine receptor ligands and antipsychotic drugs discussed below. Many patients receive lithium ion (Li^+) therapy, which dampens the manic phase. The efficacy of Li^+ has been discovered in the middle of the previous century by a single investigator using intuitive animal and human experiences (Cade, 1970). Based on animal observations suggesting sedative effects of lithium salts, Cade injected Li^+ to himself, and then to manic patients, confirming the sedative properties. The anti-manic effects were gradually confirmed by other investigators and led to the approval of Li^+ therapy several years later. Li^+ therapy requires monitoring of plasma levels, which limits its widespread use. Despite several decades of intense research, it has not been possible to identify the mechanism of action of Li^+ and to replace it with a safer drug.

Drugs for the treatment of schizophrenia, the antipsychotics, emerged from early antidepressant research programs. Some of the analogues of early antidepressants had strong calming effects in humans and were tried, with success, in schizophrenia patients. Two decades elapsed before it became clear that they are inhibitors of receptors for dopamine. All currently used antipsychotics inhibit a specific subtype of dopamine receptor, the D_2 receptor. Some of the drugs are selective inhibitors of this receptor, another group influences also serotonin and several other neurotransmitter receptors in addition to the primary effect on the D_2 dopamine receptor subtype.

Psychiatric diseases represent a particularly challenging area for drug discovery. The medical need is enormous. The emotional and economic costs for the individuals and society are immeasurable. Depression and schizophrenia have to be considered fatal diseases because of the high suicide rate. Psychiatric diseases, schizophrenia in particular, are stigmatized in most societies. The current treatment of psychiatric diseases is very inadequate. Unfortunately, drug discovery for psychiatric diseases is difficult for several reasons. The diseases are poorly defined with gradual transitions from one disease to the other. Disease mechanisms are poorly understood. Clinical trials tend to be difficult. All psychiatric diseases represent major unmet medical needs.

By necessity, the brief summary of the existing medications for psychiatric and neurological diseases paints a slightly gloomy picture. While some of the diseases can be treated with success, the existing drugs are less than perfect and many diseases remain untreatable. It takes 10 to 15 years from the moment a drug discovery project has been initiated to the approval and marketing of a new drug. This enormous time delay explains why the recent spectacular progress of neuroscience research has yet to manifest itself in new and better drugs that benefit the millions of victims of psychiatric and neurological diseases.

Fortunately, significant progress and major change are expected in the future years and decades. Drug discovery has become a unique and specialized scientific activity. It no longer is an opportunistic offshoot of basic research or incidental clinical observations. New publications and journals attest to the field's relevance and maturity. The rapid progress of both drug discovery technologies and basic neuroscience research has revolutionized neuroscience drug discovery. This book focuses on the modern approaches and provides an outlook for drugs to come. The next chapters (Chapters 2–5) describe the general principles of modern drug discovery, with emphasis on issues specific to the neuroscience area. The subsequent chapters (Chapters 6–15) give a picture of current and future treatment for each of the major nervous system diseases.

REFERENCES

Further Reading

AYD, F.J., and BLACKWELL, B. eds. *Discoveries in Biological Psychiatry.* Lippincott, Philadelphia, 1970.

CADE, J.F.J. The story of lithium. In: *Discoveries in Biological Psychiatry.* F.J. Ayd and B. Blackwell, eds. Lippincott, Philadelphia, pp. 218–219, 1970.

IVERSEN, L.L. *The Science of Marijuana.* Oxford University Press, Oxford, 2000.

PORTER, R., and TEICH, M. *Drugs and Narcotics in History.* Cambridge University Press, Cambridge, 1997.

References

BARCHAS, J.D., BERGER, P.A., CIARANELLO, R.D., and ELLIOTT, G.R. *Psychopharmacology. From Theory to Practice.* Oxford University Press, New York, 1977.

COTZIAS, G.C., PAPAVASILIOU, P.S., and GELLENE, R. Modification of parkinsonism—Chronic treatment with L-DOPA. *N. Eng. J. Med.* 280: 337–345, 1969.

DALE, H.H. The action of certain esters and ethers of choline, and their relation to muscarine. *J. Pharmacol. Exp. Ther.* 6: 147–190, 1914.

EHRLICH, P. On immunity with special reference to cell life. Croonian Lect. *Proc. R. Soc. Lond.* 66: 424–448, 1900.

GELPKE, R. *Drogen und Seelenerweiterung.* Kindler Verlag, Munich, 1975.

FINGER, S. *Origins of Neuroscience. A History of Explorations into Brain Function.* Oxford University Press, Oxford, 1994.

HORNYKIEWICZ, O. Dopamine in the basal ganglia. *Br. Med. Bull.* 29: 172–178, 1973.

HUMPHREY, P.P.A, FENUIK W., PERREN, M.J., CONNOR, H.E., OXFORD, A.W., COATES, L.H., and BUTINA, D. GR43175, a selective agonist for the 5-HT1-like receptors in dog isolated saphenous vein. *Br. J. Pharmacol.* 94: 1123–1132, 1988.

KATZUNG, B.G. *Basic and Clinical Pharmacology.* Appleton and Lange, Norwalk, CT, 6th ed., 1995.

LANGLEY, J.N. *The Autonomic Nervous System.* Heffer, Cambridge, UK, 1921.

LOEWI, O. Ueber humorale Uebertragbarkeit der Herznervenwirkung. *Pflüger's Arch. Physiol.* 189: 201–213, 1921.

Chapter 2

Drug Receptors and the Fundamentals of Pharmacology

Drug discovery for nervous system diseases is an activity at the interface between neuroscience and pharmacology. Drug discovery cannot be discussed without touching on the fundamentals of pharmacology, the science of drugs, named after the ancient Greek word pharmacon, which was used broadly for medication, potion, and poison. Modern pharmacology is an applied science built on the foundations of physics, chemistry, and molecular biology. A most useful and practical definition of pharmacology has been proposed to simply reflect the intentions of and questions asked by pharmacologists (Kuschinsky and Lüllmann, 1972). Why and how does a drug act? How do we find new and better drugs based on this knowledge? This volume addresses both questions for nervous system diseases. This chapter provides a succinct summary of the fundamental knowledge and concepts of pharmacology, as a basis for the subsequent sections on modern drug discovery.

2.1 DRUG RECEPTOR SITES AND DRUG TARGETS

The theory of drug receptors embodies the core of pharmacology. Drugs, whether small organic molecules or large biological molecules, interact in a specific way with molecules of the human body. Drugs can be artificial, newly synthesized compounds, molecules extracted from a natural source, or compounds that have been modified after extraction from a natural source. They are administered to the body and are exogenous with regard to the body. In contrast, drug receptors are endogenous molecules, in most cases proteins. Typical drug receptors are enzymes, receptors of natural signaling molecules, and transporters. In principle, every gene product and every molecule in the human body can serve as drug receptor. Most of the pharmacological theory is based on the assumption that the drug is a small organic molecule and the drug receptor a soluble macromolecule such as an enzyme. The concepts are valid, however, for more complex situations where the drug is a protein, a growth factor, for example, and where the receptor is a membrane-bound macromolecule.

Macromolecules serving as drug receptors may have different sites that can bind drugs, each defining a specific **receptor site** or receptor domain. For example, barbiturates and benzodiazepines bind the GABA-A receptors briefly introduced in Chapter 1 at different sites, although their functional effects are very similar. It is thus necessary to dis-

Drug Discovery for Nervous System Diseases, by Franz F. Hefti
ISBN 0-471-46563-1 Copyright © 2005 by John Wiley & Sons, Inc.

tinguish the barbiturate receptor site from the benzodiazepines receptor site, although the GABA-A molecule is the receptor protein for both types of drugs. To avoid confusion, the term **drug target** has become more frequently used. The GABA-A receptor is the target molecule for barbiturates and benzodiazepines drugs. It contains distinct barbiturate and benzodiazepines receptor sites. Throughout this book the terms drug target and receptor site are used as defined here. The term receptor indicates proteins that recognize naturally occurring, endogenous signaling molecules such as neurotransmitters, growth factors, and hormones. Accordingly, the following formulation represents a precise and modern formulation of the central concept of pharmacology: drugs interact specifically with distinct receptor sites on target molecules.

The currently used drugs in the neurosciences act on different types of targets. A soluble enzyme represents the target for AChE inhibitors used in Alzheimer's disease. Monoamine oxidase, the target of some antidepressant drugs, is a mitochondrial membrane-bound enzyme. The other antidepressant drugs act on transmembrane transporter proteins. The target of standard antipsychotic drugs, the dopamine D_2 receptor, belongs to the large class of G-protein-coupled receptors, transmembrane receptors that recognize many neurotransmitter and hormone signaling molecules and influence a variety of intracellular metabolic pathways. The GABA-A receptors, the target of benzodiazepines drugs used to treat sleep disorders and epilepsy, are transmembrane ion channels. Drugs outside of the neuroscience area use a yet wider spectrum of target molecules. For example, glitazones, drugs useful in diabetes to increase the response to insulin, as well as steroids for inflammation bind to intracellular regulators of transcription. It has to be emphasized that, in principle, any molecule of the body can act as drug target. Soluble enzymes, membrane-bound enzymes, transmembrane G-protein-coupled receptors, transmembrane tyrosine kinase receptors, transmembrane transporter molecules, nuclear transcription factors, and any other molecule in the body can serve as drug target. A single target can contain several drug receptor sites.

Pharmacology encompasses all steps from the administration of a drug to the body of a human or an animal, through the distribution throughout the body, the binding to a receptor site, the effects produced on the target molecule, the downstream actions on molecules, cells and organs influenced by the target to, finally, the effects on the entire body. As for any science, there is a widely accepted body of conventions and terms that serve to describe the essential observations and concepts.

2.1.1   Concentration—Binding Relationship

The specific interaction between a drug and a receptor site ideally follows the mass action law, which describes the interactions between two molecules of determined affinity. Assuming that the receptor concentration far exceeds the concentration of the drug, the following equation describes the drug—receptor site interaction:

$$B = \frac{B_{max} \cdot C}{C + K_D}$$

B indicates the concentration of receptor bound drug. B_{max} indicates the concentration of receptor sites, C the concentration of unbound (free) drug, and K_D the equilibrium dissociation constant.

The fraction of the drug bound to receptor is given by the equation:

$$D = \frac{C}{C + K_D}$$

The relationship between bound drug and receptor site is thus described by a hyperbolical curve (Fig. 2.1A). The K_D corresponds to the concentration of drug at which 50% of the receptors are occupied. Logarithmic transformation is frequently used to describe the relationship, producing the typical sigmoid curves of pharmacology that are most useful to the human eye (Fig. 2.1B).

The molecular features of a receptor site determine the ability of ligands to bind. Chemicals closely related to each other tend naturally to bind to the same binding sites. This self-evident situation provides the basis for modern drug discovery, where thousands of related molecules are evaluated toward the selection of the most potent and suitable one. The historical and technically incorrect term **structure-activity relationship** is used to describe the detailed molecular understanding of the binding of a drug to a receptor site.

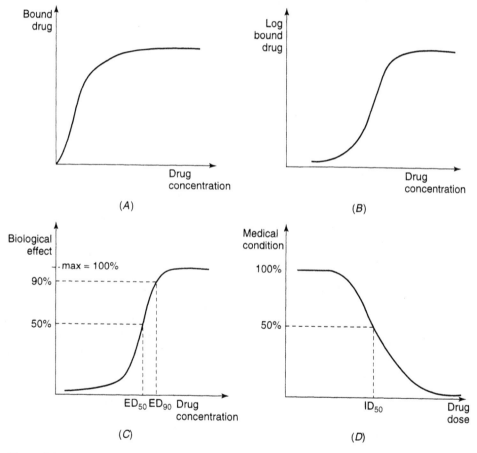

Figure 2.1　Drug concentration–receptor binding, concentration–effect, and dose–response relationship. (**A**) Linear representation of the drug concentration–receptor binding relationship. (**B**) Logarithmic representation of the drug concentration–receptor binding relationship. (**C**) Logarithmic plot of concentration–effect relationship drug stimulating a biological process. The ED_{50} indicates the drug concentration producing a half-maximal response. (**D**) Dose–response relationships observed in vivo. A parameter reflecting the disease condition is measured. The drug concentration producing 50% inhibition is indicated as ID_{50}.

The availability of radioactive high-affinity ligands has made it possible to directly measure binding of the drug to its receptor site. Ligand–receptor binding studies are a highly valuable tool of neuropharmacology and neuroscience. They have played an important part in the identification and characterization of neurotransmitter receptors. Binding of radioactive ligands has allowed the investigators to track receptor proteins during the purification process from crude membrane preparations to more and more pure preparations (Julius, 1991; Gingrich and Caron, 1993). Binding of radioactive ligands to receptors in brain sections serves to determine the anatomical localization of the receptors at the microscopical level (Kuhar et al., 1986). Receptor binding techniques are a very important instrument in modern drug discovery, since they are the simplest method to determine the selectivity of a drug candidate. In these counterscreening techniques, discussed further in Chapter 3, the ability of a drug candidate to displace receptor-specific radioactive ligands from membranes is measured to estimate the affinity to other receptors.

Modern techniques have made it possible to measure the binding of a drug to its receptor site in an intact organism. In optimal drug therapy one would like to limit the drug dose to levels that occupy the receptor sites as needed for the effect, but not beyond that. In other words optimal **receptor occupancy** is the desired goal. All techniques to measure in vivo receptor occupancy require high-affinity ligands tagged with a radioactive label or another group that can be monitored. The ability of a drug candidate to displace the labeled ligand is then being measured. In a technically simple version of these studies, the tissue containing the drug target is removed, and the amount of labeled ligand it contains is measured. With the more complex and modern imaging techniques receptor occupancy measurements can be performed in living organisms. These techniques (to be discussed in more detail in Chapter 5) have and will further revolutionize drug development in the neuroscience field.

2.1.2 Concentration–Effect Relationship

To be therapeutically useful, a drug has to change the function of its target molecule after binding to the receptor site. An inhibitor preventing the catalytic function of an enzyme represents the simplest example. Most drugs in the neuroscience area exemplify more complex circumstances. Binding of a drug to the receptor site of a target protein that functions as neurotransmitter receptor can directly activate this receptor in a similar way as the natural ligand, thus acting as an **agonist**. Alternatively, it can prevent the binding of the natural ligand, acting as an **antagonist**. The functional effect will, under ideal conditions, directly reflect the binding of the drug to the receptor site. Thus the mathematical functions describing the effect of the drug as a dependent of the drug concentration is expected to look the same as that of the concentration–binding relationship. For both, semi-logarithmic transformation is preferred for graphical visualization, and provides the typical sigmoid concentration–effect curves. The concentration at which the half maximal effect is obtained is designated ED_{50}. Sometimes ED_{10} or ED_{90} values are more useful, the concentrations at which, respectively, 10% and 90% of the maximal effect is being generated. When the effect is inhibitory, the terminology uses ID_{50} and related values (Fig. 2.1C).

Concentration–effect curves very often do not overlap with concentration–binding curves, because the relationship between binding and functional changes tend to be complex. The term **receptor–effector coupling** is used to describe this relationship. In the case of an enzyme, the receptor molecule and effector molecule are identical. In the case of a G-protein-coupled receptor the drug receptor site is located on the transmembrane protein, which is coupled by G-proteins to specific effector molecules. Binding of a drug may change the coupling in complex ways, and the response of the effector to the drug does not have to be a linear reflection of binding to the receptor site. One of several complications of the receptor–effector coupling is the phenomenon called spare receptors or **receptor reserve**. When the number of receptors in a cell is equal or even lower to that of the effectors, the number of receptors limits the response to the drug. If, however, the number of receptors is higher than that of effectors, the effector concentration becomes limiting. Only a fraction of the receptors need to be occupied for a maximal effect to occur, and lower concentrations of drugs are required to produce an effect. The concentration–effect curve is shifted to the left.

2.1.3 Dose–Response Relationship and Therapeutic Window

The functional effects of drugs can be measured at any point downstream from the target. From a medical perspective the biological response of the entire body is relevant. In human studies or parallel animal studies, the effect of the drug is measured as a function of the administered dose. The dose–response relationship is a fundamental parameter for each drug. In an ideal situation it reflects the drug concentration–effect and concentration–binding relationships and is thus visualized in a similar sigmoid curve following semilogarithmic transformation. However, as discussed later in this chapter, there are many complex steps between the moment the drug is injected or taken orally and the time an effective concentration is stimulating the receptors. Drug absorption and distribution as well as other pharmacokinetic parameters are major determinants of the resulting position and shape of the dose–response relationship. Drugs acting on the same receptor site can differ in their affinity to the binding site and in their pharmacokinetic properties, producing different dose–response curves. The term **potency** is used to define their relative ED_{50} values and relative position on the concentration axis. The term **efficacy** is used to define the maximal effect produced by any given drug (Fig. 2.1D).

No drug is perfect. Many drugs produce undesired effects at doses necessary to obtain the therapeutically useful actions. Most drugs produce adverse effects or toxic effects at yet higher doses. Some drugs can be fatal when overdosed. The concentration range between doses that produce the desired therapeutic effect and those producing the toxic effects is called the therapeutic window. Up to recent times lethality was used to quantitatively define the toxic effect. The concentration at which 50% of test animals died was determined experimentally and referred to as LD_{50}. The therapeutic window was defined as the concentration range between ED_{50} and LD_{50}. Justified concerns about animal welfare drew attention to the fact the LD_{50} determinations require large numbers of animals and cause substantial suffering. They were largely abandoned and the upper limit of the therapeutic window is now defined as the concentration producing unacceptable toxicity from a human perspective.

2.1.4 Competitive Antagonists and Direct Agonists

Most drugs that inhibit enzymes bind to the natural binding domain of the substrate. They prevent the enzyme from working by competing with the natural substrate. Such drugs are competitive antagonists. A similar situation exists for many G-protein-coupled receptors. For example, the dopamine D_2 antagonists used for the treatment of schizophrenia bind to

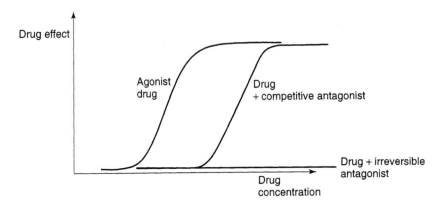

Figure 2.2 Direct agonism and antagonism at a receptor site. The action of an antagonist, given at a single concentration can be overcome by increasing the concentration of the agonist. It is not possible to overcome the inhibition of an irreversible antagonist.

the same binding site as the natural ligand dopamine and prevent dopamine from binding. They are competitive antagonists. Under normal circumstances the action of a competitive antagonist can be overcome by higher concentrations of agonists (Fig. 2.2). In the case of the dopamine receptors, it is possible to replace the natural ligand with drugs that mimic the stimulatory action of dopamine. Such drugs are direct agonists. The dopamine D_2 agonists used in the treatment of Parkinson's disease mimic the action of the natural ligand, dopamine, at the dopamine binding site.

Two special situations are worth mentioning. The first is that of an **irreversible antagonist**. Some antagonists have affinities much higher than that of the natural ligand, making them impossible to displace and rendering them nearly irreversible. Other antagonists may have relatively low affinities but form covalent bonds with molecules at the receptor site, thus permanently blocking the receptor site. The second special case is that of **partial agonists**. The maximal effect product by natural and exogenous agonists does not have to be identical. They can differ in their maximal efficacy produced at concentrations that fully occupy all available receptors. Agonists with a maximal efficacy below that of the natural ligand are called partial agonists.

2.1.5 Allosteric Agonists, Noncompetitive Antagonists, and Inverse Agonists

It is possible to influence the function of a target molecule by acting on receptor sites that are not identical to those recognizing the natural ligand. These binding sites are referred to as allosteric binding sites. The drugs acting on them are allosteric or indirect agonists, or if they have a negative influence, allosteric or noncompetitive antagonists. Several G-protein-coupled receptors are known to bind molecules outside of the natural binding pocket (Fig. 2.3). These allosteric binding sites provide many opportunities for drug discovery and make it possible to identify compounds that influence the function of these receptors in subtle ways.

Allosteric regulates of constitutively active receptors or of ion channels may increase or decrease the downstream signaling. GABA-A receptors, the targets of the benzodiazepines and barbiturate drugs, provide a well-studied example. The neurotransmitter GABA is the natural ligand of the GABA-A receptors, whereas barbiturates and benzodi-

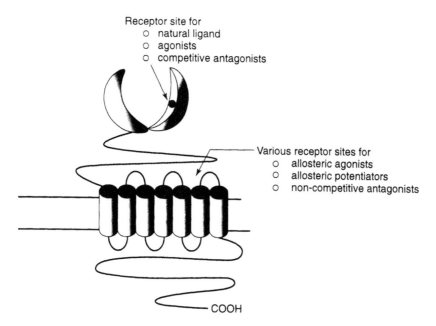

Receptor site for
o   natural ligand
o   agonists
o   competitive antagonists

Various receptor sites for
o   allosteric agonists
o   allosteric potentiators
o   non-competitive antagonists

COOH

Figure 2.3   Binding sites for agonists, competitive agonists, allosteric agonists and potentiators, and noncompetitive antagonists at a G-protein-coupled receptor. (Reprinted with permission, Conn, 2003).

azepines bind each at a specific barbiturate receptor site or benzodiazepines receptor site. Both binding sites are located far from the binding site for GABA. Binding of the clinically used benzodiazepines drugs to the benzodiazepines binding site facilitates the action of the natural ligand GABA. The ion channel opens more frequently and its function is enhanced. The drugs potentiate the action of GABA. They are allosteric agonists acting at the benzodiazepines receptor site. As for every drug receptor site, it is possible to design molecules that inhibit the binding of benzodiazepine site ligands in a competitive way, so-called benzodiazepine receptor antagonists. For this receptor site, they are competitive antagonists. However, for the functionally relevant site, the GABA binding site, they have no functional consequence. It is possible to design ligands for the benzodiazepine receptors site that influence the GABA receptor in the direction opposite that of the allosteric agonists. Such molecules diminish the action of GABA so that the channel opens less frequently. In absence of a better term, the term **inverse agonist** is typically used for these molecules. The terminology, unfortunately, often generates confusion, in particular, related to the GABA-A receptors. Since GABA is an inhibitory neurotransmitter, benzodiazepine receptor agonists, which increase its action, typically inhibit neuronal activity. Inverse agonists, which reduce the inhibitory action of GABA-A receptors, typically stimulate neuronal activity. It is important to remember that inverse agonists are not antagonists at the GABA receptor site. However, inverse agonists can have similar actions as competitive antagonist at the GABA binding site. Figure 2.4 illustrates this somewhat confusing situation.

The discovery of an allosteric binding site typically triggers the search for a natural ligand to this site. Very often this search is not successful. It does not have to be. The interaction between drug and receptor site can reflect an entirely artificial situation that has no counterpart in physiology. The pharmacological and therapeutic value of the binding site is not diminished by the absence of a physiological role.

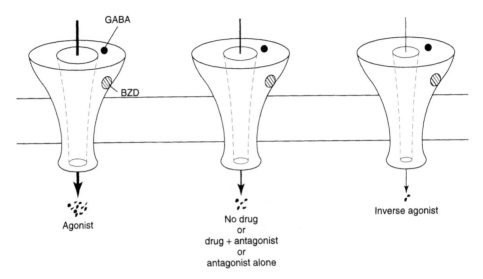

Figure 2.4 Agonism, antagonism, and inverse agonism at an allosteric binding site of an ionotropic receptor. The GABA-A receptor serves as an example. The benzodiazepine receptor site modifies the action of the natural ligand of GABA. Benzodiazepine receptor site agonists increase ion flux through the channel, and so increase the GABAergic inhibition. Inverse agonists decrease channel function and the GABAergic inhibition. Benzodiazepine receptor antagonists block the actions of agonists and inverse agonists, and have no effect on the channel by themselves.

Very often the term antagonism is used in a broad and poorly defined way. We speak of **chemical antagonism** when a compound interferes with another by inactivating it through a chemical reaction. For example, arsenic or mercury poisoning is treated with dimercaprol, which inactivates the metal by forming stable organometallics. Dimercaprol is a chemical antagonist or antidote in such a situation. The term functional antagonism or **physiologic antagonism** is used to describe biological systems with opposite effects. In the nervous system, glutamate and GABA often are functional antagonists to each other, since they exert excitatory and inhibitory effects on postsynaptic neurons, respectively.

2.2 ABSORPTION, DISTRIBUTION, METABOLISM, AND EXCRETION OF DRUGS (ADME)

Oral administration is the most convenient way of drug administration to patients. Many individual steps have to happen between swallowing a pill and the binding of the drug to its receptor site. In the case of drugs for schizophrenia, depression, and many other diseases of the nervous system, the receptor sites are located in the brain. Drugs for these diseases have to be absorbed in the intestine, pass liver metabolic enzymes, reach the blood stream, pass through the blood-brain barrier, and, once in the brain, reach the receptor. The general science describing these events is called pharmacokinetics. More recently the term ADME has received wide acceptance to summarize these processes, since it includes the important metabolic conversions. The following paragraphs provide a backbone description of these processes, the minimal necessary for a discussion of drug discovery. Figure 2.5 illustrates the basic concepts. Many textbooks of pharmacology cited at the end of the chapter provide thorough descriptions.

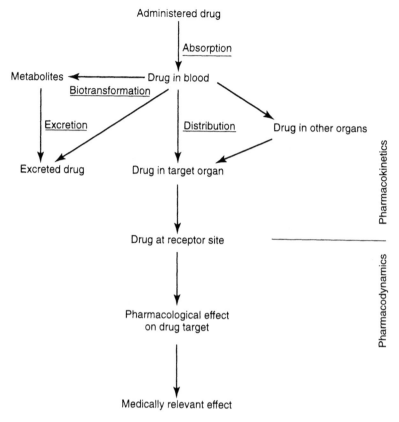

Figure 2.5   Fate of a drug following administration.

2.2.1   **Absorption and Distribution**

Drug absorption is influenced by many factors, the route of administration being the major determinant. For drugs used chronically, oral (enteral) administration is preferred. For drugs used in the hospital, intravenous (a form of parenteral) administration is more convenient. Other forms of parenteral administration, beside the intravenous (i.v.) route, are subcutaneous (s.c.), and intramuscular (i.m.) injections. When a drug is given orally (per os, p.o.) it has to dissolve properly in the gastrointestinal tract and reach the portal vein either through passive diffusion or active transporter processes. Absorption rates can differ at specific levels of the gastrointestinal tract, reflecting changes in pH or the differential distribution of transporter proteins from stomach to the lower intestine. It is possible to influence the rate of absorption by packaging the drug into special capsules that delay its release. Such slow-releasing formulations play a major role in modern drug development and often make the difference between an optimal drug and an efficacious but inconvenient drug. Not surprisingly, drug formulation has evolved into a major field of applied science by itself.

Intramuscular and subcutaneous administrations pose specific and unique absorption issues. Both are incompatible with large injection volumes. Intramuscular administration is preferred for substances causing irritation to epithelial cells. Subcutaneous administration is useful for highly insoluble molecules that have to be given as suspension. Distribution to the blood is difficult to predict in both cases. A further method of parenteral administration, injections into the peritoneal cavity, is the easiest route of administration to animals. Absorption is particularly complex following such intraperitoneal (i.p.) administration, since many different surfaces are involved in absorbing the drug. This route of administration is only rarely used in humans, thus reducing the predictive power of the animal studies. Intravenous administration bypasses the absorption problems. It is the preferred route of administration during hospital care because most patients are given intravenous lines, and drugs are easily added to the drip solution. Intravenous administration is a necessity in pharmacokinetic studies to measure the distribution of a drug in the body in absence of the complicating factors caused by parenteral administration.

Once it reaches the blood, a drug is distributed throughout the body. The blood stream brings it first to the best perfused organs such as heart, liver, and kidney. Muscle, skin, and viscera are less well perfused and tend to receive the drug with a delay. The brain is in a unique situation. It is very well perfused however protected by the blood-brain barrier. The cerebrospinal fluid represents an additional compartment within the brain, to which and from which a drug can flow. The special situation of the brain is discussed in more detail in Chapter 5.

Some drugs accumulate in specific parts of the body. Specific molecules, cellular compartments, cells, or organs can form reservoirs for specific drugs. Albumins, the blood plasma proteins, are the most important drug reservoir. For specific drugs, close to 100% of the drug in the blood can be albumin bound. Plasma protein-bound drug is in equilibrium with the free drug. Cellular reservoirs can be formed by specific cells of muscle, liver, and other organs, reflecting binding or accumulation through transporters. Fat tissue is an example of organ reservoir, since lipophilic drugs often accumulate there. Most of the accumulation in reservoirs is reversible, but there are rare exceptions to this rule.

2.2.2 Metabolic Transformation

With very few exceptions, all drugs undergo metabolic transformation in the mammalian body. One typically distinguishes between phase I and phase II biotransformations. Phase I transformations introduce functional groups into the drug. Hydroxylation, dealkylation, and hydroxylations are frequent phase I reactions. They tend to inactivate the drugs and generally make them more hydrophilic, facilitating excretion. Phase II transformations are conjugation reactions that covalently link the drug to compounds such as glutathione, glucuronic acids, amino acids, and other compounds naturally occurring in the body. Enzymes in the liver catalyze the metabolic transformations. The family of the liver cytochrome P450 monooxygenases is the most important contributor to drug metabolism. It is believed that these enzymes evolved to protect the mammalian body from toxins in plant foodstuff. Several families and subfamilies of cytochrome P450 enzymes have been characterized. Members of the CYP1, CYP2, and CYP3 enzyme families catalyze most drug transformations. In the human body the specific enzymes CYP3A, CYP2D6, and CYP2C metabolize the vast majority of the existing drugs.

Understanding and control of metabolic transformation is a highly important part of the modern drug discovery process. The rate of metabolic transformation determines how rapidly a drug disappears from the blood stream and thus controls its duration of action. Small chemical variations with little impact on the binding to the drug receptor site can radically change the metabolic transformation. The understanding and ability to manipulate these independent structure-activity relationships drive the success of most small molecule drug discovery programs. Metabolic transformation of drugs, through phase I reactions, in particular, sometimes generates unexpected toxic products. In every drug discovery project it is thus necessary to characterize at least the major metabolites and assess their toxic potential. Very often metabolic transformations vary from species to species, rendering this a very complex task.

Metabolic transformation determines the potential of a drug candidate to interfere with the function of another drug. Such drug–drug interactions are a common issue in the current medical practice, since many patients, especially the elderly, use many drugs at the same time. If the same enzyme metabolizes the various drugs, they compete with each other and alter each other's metabolic transformation. Some drugs inhibit specific CYP450 enzymes that convert other drugs, without being a substrate for this enzyme themselves. Some drugs alter the expression of CYP450 enzymes. Since drug–drug interactions often determine the success of a drug in medical practice, it is necessary to understand in detail their effects on metabolic enzymes in addition to the study of their own transformation. All too many drug candidates had to been abandoned because of their effects on the CYP450 enzymes.

Excessive metabolism in the liver can be a significant obstacle for some of the drug discovery projects. Following oral administration and absorption by the gastrointestinal walls, a drug reaches the portal vein and the liver before the general circulation. If the metabolic transformations or extraction into the bile are highly effective, there is a significant concentration gradient between the blood in the portal vein and the general circulation. This phenomenon is referred to as **first-pass effect** and can be difficult to overcome in the drug discovery process. If not possible through drug design, administration routes other than oral have to be considered.

Most small molecule drugs are metabolically transformed in complex ways. In contrast, biologics, peptides, proteins, and antibodies tend to have simpler, and more predictable, metabolic pathways and pharmacokinetic properties in general. Peptides and proteins are cleaved by blood-borne and intracellular peptidases. Antibodies are taken up by cellular receptors for intracellular degradation. Antibodies offer the special advantage of metabolic stability and long half-life in the blood. In the neuroscience area the biologics tend to play a minor role in drug discovery because of their inability to cross the blood-brain barrier.

2.2.3 Excretion

Most drugs are removed from the body as metabolites; only few are excreted unchanged. The kidney is the major excretory organ. Polar compounds are more readily excreted by the kidney than nonpolar ones. Most phase I and phase II biotransformations increase the polarity of the compounds, thus facilitating renal excretion. Besides renal removal, drugs can be excreted through the bile or feces. The routes of metabolic transformation and excretion can be astonishingly complex. It is possible for a drug to be transformed in the liver, its metabolite transported through the bile into the intestinal tract from where it is reabsorbed into the blood stream for ultimate excretion by the kidneys. Excretion pathways for the drug and its metabolites are important determinants for the duration of action and potential toxicity of a drug candidate.

2.2.4 Pharmacokinetic Parameters

Quantitative measurements of ADME parameters are difficult to obtain, since many of them require invasive surgical procedures. However, there is a well-accepted system of quantitative parameters that is generally used to describe these events in a summary way. These parameters reflect practical considerations rather than pure science. They are based on measurable parameters in humans, blood levels in particular. These pharmacokinetic parameters are determined for every drug candidate and make possible the comparison with existing drugs. Figure 2.6 illustrates some of the terms introduced below on the basis of a simple graph showing the drug concentration in the blood as a function of time after injection.

Volume of distribution is the first of these pharmacokinetic parameters. It is defined as the ratio of the total amount of drug in the body to its concentration in the blood (C_b):

$$V_D = \frac{\text{Amount of drug in body}}{C_b}$$

The volume of distribution does not relate to a physically existing volume. It indicates the blood volume that would contain all the drug existing in the body. A drug that does not distribute outside of the blood has a volume of distribution close to the actual blood volume of a person, about 5.5 L for the typical 70 kg person or 0.08 L/kg. A drug that accumulates in tissue may have a value much higher than that. The volume of distribution of the antidepressant imipramine, for example, is 1600 L/70 kg. For clarity, all pharmacokinetic parameters are expressed per volume of blood in this volume. In general drug discovery practice, they are often calculated for blood plasma rather than total blood. For the experimental measurement of the volume of distribution in humans and animals, a known amount of drug is injected intravenously, and blood levels are then measured sequentially. Extrapolation to time zero generates a theoretical blood level at the time of injection that can be compared with the dose injected, thus allowing the calculation of the volume of distribution.

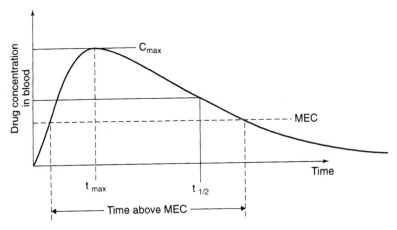

Figure 2.6 Blood concentration–time relationship. C_{max}: maximal blood concentration reached; t_{max}: time from administration to C_{max}; $t_{1/2}$: elimination half-life: MEC: minimal effective concentration, the concentration minimally needed to produce a biological effect; Exposure is determined by calculating the area under the curve (AUC).

Clearance is the second useful pharmacokinetic term. Clearance is defined as the ratio of the rate of elimination of drug to its concentration in the blood:

$$Cl = \frac{\text{Rate of elimination}}{C_b}$$

Clearance is measured as blood volume per time for the entire body (L/h/70 kg) or per unit of weight (L/h/kg). As the volume of distribution, clearance is an imaginary measure, not reflecting a physically existing phenomenon. It indicates the blood volume that would have to be cleared from drug during the time unit to eliminate the drug completely. Thus the highest clearance rates are similar to the actual blood flow 18 L/h for a 70 kg person. Most drugs have clearance rates much lower than this. For example, the clearance of anxiolytic drug diazepam is 1.6 L/h/70 kg.

Half-life ($t_{1/2}$) is the term most easily amenable to intuitive understanding. It indicates the time necessary for the reduction of the plasma concentration of a drug to half of its initial value. The half-life can be easily measured by sequential determinations of plasma drug levels.

Volume of distribution, clearance, and half-life are related to each other. Accumulation of drug outside the blood delays elimination, thus increasing the half-life. Since the volume of distribution mirrors the accumulation in the body, there is a proportional relationship between volume of distribution and half-life. The opposite is true for clearance. Clearance mirrors the rate of elimination of a drug; there is an inverse relationship between clearance and half-life. The following equation describes the relationship under the assumption of ideal conditions of a single compartment:

$$t_{1/2} = \frac{\ln 2 \cdot V_d}{Cl}$$

or

$$t_{1/2} = \frac{0.693 \cdot V_d}{Cl}$$

It has to be emphasized that many drugs do not follow the ideal conditions of a single compartment. Both accumulation and elimination rates can be nonlinear. Many drugs have biphasic elimination characteristics that are not adequately reflected by a single half-life measurement. To overcome this problem, it is sometimes necessary to separately define initial half-life and terminal half-life values.

Bioavailability is defined as the fraction of a dose of drug that reaches the blood. For intravenous administration this value is, by definition, 100%. For all other routes of administration, oral administration, in particular, it can be far less than 100% because of incomplete absorption. Bioavailability is practically determined by estimating the area under the curve (AUC) from sequential measurements of blood levels until all the drug has been excreted (Fig. 2.6). Bioavailability is theoretically not a significant issue in drug discovery, since low bioavailability can be simply overcome by giving more drug. However, from a practical point of view bioavailability can be a major issue. Patients find it inconvenient to swallow large pills. High drug levels in the intestine increases the probability of local toxicity. Finally, the production and handling costs associated with large drug amounts may reduce the commercial attraction for a drug development project.

Exposure is a term particularly important from a point of view of drug safety and long-term adverse effects. It attempts to capture the total amount of drug a body or an organ has been exposed to over time. It is typically defined as the AUC of the blood concentration curve over a single or over repeated administration (Fig. 2.6). This value can also be interpreted as a reflection of the average blood concentration of a drug over repeated administration. The term has its origins in toxicology, but has found its way into the general vocabulary of pharmacokinetics. It plays an important role in studies of drug safety, where it is necessary to have comparative exposures between test animals and humans to make predictions meaningful.

2.3 CONCLUSIONS

Pharmacokinetics and pharmacodynamics provide a generally accepted concept and vocabulary to capture the steps between administration of a drug to a patient and the appearance of clinically manifest consequences. The processes including absorption, distribution, biotransformation, and elimination determine the pharmacokinetic properties of a drug. They present challenges and hurdles in every drug discovery program. Pharmacodynamics, the science of the molecular interactions between a drug and its receptor site, provides quantitative descriptions of the binding of a drug to its target and the resulting downstream events. Pharmacokinetic and pharmacodynamic parameters are direct functions of the drug dose and tissue concentration. These associations are described as concentration–binding, concentration–effect, and dose–effect relationships. The chemical nature of the drug and the dose at which it is given determine the effects. Humankind since the beginnings has known the crucial importance of the dose. Paracelcus, a pharmacists who lived 500 years ago, is believed to be responsible for the frequently invoked saying "It is the dose that makes the poison" (Montague, 2003).

REFERENCES

Further Reading

BIRKETT, D.J. *Pharmacokinetics Made Easy*. McGraw-Hill, New York, 2003.

HARDMAN, J.G., LIMBIRD, L.E., MOLINOFF, P.B., RUDDON, R.W., and GILMAN, A.G. *Goodman & Gilman's The Pharmacological Basis of Therapeutics*. McGraw-Hill, New York, 9th ed., 1996.

KATZUNG, B.G., ed. *Basic and Clinical Pharmacology*. Appleton and Lange, Norwalk, CT, 8th ed., 2001.

KENAKIN, T.P., and KENAKIN, T. *Pharmacologic Analysis of Drug-Receptor Interaction*. Lippincott Williams and Wilkins, 3rd ed., 1997.

KENAKIN, T., and KENAKIN, T.P. *Molecular Pharmacology*. Blackwell Science Cambridge, MA, 1997.

MELMON, K.L., ed. *Clinical Pharmacology: Basic Principles in Therapeutics*. McGraw-Hill, New York, 3rd ed., 1992.

SHARGEL, L., and YU, A.B.C. *Applied Biopharmaceutics and Pharmacokinetics*. McGraw-Hill/Appleton and Lange, 3rd ed., 1996.

Citations

CONN, P.J. Physiological roles and therapeutic potential of metabotropic glutamate receptors. *Ann. NY Acad. Sci.* 1003: 12–21, 2003.

GINGRICH, J.A., and CARON, M.G. Recent advances in the molecular biology of dopamine receptors. *An. Rev. Neurosci.* 16: 299–322, 1993.

JULIUS, D. Molecular biology of serotonin receptors. *An. Rev. Neurosci.* 14: 335–360, 1991.

KUHAR, M.J., DE SOUZA, E.B., and UNNERSTALL, J.R. Neurotransmitter receptor mapping by autoradiography and other methods. *An. Rev. Neurosci.* 9: 27–59, 1986.

KUSCHINKSY, G., and LÜLLMANN, H. *Kurzes Lehrbuch der Pharmakologie*. Georg Thieme Verlag, Stuttgart, 5th ed., 1972.

MONTAGUE, P. Paracelcus Revisited. In "Rachel's Environment and Health News 755." *http://www.rachel.org*, 2002.

Chapter 3

Drug Discovery

Modern drug discovery aims at using scientific and rational technology to produce a steady stream of new and effective drugs. Drugs found by the science-based approach will gradually replace the current ones that, in their majority, came to life due to incidental discoveries. If the modern, scientific approach is successful, it will re-discover drugs provided by nature a long time ago, a high hurdle. Is modern, industrialized drug discovery able to find morphine? Only an affirmative "yes, certainly!" will constitute a satisfactory answer for the ongoing technology-driven drug discovery efforts.

3.1 THE PROCESS OF DRUG DISCOVERY AND DEVELOPMENT

Drug discovery and development are complex and time-consuming endeavors. Many steps and many years intercalate between the start of a drug discovery research project and the delivery of a new drug to patients in need. Very often it is difficult to precisely define the moment a drug discovery project has been initiated. They often emerge gradually from the basic scientific investigations. The endpoint, however, is defined with precision, by the formal approval of a new drug by a regulatory agency such as the Federal Drug Administration (FDA). Figure 3.1 shows an often-used diagrammatic illustration of the drug discovery process. Early research gradually focuses on a specific path that generates a drug candidate. Such a drug candidate will then be subjected to general safety testing in animals, followed by the various phases of clinical evaluation. During the past decades the process from project initiation to the approval of a new drug has taken 10 to 15 years. Sometimes hundreds of scientists are involved at specific time points during this long process.

While useful, the graphical rendering of the drug discovery and development process in Figure 3.1 depicts a superficial view only. It fails to indicate some of the major decision points during the process. A more appropriate representation is given in Figure 3.2. It organizes the process around two major decision points, first, the selection of the drug target and, second, the selection of the drug candidate. Both decision points are precisely defined in physical and temporal terms. The two decision points define three stages of the drug discovery and development process. During the first stage, various molecules of the human body are explored as possible drug targets. Researchers attempt to find sufficient supportive evidence from in vitro investigations, animal studies, and human observations

Drug Discovery for Nervous System Diseases, by Franz F. Hefti
ISBN 0-471-46563-1   Copyright © 2005 by John Wiley & Sons, Inc.

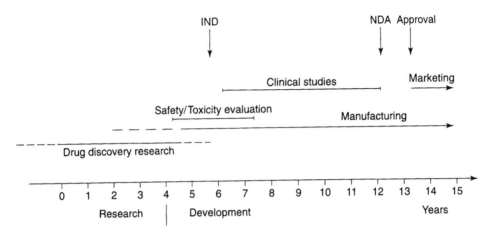

Figure 3.1 Typical time lines in the identification of a new drug. IND: Application to Regulatory Agency for Investigational New Drug; NDA: New Drug Application. (terminology used by the US Federal Drug Administration)

that a putative target molecule plays a crucial role in the disease process, and that altering its function with a drug might benefit the patients. Once a target has been selected, at the beginning of the second stage, the nature of drug discovery research changes drastically. The optimal drug candidate has to be identified. Medicinal chemistry becomes the driving force in a small molecule drug discovery program. In an iterative way, more and more selective, potent, and safe molecules are being produced, until a molecule with appropriate attributes to serve as drug candidate can be identified. In a program for biological drugs, such as modified antibodies or growth factor receptors, molecular biological techniques take the place of medicinal chemistry in the optimization of the drug candidate. During the third stage, safety and clinical efficacy of the selected drug candidate have to be demonstrated. Extensive safety studies in animals precede carefully designed human studies that minimize the risk to volunteers and patients. Typically a large-scale human study concludes the third stage and, if successful, culminates in the approval and clinical use of the new drug.

The three stages will be discussed in detail below. There is no standardized terminology about these various stages as yet, although many drug discovery researchers honor conventional terms. Stages one and two, the time interval before selection of a drug candidate, are typically referred to as **drug discovery**. Stage three, the time interval between selection of a drug candidate and its formal approval as a drug is referred to as **drug development**. Quite appropriately, efforts during stage one are sometimes referred to as exploratory drug discovery projects. When moving to the second stage, they become mature or full-blown drug discovery projects. In absence of a commonly used terminology, the decision points separating the stages are used in this book to subdivide the process.

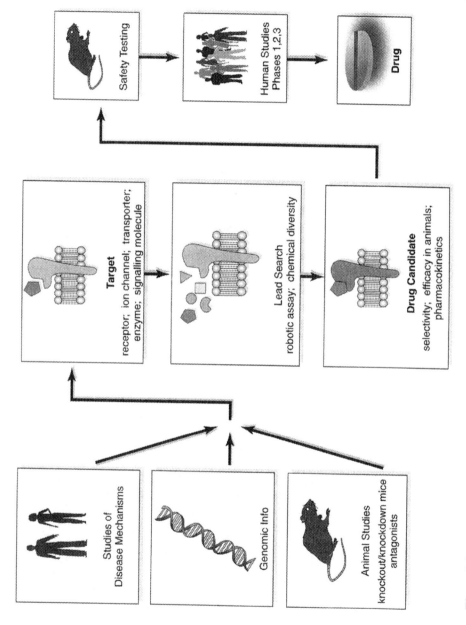

Figure 3.2 Phases and decision points in drug discovery and development. The selection of the drug target and the selection of the drug candidate are the two major decision points that separate three distinct phases.

27

3.2 FROM EXPLORATION TO TARGET SELECTION

In principle, every gene product synthesized in human cells, according to current estimates 30,000 to 100,000 molecules, can serve as drug targets. Some are more promising than others, but the number of possibilities is high even when rigorous selection criteria are applied. Since the capacities of the advanced stages of the drug discovery process are limited, those of clinical development in particular, the selection of the drug target is arguably the most critical step in the entire process. The following paragraph discusses the various approaches available to select a target from a general perspective. Chapter 4 will provide a comprehensive overview of targets and target opportunities and selection criteria for the neuroscience area.

3.2.1 Validated Targets

Selective antagonists of the dopamine D_2 receptor alleviate the symptoms of schizophrenia, giving the D_2 receptor the status of a validated drug target. The insulin receptor is an obvious validated drug target since insulin injections lower blood sugar levels. The number of validated drug targets is rather small, a recent estimate has put the number at about 500 (Drews, 2000). As discussed in more detail in Chapter 4, there are only about 15 validated drug targets in the neuroscience area. The very small number of validated targets as compared to the number of gene products leads to the obvious conclusion that they represent only a very small fraction of the ultimately useful drug targets. Nevertheless, validated targets are uniquely attractive for drug discovery researchers. They provide an assured way toward an efficacious drug. They avoid the agony of waiting for many years for conclusive clinical results and abolish the huge financial risks, which have to be taken when moving through the clinical trials with a drug acting on a speculative target. Since no drug is perfect, it is always possible to improve on existing drugs that act on the validated targets. Minor changes can translate to major advantages in clinical practice. Improvements in half-life alone can have major impact, since, for example, patients will prefer a drug that can be taken once a week over a drug to be taken twice daily and specifically linked to meals. Drugs with minimal potential for drug–drug interactions are favored, since physicians will prefer drugs without such complications. Generating drugs with such incremental improvements brings little intellectual and scientific satisfaction and is often decried as a "me-too" effort. It needs to be emphasized, though, that many of the medically and commercially most successful drugs fall into this category. "Best beats first" is the rule often invoked in the companies. Similar to the computer industry, the pharmaceutical industry abounds in stories of impressive innovations scooped by savvy competitors who turned them into commercial successes with incremental improvements. Not surprisingly, clinical validation remains the strongest argument in the selection of a drug target.

   Drug targets are objects of scientific investigation, and the understanding of their properties increases over time. The information often generates opportunities for new drug discovery projects. The full conformational description of a drug target protein may suggest new receptor sites. Complex transmembrane ion channels are most likely to offer many drug receptor sites. The example of the GABA-A receptors vividly illustrates this point. They harbor distinct binding sites for barbiturates, benzodiazepine drugs, and neurosteroids. Drugs acting on the benzodiazepine receptor site have gradually replaced those acting on the barbiturate receptor site, and the benzodiazepine receptor site continues to offer new possibilities for more selective and improved drugs. There are several ways to identify novel receptor sites on validated targets. Conformational analysis may indicate attractive binding pockets in strategic locations, for example, at the interface of protein subunits of a multimeric molecule. New receptor sites may be identified by gradually exploring the areas surrounding the known receptor sites of existing drugs. In this approach molecules are designed as hybrids between existing drugs and moieties believed to bind to adjacent areas (Burley and Bonnano, 2002). The iterative approach leads to the definition of overlapping novel receptor sites that ultimately may become separate enough to qualify as independent and novel.

Many of the current drug targets received clinical validation before the sequencing of the human genome was completed. The complete information revealed that many drug targets were a family of proteins rather than being singular molecular units. These discoveries open complex and exciting questions. Is binding to all family members necessary or, alternatively, are single subunits mediating the therapeutic effects? Are desired effects and adverse effects mediated by different subunits? If yes, it should be possible to design highly selective drugs that bind to the subunit mediating the desired effects only. The antidepressant, anxiolytic, and analgesia fields provide examples for this approach to be discussed in more detail later. In each case the drug discovery efforts have focused on the receptor subtype believed to mediate the desired therapeutic response. Recent developments in the NSAID area serve as the best example for this approach. NSAIDs inhibit the formation of pain-mediating molecules, the prostanoids, by inhibiting the enzyme cyclo-oxygenase (cox). Molecular biological advances revealed the existence of two different isoforms, cox-1 and cox-2. Cox-2 levels are elevated in inflamed tissue where the pain occurs, whereas cox-1 is expressed in the gastrointestinal tract. The selective localization strongly suggests that inhibition of cox-1 mediates the adverse effects on the gastrointestinal tract, whereas the desired analgesic effects are mediated by cox-2. These considerations triggered a worldwide competitive race to make selective inhibitors for cox-2. Indeed, these selective cox-2 inhibitors have reached clinical practice during recent years and have started to replace the nonselective NSAIDs in the treatment of patients with gastrointestinal adverse effects.

The approach to identify drug targets from existing drugs is sometimes referred to as **reverse pharmacology**, a suggestive but rather imprecise term. It also encompasses the so-called **orphan drugs**, clinically effective molecules whose mechanism of action and target has remained obscure. Gabapentin provides the best example of an orphan drug in the neuroscience area. It is medically and commercially successful for the treatment of chronic pain. Low potency, limited efficacy, and adverse effects make it a primary target for attempts to displace it with a better drug. Despite years of research efforts, the target has remained obscure. Whoever cracks this nut will reap large benefits. The example of gabapentin best illustrates the attraction of reverse pharmacology approaches.

3.2.2 Evaluating Putative Targets

Certain groups of molecules are intuitively attractive as potential drug targets. Soluble enzymes with a critical function in the metabolic process belong to this category. The binding pockets for their substrates present natural receptor sites for drugs. Hormone receptors and G-protein-coupled receptors are attractive for the same reasons. Their natural ligands are key regulators of biological processes and the binding pockets offer putative drug receptor sites. Many pharmaceutical and biotech companies have taken the route to systematically evaluate G-protein-coupled receptors and other receptors for suitability as drug targets for these reasons. Additional, practical reasons explain the enthusiasm in support for the "receptor to drug approach" found in many companies. Academic research groups, from which the companies recruit their drug discovery scientists, tend to focus on molecular mechanisms of receptor functions and create a natural tendency for the scientists to be knowledgeable in subgroups of receptors. More important, the research tools, such as clones and assays, are unique for specific groups of proteins, generating a natural tendency to stay with the known and doable. The business plans of many biotech companies state the intention to fully evaluate the platform of a receptor group as potential drug targets.

The recent discovery of the melanocortin 4 receptor (MC4R) as a drug target for obesity beautifully illustrates the power of the receptor to drug approach. This receptor binds α- and β-melanocyte-stimulating hormones (MSH), two fragments of pro-opiomelanocortin and, in addition, agouti-related protein (AGRP), a natural antagonist to α- and β-MSH. MC4R is expressed at highest levels in the hypothalamus, suggesting a role in endocrine regulation. The anatomical observations triggered further functional studies. Mice with a deletion of the MC4R gene (MC4R knockouts) have been found to eat excessive quantities of food and become obese. Several human mutations of MC4R have been detected that are linked to obesity. The human findings validate the MC4R receptor as drug target and suggest that MC4R agonists may become effective therapeutic agents for obesity and the associated metabolic diseases (Zimanyi and Pelleymounter, 2003; Crowley et al., 2002; Farooqi et al., 2003).

The example of the MC4R illustrates the stepwise progression from receptor to drug target. The process starts with the cloning of a new receptor and the localization of its expression. Interpreting the location in the context of functional neuroanatomy then suggest tentative functional roles of the receptor. If interesting, they will trigger the rapid generation of gene knockout animals in which this receptor is lacking. Alternatively, gene silencing strategies with antisense or small interfering RNA (siRNA) are utilized. Very often knockout animals have been generated earlier and the information is available immediately from publications or commercial databases. If the phenotype of the mice with gene deletion, or gene silencing, is in line with the functional speculations made from the localization studies, and if this function is related to a disease process, it may be possible to make a case for the use of the receptor as a drug target. Figure 3.3 provides an illustration of the approach. Several companies have made this strategy into a general method for the identification of new drug targets. The publication of the human genome sequence has made it possible to fully cover groups of genes, such as G-protein-coupled receptors or transmembrane tyrosine kinase receptors. The complete sequence of the human genome provides a survey of all possible drug targets. Companies have emerged that generate a full set of knockout mice of gene groups with high probability to become drug targets. Indeed, the knockout technology is a very powerful tool in the drug discovery process. However, it is important to emphasize its limitations. Some of the knockouts are embryonic lethal and not available for analysis. In some gene knockout animals, related genes can be upregulated and compensate for the missing one. Adult functions of a gene, the really important function from a drug discovery perspective, can be masked by developmental functions. Secondary effects on neighboring genes may occur. There are several known examples where different strains of knockout mice with deletions of the same gene were found to have different phenotypes (Zambrowicz and Sands, 2002).

Knockout data and their interpretation play a significant role in modern drug discovery and are often mentioned throughout this book. Limitations will be made apparent

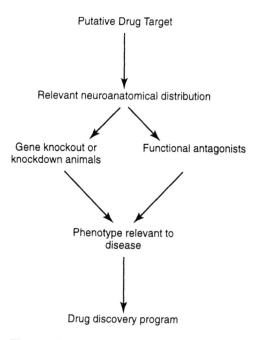

Figure 3.3 Receptor to drug approach. The strategy is widely used to evaluate G-protein-coupled receptors and ion channels for target utility. The selection of drug targets relies on the anatomical location of the protein and the tentative association of the animal phenotype to the human disease.

whenever possible. Gradually advances in conditional knockout methods and gene silencing technologies will replace the simple gene knockout technologies. The ability to generate conditional knockouts, animals in which a specific gene can be silenced transiently during adult life, will have enormous utility in the drug discovery process (Seibler et al., 2003). The power of the more recently discovered RNA interference technologies has not been fully explored as yet. They have the potential to live, up to earlier promises made by antisense technologies to selectively silence specific genes in specific locations. The siRNA molecules exert such a function under natural conditions and thus are effective. Expression of siRNA in specific cells at specific developmental times will make it possible to rapidly analyze gene functions in an adult organism (Hannon, 2002; Thompson, 2002). Inactivation of genes at specific times and select locations will make it possible to quickly define their functions. These methods will further increase the power of the receptor to drug target approach. In the neuroscience area, the receptor to drug approach has played and continues to play a very prominent role. It will be discussed in detail in Chapter 4.

3.2.3 Rational Target Identification from the Study of Disease Mechanisms

When the biotech industry was born two decades ago, it quickly directed its attention to obvious drug products such as insulin, growth hormone, and other growth factors. They were considered the low-hanging fruits easily collected first, because it was well known that absence of insulin causes diabetes and the absence of growth hormone causes dwarfism. The molecules were known to play a crucial role in the disease mechanisms or pathophysiology of these diseases. In more modern words, we would say that the insulin receptor and the growth hormone receptor are drug targets identified through studies of the disease mechanism and later validated through the use of their natural ligands as drugs. In a similar way the thyroxine receptor can be considered a drug target identified from the study of a disease mechanism of thyroid disorders.

The examples above illustrate that understanding of the disease mechanisms provides a direct and effective way forward to identify drug targets and to fish out the crucial ones from the total pool of gene products. There are several examples from outside of the neuroscience area that illustrate the power of this approach. In the diabetes area the evaluation of the metabolic steps surrounding the action of insulin has led to the identification of further targets. Upstream of the insulin receptor the secretion of insulin is regulated by glucagon-like peptide-1 (GLP-1), making its receptors an attractive drug target. GLP-1 is degraded by dipeptidyl peptidase IV, so specific inhibitors of this enzyme prolong the duration and magnitude of the GLP-1 action (Drucker, 2001). Downstream of the insulin receptor there are additional points for pharmacological interference. Binding of insulin to the receptor results in phosphorylation and activation of the receptor. A specific phosphatase has been identified, protein tyrosine phosphatase 1B (PTP1B), that selectively dephosphorylates the insulin receptor and blocks signaling and further downstream events. Inhibitors of this phosphatase will prolong and enhance the activation of the insulin receptor by insulin (Johnson et al., 2002).

Array technologies, providing a sweeping overview of gene expression at the mRNA or protein level, may be particularly useful in the quest to identify disease mechanisms and novel drug targets. Events upstream and downstream from a disease-causing gene can be quickly explored when a transgenic animal is available that replicates the disease. In an alternative approach, it may be possible to utilize the existence of drugs alleviating the same disease through different mechanisms of action. For example, several different types of drugs are used for the control of blood pressure. Comparison of their effects using genomic or proteomic technologies might be able to identify common pathways that determine the blood pressure. Insight in common pathways may lead to novel drug targets more central to the disease mechanism. Gene array or protein array approaches are conceptually very exciting and likely to produce tangible results in the foreseeable future.

At the present time the anti-parkinsonian drug L-DOPA, is the only successful example of drug discovery derived from the study of disease mechanisms in the neurosciences. However, as discussed in detail in later chapters, the disease-driven drug discovery approach is likely to become the rule rather than the exception in the future. The recent developments in the Alzheimer field are the best example in support of this optimistic view. The earlier discovery of the genetic deficit of Huntington's disease has guided researchers to concepts that may become useful for target identification. Genes causing familial Parkinson's disease have pointed the field to approaches that may generate drugs able to slow down the progression of the disease. Other diseases of the nervous system are likely to follow the investigational strategy outlined by the research on these neurodegenerative diseases.

3.3 FROM TARGET TO DRUG CANDIDATE

Selection of a target for further efforts is one of the most significant decisions taken in biopharmaceutical companies. The "go" decision triggers major commitments of human and material resources. It is therefore not surprising that most established companies have formal decision-making processes for this stage. Corporate strategy, considerations of medical need, and market opportunity typically are taken into consideration. Small companies that have not yet reached the stage of profitability typically inform investors and the public of the major project decisions taken at this stage. The magnitude of the commitment explains why many people have attempted to find rational and quantitative rules to help with this stage (Knowles and Gromo, 2002). Up to the present time these efforts tend to be futile though. They have not been substantiated by retrospective analysis, in part because the number of drug candidates that actually reach the market continues to be very low. Target validation and predicability remain too poor and mercurial. Medical practice changes over the many years of a drug development process so that the drug faces a situation not accurately predictable at the time of target selection. Thus intuition and experience continue to play a major role in target selection processes. It is one of the prime responsibilities of R&D management in biopharmaceutical companies. Unfortunately, the time interval between decision and outcome most often exceeds the tenure of the decision-makers in these positions. This creates the unique situation that people having made the wrong decisions often are not accountable and, in the case of success, people who had not participated in the crucial decision often enjoy the benefits.

The road from target selection to drug candidate follows a well-delineated path. However, the path is by no means easy or guaranteed to be successful. Sometimes the voyage has to be abandoned because insurmountable obstacles are encountered. The goal of the journey is precisely defined. A drug candidate is to be identified, a molecule that is suitable for large-scale safety testing in animals and testing for safety and efficacy in humans. Such a drug candidate has to bind to the receptor site on the target with high affinity and elicit the desired functional response. It has to be selective for the chosen receptor site, to minimize undesired and adverse effects. It must have sufficient bioavailability and distribution to reach the receptor site following systemic administration, and finally, it has to elicit the desired responses in vivo, in animal models of the human disease. The principles are the same for small molecule drug candidates or biological drugs. Specific aspects of the pathways differ between small organic molecules and biologics. The pathway for small molecules tends to be more complex and elaborate and is described first in the subsequent paragraphs.

3.3.1 Lead Screening

Synthetic efforts for small molecule drug candidates are most effective when they start with compounds that already have some of the desired features. Affinity to the receptor site typically serves as initial criterion for consideration of a compound as starting point for a further chemical optimization program. Compounds chosen as starting points for medicinal chemistry programs are referred to as leads. Sometimes leads are available for obvious reasons. Existing drugs can serve as leads in a program on a previously validated drug receptor. Natural receptor ligands provide leads when the drug target is a receptor, such as a neurotransmitter or hormone receptor. Obvious leads are rare, however, so a broad search for leads is the first step of most drug discovery programs.

In recent years the broad search for lead compounds, lead screening, has evolved from a relatively simple benchtop activity to a highly organized and technically sophisticated effort. The number of molecules available for lead screening is one of the determinants of success. The large pharmaceutical companies have thus increased the size of their compound collections into the range of one to five million. Such numbers require full automation. In a modern lead screening operation, advanced robots that handle every step from sample dispersion to data analysis carry out current screening procedures. Highly specialized scientists run highly complex equipment. The high-throughput screening (HTS) technologies continue to evolve rapidly and seem to improve month by month. Scientists running these robotic facilities are typically very motivated and show the excitement of automated biotechnology and, fortunately, the specter of boring repetitive screening work that haunted the pharmaceutical industry now belongs to the past.

Assay development is a major feature of HTS technologies. The assays for robotic runs must be robust, reproducible, and miniaturizable. Simple assays, with few steps and very small incubation volumes, are required. HTS assay volumes are a few microliters, and the emerging ultra-HTS technologies utilize nanoliter assay volumes. While simple competition binding assays can be miniaturized with relative ease, cell-based assays with an optical endpoint offer the most technical advantages for HTS. In such assays a drug target of interest is coupled functionally to a pathway that can be linked to an optical signal from a special dye. Fluorescent readouts are the most desired endpoints. In the neuroscience area the availability of dyes has made it possible to run HTS assays on ion channel drug targets. Ionotropic receptors and neuronal ion channels used to be considered difficult drug targets because time- and labor-intensive electrophysiological methods were the only tools to measure drug effects. Because of the new optical assays that are very often based on calcium-sensitive dyes, ion channels are now at the same level of technical feasibility as G-protein-coupled receptors. In the modern world of screening, assay development is the key to success. For ultra-HTS in particular, assay development is the limiting step rather than the screening runs themselves. The former can take months, the latter a few days or weeks (Wolcke and Ullmann, 2001; Gonzalez et al., 1999).

The size and quality of the chemical sample collection used in the HTS runs is an obvious determinant of the lead search. In pharmaceutical companies with a long tradition, sample collections comprise all compounds ever synthesized inhouse, and they tend to reflect earlier programs. In every program a few thousand compounds are being synthesized before the right drug candidate emerges. All these molecules will be part of the sample collection. Thus, in a company that specializes in G-protein-coupled receptor targets, the sample collection is likely to contain leads for other G-protein-coupled receptor drug discovery programs but will probably not contain useful leads for ion channel targets. To overcome this bias problem and to increase the breath of the sample collection, many companies have started to synthesize or acquire additional libraries of chemicals. Core structures are chosen and are then diversified with combinatorial chemistry methods (Geysen et al., 2003). Over a time period of just a few years, it is possible to enlarge the sample collection by hundred thousands of new molecules with such an approach.

Organic chemistry offers almost infinite possibilities to create new molecules. Is it thus necessary, and beneficial, to synthesize more and more molecules and to increase the sample collections indefinitely? While this is a possible scenario, at least some of the companies attempt to create more suitable, "smarter," chemical libraries rather than just bigger ones. As a first step in this direction chemicals are removed from the collection that are proved unsuited as leads, as judged from multiple assay experiences. Some molecules give positive signals in many assays and thus lack appropriate selectivity. Groups of compounds may show up as positives in the same assay because they bind to the same receptor site subspaces. A single compound may adequately represent such a group. Information on pharmacokinetic properties on lead compounds will gradually accumulate when molecules are chosen as leads, or such information can be generated for entire subgroups of the sample collection. Such information will make it possible to identify and remove molecules that have poor bioavailability or half-life, or that bind to or induce CYP450 enzymes. From the neuroscience perspective, it would be particularly useful to exclude molecules unable to pass the blood-brain barrier. Practical rules reflecting heuristic experiences are sometimes applied in the selection of compounds for inclusion in the sample collection. Chemists at Pfizer developed the so-called rule of five that molecules have to fulfill to be useful for drug discovery processes (Lipisnki, 1997). The rule stipulates that molecules must have a molecular weight less than 500, log P less than 5, no more than 5 hydrogen bond donors, and no more than 10 hydrogen bond acceptors. Log P is used as a measure of lipophilicity, determined as distribution coefficient of a compound between *n*-octanol and water. Modern sample collections contain many molecules that violate the rule of five. Keeping the molecular weight under 500 has become particularly difficult because broad synthetic efforts naturally tend to increase the size of the chemicals. However, most successful drugs have molecular weights below 500 and log P values below 5, and failed compounds tend to fall outside this range (Wenlock et al., 2003).

Adopting a purely theoretical standpoint, one could argue that a rational chemical design process should replace the practical trial and error approaches described above. Receptor sites on target proteins typically span about 1 to 10 nm. The optimal sample collection would thus include all molecules necessary to occupy all possible chemical configurations in a three-dimensional space of 1000 nm^3. It is not clear at the present time how many molecules would be minimally necessary to satisfy all three-dimensional properties. While these considerations are highly interesting from a theoretical point of view, they currently do not seem to play a relevant part in the design of the sample collections used in HTS.

Data handling and computer technologies have contributed massively to the advances of modern screening technologies. HTS with millions of compounds not only generates a massive problem with logistics of sample handling but also a massive problem for data analysis. The attempts described above to improve the quality of the sample collection require rapid incorporation of data from downstream assays. Downstream assays by themselves require major efforts at the scale of primary HTS just a few years ago. With a 2 million compound library and a hit rate of 0.1% that is considered reasonable, a HTS run will generate 2000 compounds for further analysis. Visual analysis of hits by trained chemists is not adequate for such numbers. Thus HTS is the first step only, and it has to be followed by theoretical and practical steps for further selection. Modern computer technologies make it gradually possible to substitute virtual screening for actual screening. The chemical space of organic molecules can be described in mathematical terms as well as the known drug receptor sites. With this information advanced computer programs can help to identify the optimal molecules among the large number of hits in the first HTS run. At the present time such virtual screening does not play a major role in hit analysis. However, with increasing optimization and standardization of sample libraries it seems that virtual screening will gradually become more influential in the lead search process (Bajorath, 2002).

3.3.2 Medicinal Chemistry

The selected lead compounds bind with reasonable affinity to the drug receptor, but all other properties have yet to be optimized. Thus a synthetic medicinal chemistry program is initiated. Typically the selectivity of the leads is assessed and addressed first. Leads are evaluated in a broad counterscreening program, in which they are tested for affinity to most of the known drug receptor sites. At the present time the majority of them are receptor sites on G-protein-coupled receptors, but ion channels and tyrosine kinases are increasingly added to the counterscreen palettes. Some companies run these counterscreens in-house, others outsource them to specialized companies. The broad counterscreen typically identifies a small number of undesired binding affinities that need to be worked out through chemical modifications. If a large number of additional affinities are discovered, the lead compounds may be discarded in favor of more selective available ones. Counterscreen assays for the undesired affinities in a lead compound often remain an issue for the subsequent series of chemical derivatives, and they become part of the routine assays used in support of the further medicinal chemistry program.

Increasing the affinity to the receptor site is the next main goal of the medicinal chemistry program. To reach adequate selectivity and potency in vivo, it is necessary to find compounds with binding affinities in the low nM or even pM range. Binding assays are relatively simple and highly suitable for determining the affinity. In a typical medicinal chemistry program, the binding assays are at the direct interface between biology and chemistry, and they represent one of the most critical interactions in the drug discovery process. Very often these assays are done in a highly automatic way, using robotic setups that are smaller variants of HTS. Rapid chemical synthesis techniques allow small group of chemists to produce up to several hundred new compounds per months that line up for testing. Compounds with sufficiently high affinity move to further assays that determine the functional effects on the target molecule, to distinguish agonist from antagonistic responses. Binding and functional assays define the in vitro segment of the medicinal chemistry selection process. Compounds with sufficient binding affinity, selectivity and functional efficacy are taken forward into further in vivo selection processes.

The in vivo assays serve to select compounds with satisfactory pharmacokinetic properties to reach the receptor site and to elicit the desired effect in animal models of the disease. There is a high degree of variability among drug discovery projects in the specific way this is handled. In the simplest possible case a single animal model can satisfy all these needs. For example, in programs for new pain drugs, simple rodent assays are available that allow testing of 10 or more compounds per week by a single investigator. Biological efficacy of a compound in such a model by oral administration implies sufficient bioavailability, receptor occupancy, as well as appropriate effects on the receptor. For most drug discovery projects, however, these different steps are evaluated with individual assays. Standard pharmacokinetic methods described in Chapter 2 are used to measure bioavailability and to select compounds with satisfactory properties. In vivo receptor occupancy assays determine adequate binding to the receptor. Finally, a functional model of the disease serves to measure the appropriate biological response. The level of difficulty and capacity of the available in vivo models drive these decisions. Very often animal models of specific diseases are complex and require treatment durations of several months. Generalization inappropriately blurs the large differences among drug discovery programs. The practical examples to be discussed in later chapters will provide a more accurate picture.

Many companies have started to incorporate early in medicinal chemistry programs assays that address specific safety concerns. Cardiovascular effects, for example, even when minor, represent major problems for a drug candidate, since they can lead to sudden death in patients. Of particular concern are drugs that increase the QT-interval in the sequence of cardiac contractions, since they predict increased risk of heart attacks. The hERG ion channel has been identified as determinant of the QT-interval, and unfortunately, this channel has a binding site with significant structural overlap with many G-protein-coupled receptor drug receptor sites. Thus hERG receptor site-binding assays are often incorporated in routine in vitro counterscreening batteries. During the more advanced stages they are supplemented by in vivo evaluations of cardiac functions. In a similar way inhibition and induction of CYP450 enzymes are often monitored early with in vitro systems. More advanced molecules are sometimes evaluated in exploratory safety studies in which the liver function of rodents are measured in vivo.

Drug discovery projects evolve with time in distinct patterns. During the early stages the biological assays are adjusted and optimized. Redundant steps are omitted. Mature drug discovery programs have a well-established **critical path** of in vitro and in vivo biological assays by which chemicals are selected. Minimizing and optimizing the steps of the critical path is one of the keys to success in drug discovery. An optimized critical path allows the drug discovery researcher to select the best compound at each step without redundancies. The selection process of an optimized medicinal chemistry program and critical path has similarity to the Darwinian selection process of biological evolution. However, chemicals are not randomly generated as the mutations in biology but are designed based on rational considerations. The path from target selection to identifying a drug candidate is long and complicated. Anecdotal information suggests that several thousands of molecules have to be synthesized before an acceptable drug candidate emerges. Several years and large groups of chemists and biologists are often necessary to achieve the goal.

3.3.3 Biologics

Biological drugs for diseases other than those of the nervous system have been successfully introduced during the past decade. Examples include growth factors, such as human granulocyte colony-stimulating factor to treat blood cell loss during cancer chemotherapy, and antibodies such as anti-tumor necrosis factor-α for rheumatoid arthritis. For nervous system diseases biologics are far less attractive because they do not cross the blood-brain barrier in sufficient quantities to make effective drugs. However, they can be useful for diseases of the peripheral nervous system such as neuropathies and peripheral forms of pain. Growth factors have been tested clinically, without clear success. Antibodies for pain are likely to reach clinical testing soon. For severe and fatal diseases intracranial administration may be used in absence of other attractive options. The ongoing clinical evaluation of growth factors in Parkinson's disease provides an example.

When natural growth factors are used as drugs, high potency and good efficacy are a given, and no attempts are made to optimize them. However, other standard issues of drug discovery process remain. Most important, the natural function of the molecule does not assure appropriate pharmacokinetic properties for the same molecule following administration from an external source. Most proteins, many growth factors in particular, disappear from the circulation within minutes after administration. It is thus necessary to ascertain that sufficient quantities of growth factors reach the receptor sites on the target molecules. A natural growth factor, injected at high doses to overcome the pharmacokinetic problems, may bind to other receptors and mediate adverse effects. Safety considerations are thus very similar to those in a small molecule drug discovery program.

Antibodies can serve as drugs by removing key players in a pathological process. Mediators of pain could be captured by antibodies and denied the ability to stimulate their functional receptors. Long half-lives is a key advantage of antibodies making pharmaco-kinetic considerations a secondary issue. Antibodies generated in animals are not useful as drugs because they generate immune reactions in the human patients. Human anti-bodies or humanized antibodies are produced to successfully overcome this problem. During humanization, all amino acids except those responsible for the actual binding are changed to those of human antibodies. Antibodies can be modified to increase their affin-ity and selectivity. The sequential steps by which molecular biological methods are used to improve the antibodies are analogous to those of a medicinal chemistry program. The critical path of in vitro and in vivo assays is closely similar. Selectivity, potency, and effi-cacy have to be established in the selection of the final drug candidate.

3.4   FROM DRUG CANDIDATE TO DRUG

The declaration of a drug candidate is the second major decision step in drug discovery and development. It automatically triggers the onset of a new set of procedures and for-malities. All further steps are monitored or even controlled by regulatory agencies such as the Federal Drug Administration (FDA) in the United States.

3.4.1   Safety Testing

Drug candidates are subjected to formalized testing procedures in animals before they can be given to humans. Typically the time period of administration to animals has to exceed the intended treatment duration in humans. For short-term administration it is usually required to assess toxicity by treating animals from two species during a few weeks. Rats, rabbits, dogs, and monkeys are the most frequently used test species. Pharmacokinetic properties, which can vary massively from species to species, drive the species selection. Plasma levels have to reach sufficiently high levels to yield sufficiently high exposure to the tested drug candidate. A wide range of doses is administered. Typically, during the course of the safety studies, toxic effects become apparent at the higher dose levels. These easily observable high-dose effects then guide the investigators in the search for less obvious toxic effects at lower doses. Besides behavioral observations, body fluid compo-sition is being analyzed for abnormalities, and at the end of the study, the organs of the test animals are weighted and the tissues processed for histological analysis. The safety studies provide an initial definition of the therapeutic window for a drug candidate. A factor of 20 or higher is typically desired between plasma concentrations and exposures expected to be clinically efficacious and those producing toxicity in animals.

When a drug candidate is intended for chronic use, longer toxicity studies are neces-sary. Six months long safety studies are typically required to support phase II clinical studies. For regulatory approval safety studies of two-year duration may be necessary. Besides simply extending the exposure time, the long-term studies are more likely to reveal rare events such as carcinogenicity. All drug candidates have to be evaluated in the stan-dard Ames in vitro mutagenicity test. However, the test does not have sufficient predic-tive power for carcinogenic events occurring at low doses over prolonged periods of time, thus justifying the long-term in vivo testing. Additional animal testing is required for drugs intended to be prescribed for children or women at reproductive ages. Effects on repro-ductive behavior and performance are typically evaluated in special studies for which rabbits are being used.

Safety testing is currently the most unpredictable and most frustrating step in drug discovery and development. Most pharmaceutical companies share the experience that about three out of five drug candidates fail in safety for unpredictable and unknown reasons. Examples of insurmountable problems include organ toxicity at therapeutic concentrations, fatal events such as heart failure or ischemic stroke at doses not much higher than those needed for the therapeutic effects, crystalline precipitation of the drug or a metabolite in the kidney, and many others. The list of toxicities observed is remarkably astonishing and depressingly long. Different and idiosyncratic toxicities are often observed for compounds that differ only slightly with regard to their chemical structure. The idiosyncratic nature of most toxic events makes it worthless to investigate the mechanism of toxicity,. Moving a different compound into development most often is easier and more cost effective than investigating the mechanism of toxicity, since such an effort can easily take many years. Compounds are thus simply abandoned, a most frustrating event for the scientists that worked several years to generate the drug candidates.

The high attrition rate of compounds in safety testing observed with small organic compounds emphasizes the main advantage of biological drugs. Natural proteins and specific antibodies are less likely to produce fatal insurmountable toxic events than small molecules of xenobiotic origin. While statistics are not publicly available, anecdotal information strongly supports the view that antibodies fare particularly well in safety testing. To improve the difficult situation with small molecules, many pharmaceutical companies have started to invest substantial efforts to improve toxicity predictions. Gene array technologies offer one possible approach. They are based on the hope that toxic events occurring after long periods of administration can be predicted from patterns of gene expression changes occurring after single administration. This approach may not be able to exclude all toxic compounds, but it offers the potential to identify patterns that correlate with toxicity. Gradually increasing experience with existing drugs and novel drug candidates may lead to a high degree of predictive power. Given the high costs of drug development, a significant fraction of which reflects the loss of compounds in safety, efforts are clearly warranted that may predict adverse events in the safety studies.

Even the most rigorous safety testing in animals cannot exclude all toxicity in humans. There may be species-specific events that only occur in humans. There may be very rare events that are only observed when large numbers of patients have been exposed to new drugs. In rare cases drugs have to be withdrawn after approval because of such events. In more benign situations patients and physicians have to be made aware of additional safety precautions. Patient safety is an absolute and primary concern in drug discovery, and development and the medical oath of not doing harm applies rigorously. Further clinical development is guided by these principles even when animal studies have not raised significant safety issues.

3.4.2 IND Filing and Phase I Human Safety Studies

After satisfactory completion of animal safety studies and before the start of human experimentation it is necessary to file a Notice of Claimed Investigational Exemption for a New Drug (IND) with the FDA and to obtain the agency's approval to proceed. The IND application describes the composition and synthesis of the drug candidate, all data from in vitro studies and animal experimentation, as well as the clinical plans. Following IND approval, phase I clinical studies may initiate. Their aim is to determine safety in a small number of human volunteers. Very low doses, 1/10 or less of the anticipated effective dose, are administered, and patients are carefully monitored for signs of discomfort and toxicity. Gradually, over many sessions, the dose is increased until the first, even very mild signs of adverse effects appear, such as behavioral or cardiovascular changes. The dose just below that creating the first sign of adverse effects will be the maximally permissible dose in further studies. For drugs intended for chronic use, the single-dose phase I studies are followed by multiple-dose studies, again starting at very low doses. The phase I studies define the upper level of the therapeutic window of a drug candidate. In rare situations no adverse effects are observed even at high doses, substantiating the hope for a broad therapeutic window of the future drug.

Phase I studies lack adequate controls to evaluate efficacy. However, it is often attempted to get initial hints for efficacy in these studies. Obvious examples are signs of sedation for drug candidates intended to stimulate sleep. More often it is attempted to obtain a biological signal that reflects a measurable action of the drug, a so-called pharmacological readout of drug action. Determination of receptor occupancy with imaging methods represents a sophisticated version of this approach. These approaches are becoming increasingly important in the neuroscience area and will be discussed in detail in subsequent chapters.

3.4.3 Proof of Efficacy Phase II Studies

During phase II, medical efficacy of a drug candidate is tested in patients suffering from the targeted disease. One or two doses are typically used. They can be based on receptor occupancy data obtained in phase I or, traditionally, simply represent the maximally permissible dose established in the phase I studies. Phase II efficacy trials, to be reliable, must be designed as double-blind studies, so that neither the patient nor the treating physician knows whether a patient receives the actual drug. They must contain a placebo control group or a group of patients treated with a drug previously approved for this clinical condition. Placebo controls are particularly important in psychiatric diseases where the perception of being treated tends to elicit very significant beneficial effects in patients. In case of a positive result, the initial phase II studies are often followed by additional studies with small numbers of patients to get a better understanding of the dose–response relationship. Such phase IIb dose-ranging studies help to determine the optimal dose for the large-scale phase III evaluations.

The disclosure of phase II results is a determining, and perhaps the most emotional, moment in the drug discovery and development process. Success in phase II validates the drug target. Success in phase II provides a high probability of success for the specific drug candidate in phase III. The efforts over many years become justified as well as future efforts on the mechanism of action and related drugs. Failure in phase II dooms the drug candidate and, most likely, any further attempts on the target molecule. Unfortunately, too often scientists see years of dedicated effort rendered pointless because of a negative result in a phase II study.

3.4.4 Phase III Studies, NDA, Regulatory Approval, and Marketing

Phase III studies serve to confirm efficacy in larger patient populations and to obtain additional safety data. Hundreds, sometimes thousands, of patients participate in these studies that generate better understanding of the spectrum of efficacy and adverse effects over a wide range of individual patients. Double blinding is a necessity for these studies. If the phase III results confirm efficacy of the drug candidate, a New Drug Application (NDA) is filed with the FDA. The agency has established approval procedures that distinguish between truly novel drugs and drugs that are similar to previously approved compounds. A decision can take several months, but legislative changes during recent years have made unjustified delays a problem of the past. Modern regulatory agencies are staffed with dedicated professionals who share the goal to bring safe and effective medication to patients in need.

3.5 CONCLUSIONS

The drug discovery and development process is divided into three distinct stages by two key events, the selection of a target and the identification of a drug candidate.

Target selection remains an empirical process that overlaps substantially with basic research. Three general approaches can be defined. First, existing validated targets are explored, since they provide a relatively assured way to improved drugs. However, only a very small number of biological molecules are validated drug targets, those that mediate the actions of approved and clinically efficacious drugs. In the second strategy, all biological molecules are broadly assessed for suitability as drug targets. All biological molecules can serve as drug targets in principle, but molecules with crucial regulatory functions such as enzymes, hormones, and neurotransmitter receptors have a higher likelihood to be useful. Select groups of such molecules are evaluated for target suitability using in vivo animal studies. Classic knockout technologies and more advanced conditional knockout and knockdown strategies help to select the most promising ones. In the third strategy, potential drug targets are selected from a detailed analysis of disease mechanism. This strategy has the highest probability of success and is likely to become the dominant one in the foreseeable future.

Selection of a target triggers a sequence of determined events toward the goal of identifying a suitable drug candidate. For small organic molecule drugs, the process starts with the search for lead compounds using advanced HTS technologies. This is followed by medicinal chemistry efforts to optimize affinity to and selectivity for the receptor site, pharmacokinetic properties, and efficacy in animal models of the disease. For a biologics drug discovery program, natural molecules or modified natural molecules are optimized toward acceptable pharmacokinetic properties and adequate safety. In both cases the process culminates with the selection of a single molecule as a drug candidate.

Drug candidates undergo rigorous safety testing in animals. At doses identified as safe in animals, the drug candidates are then evaluated for safety in human phase I studies. At doses that do not produce any adverse effects or risks, the drug candidate is then evaluated for efficacy in a double-blinded phase II study in the appropriate patient population. If positive, large-scale phase III studies establish safety and efficacy in broad patient populations and lead to final approval for general use.

The process of discovering and developing new drugs is complex and long. Failures are the routine rather than the exception. Given the massive cost and effort, it is important to optimize every step individually to increase the probability of success of the entire program. Modern drug discovery is a unique process at the interface of basic science and organized development. Modern drug discovery is very different from the empirical and heuristic approaches just a few decades ago, and it now represents a mature and self-standing discipline.

REFERENCES

Further Reading

ABRAHAM, D.J., ed. *Burger's Medicinal Chemistry and Drug Discovery*. Wiley, New York, 6th ed., 2002.

BLADON, C. *Pharmaceutical Chemistry: Therapeutic Aspects of Biomacromolecules*. Wiley, New York, 2002.

BLEICHER, K.H., BOHM, H.J., MULLER, K., and ALANINE, A.I. Hit and lead generation: Beyond high-throughput screening. *Nature Rev. Drug Disc.* 2: 369–378, 2003.

DREWS, J. Drug Discovery: A historical perspective. *Science* 287: 1960–1964, 2000.

GAD, S.C. *Drug Safety Evaluation*. Wiley, New York, 2002.

HO, R.J., and GIBALDI, M. *Biotechnology and Biopharmaceuticals*. Wiley, New York, 2003.

HANNON, G.J. RNA interference. *Nature* 418: 244–251, 2002.

WALTERS, W.P., and NAMCHUK, M. Designing screens: How to make your hits a hit. *Nature Rev. Drug Disc.* 2: 259–266, 2003.

Citations

BAJORATH, J. Integration of virtual and high-throughput screening. *Nature Rev. Drug Disc.* 1: 883–894, 2002.

BURLEY, S.K., and BONANNO, J.B. Structural genomics of proteins from conserved biochemical pathways and processes. *Curr. Opin. Struct. Biol.* 12: 383–391, 2002.

CROWLEY, V.E.F., YEO, G.S.H., and O'RAHILLY, S. Obesity therapy: Altering the energy intake-and-expenditure balance sheet. *Nature Rev. Drug Disc.* 1: 276–286, 2002.

DRUCKER, D.J. Development of glucagon-like peptide-1-based pharmaceuticals as therapeutic agents for the treatment of diabetes. *Curr. Pharm. Des.* 7: 1399–1342, 2001.

FAROOQI, I., KEOGH, J.M., YEO, G.S.H., LANK, E.J., CHEETHAM, T., and O'RAHILLY, S. Clinical spectrum of obesity and mutations in the melanocortin 4 receptor gene. *N. Eng. J. Med.* 348: 1085–1095, 2003.

GEYSEN, H.M., SCHOENEN, F., WAGNER, D., and WAGNER, R. Combinatorial compound libraries for drug discovery: An ongoing challenge. *Nature Rev. Drug Disc.* 2: 222–230, 2003.

GONZALEZ, J.E., OADES, K., LEYCHKIS, Y., HAROOTUNIAN, A., and NEGULESCU, P.A. Cell-based assays and instrumentation for screening ion-channel targets. *Drug Disc. Today* 4: 431–439, 1999.

JOHNSON, T.O., ERMOLIEFF, J., and JIROUSEK, M.R. Protein tyrosine phosphatase 1B inhibitors for diabetes. *Nature Rev. Drug Disc.* 1: 697–709, 2002.

KNOWLES, J., and GROMO, G. Target selection in drug discovery. *Nature Rev. Drug Disc.* 1: 63–69, 2002.

LEWANDOSKI, M. Conditional control of gene expression in the mouse. *Nature Rev. Genet.* 2: 743–755, 2001.

LIPINSKI, C.A., LOMBARDO, F., DOMINI, B.W., and FEENEY, P.J. Experimental and computational approaches to estimate solubility and permeability in drug discovery and development settings. *Adv. Drug Del. Rev.* 23: 3–25, 1997.

THOMPSON, J.D. Applications of antisense and siRNAs during preclinical drug development. *Drug Disc. Today* 7: 912–917, 2002.

WENLOCK, M.C., AUSTIN, R.P., BARTON, P., DAVIES, A.M., and LEESON, P.D. A comparison of physiochemical property profiles of development and marketed oral drugs. *J. Med. Chem.* 46: 1250–1256, 2003.

WOLCKE, J., and ULLMANN, D. Miniaturized HTS technologies—uHTS. *Drug Disc. Today* 6: 637–646, 2001.

ZAMBROWICZ, B.P., and SANDS, A.T. Knockouts model the 100 best-selling drugs—Will they model the next 100? *Nature Rev. Drug Disc.* 1: 38–51, 2002.

ZIMANYI, I.A., and PELLEYMOUNTER, M.A. The role of melanocortin peptides and receptors in regulation of energy balance. *Curr. Pharm. Des.* 9: 627–641, 2003.

Chapter 4

Drug Target Selection for Nervous System Diseases

Target selection is the most critical issue and most difficult decision in drug discovery for neurologic and psychiatric diseases. There are more than a thousand highly promising, putative drug targets. However, the vast majority of them are very poorly or not at all validated. The total worldwide capacity of all biopharmaceutical companies is not sufficiently large to explore all target opportunities. The patient populations are too small to allow the clinical investigators comparative testing of all the drug candidates within a reasonable period of time. While target selection is a difficult issue for all indications, it is particularly severe a problem in the neurosciences. Other organ systems are less complex and are better understood. The diseases related to them are often covered fairly well by the existing drugs. A mature field such as the cardiovascular area is served by many classes of existing drugs that provide a good number of clinically validated drug targets. Given the special situation of the neuroscience area, it is well justified to devote an entire chapter to the difficult problem of target selection. The structure of the chapter follows that of the previous one. It discusses sequentially the further exploration of validated targets, the evaluation of putative and speculative targets, and the identification of suitable targets through the study of disease mechanisms.

4.1 VALIDATED TARGETS AND REVERSE PHARMACOLOGY

The total number of clinically validated targets in the neuroscience area is only 14. This number is based on the drugs that are currently approved and generally used in the medical treatment. Of the 14 validated targets, 3 are enzymes involved in neurotransmitter degradation, 4 are G-protein-coupled receptors for neurotransmitters, 2 are ion channel receptors for neurotransmitter, 3 are neurotransmitter transporters, 1 is a voltage-gated ion channels, and 1 is a temperature-gated ion channels (Table 4.1). Adding the targets validated through the drugs of abuse nicotine and arecoline, which act on acetylcholine receptors, cocaine that acts on the dopamine transporter, and cannabis acting on its specific receptor the total number of validated targets rises to 17. The number becomes slightly higher if drugs influencing the actions of the autonomous nervous system are included in the list. In their majority these are agonists or antagonists for acetylcholine and norepinephrine receptors. Whatever detailed criteria are applied, the number of validated targets is incredibly small when compared with the total number of genes expressed in the nervous system. The number of proteins ultimately useful as drug targets must be much higher.

Drug Discovery for Nervous System Diseases, by Franz F. Hefti
ISBN 0-471-46563-1   Copyright © 2005 by John Wiley & Sons, Inc.

Table 4.1   Clinically validated targets of drugs for nervous system diseases

Target	Drug	Effect
Enzymes		
Monoamine oxidase (MAO-A and MAO-B)	Pargyline and related antidepressants	Inhibition of monoamine transmitter degradation
Catechol-*O*-methyltransferase	Tolcapone and related anti-Parkinson drugs	Inhibition of dopamine degradation
Acetylcholinesterase	Tacrine and related anti-Alzheimer's drugs	Blockage of acetylcholine degradation
G-Protein-Coupled Neurotransmitter Receptors		
D_2 receptor	Haloperidol and all antipsychotics	Antagonists
	Bromocriptine and related anti-Parkinson drugs	Agonists
$5\text{-HT}_{1B/D}$ receptors	Sumatriptan and related antimigraine drugs	Agonists
GABA-B receptor (GABA-B$_1$ and -B$_2$)	Baclofen (antispasticity drug)	Agonist
μ Opioid receptor	Morphine and related opioid drugs for pain	Agonists
Ionotropic Neurotransmitter Receptors		
GABA-A receptor	Diazepam and related benzodiazepine drugs Barbiturates	Allosteric agonists
NMDA receptor	Ketamine used as anesthetic Memantine for Alzheimer's disease	Antagonists
Neurotransmitter Transporters		
NE transporter (NET)	Imipramine and related antidepressants	Blockage of NE reuptake
5-HT transporter (SERT)	Paroxetine and related antidepressants	Blockade of 5-HT reuptake
GABA transporter (GAT-1)	Tiagabine (anti-epilepsy drug)	Blockade of GABA reuptake
Voltage-Gated Ion Channels		
Na^+ channels	Lidocaine and other local anesthetics	Blockade of channel function
Temperature-Gated Ion Channels		
TRPV1 channels	Capsaicin for local pain control	Desensitization of channel

Clinically validated targets are attractive because they offer a direct way to new drugs through reverse pharmacology approaches. Most of the validated targets are molecules related to neurotransmitter mechanisms, in particular those of the classical transmitters GABA, glutamate, acetylcholine, dopamine, norepinephrine, and serotonin. In the strict sense the reverse pharmacology approaches concentrate on a single target molecule. However, in the case of neurotransmitter receptors, it seems more useful to broaden the horizon to the entire synapse. Stimulating the synthesis, enhancing the release, blocking the reuptake, or directly mimicking the transmitter action are parallel ways to achieve increased postsynaptic action. For these reasons the following section discusses the transmitter mechanisms of the major transmitter. Some of the targets discussed in the reverse pharmacology section could equally well be considered in the subsequent section on speculative targets. It seems more useful though to keep together the targets related to a specific neurotransmitter.

4.1.1 GABAergic Mechanisms

It has been estimated that more than half of the synapses in the brain use GABA as their transmitter. Since GABA elicits an inhibitory response in almost all the cases, GABA is considered the dominant inhibitory central neurotransmitter. GABAergic interneurons are ubiquitously distributed in the brain and spinal cord. In addition there are groups of long GABAergic projection neurons, among them the descending pathways of the extrapyramidal motor system and the projections of the cerebellar Purkinje cells.

Figure 4.1 shows a diagram of the structure of a GABAergic synapse. The metabolic neurotransmitter pathways are relatively simple. Glutamic acid decarboxylase (GAD) catalyzes the synthesis of GABA from glutamate, which is derived from the general metabolism related to the Krebs cycle. It is predominantly located in the central nervous system and serves for mapping GABAergic neurons in immunohistochemical procedures. A second enzyme, GABA-transaminase (GABA-T), is responsible for the catabolic step and the formation of the metabolite succinic semialdehyde, which is then reintegrated into the general metabolism. Inhibitors of GAD and GABA-T have been explored as drug candidates. They, respectively, reduce and elevate the levels of GABA, and they decrease and increase the inhibition in a general way. They may thus have utility as general stimulants or anti-epileptic drugs. However, these efforts have been largely abandoned in favor of drug discovery research on GABA receptors. The receptors offer a much wider spectrum of diversity and have become favorite objects in the drug target search.

Two groups of receptors mediate the actions of GABA. The GABA-A receptors are ion channels, ionotropic receptors, and they play the dominant role. The GABA-B receptors belong to the group of G-protein-coupled receptors and are referred to as metabotropic receptors. (The term metabotropic does not adequately reflect the function of these receptors, which mediate changes in intracellular metabolism as well as ion flux. However, the term is frequently used for G-protein-coupled receptors for molecules that also act on ionotropic receptors.) The GABA-A receptors are the target for the benzodiazepine-type drugs and barbiturates, and thus represent a highly validated drug target. They offer the best example for the power of the reverse pharmacology approach. The GABA-B receptors are the target of baclofen, a drug used for the treatment of spasticity and specific forms of pain.

The synaptic action of GABA is terminated by specific transporter proteins, located on the glial cells or the GABAergic neurons themselves. The easy ability to manipulate

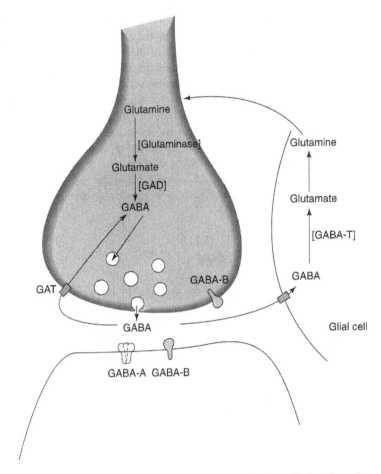

Figure 4.1 Diagram of the GABAergic synapse. GABA is synthesized from glutamate by glutamic acid decarboxylase (GAD). Metabolism in neurons in glial cells is catalyzed by GABA-transaminase (GABA-T). GABA-A ion channel and GABA-B G-protein-coupled receptors mediate post- and presynaptic actions of GABA. The synaptic action of GABA is terminated by several GABA transporters (GAT).

the function of the GABAergic synapse with drugs acting on GABA-A receptors has masked the potential of the transporters as drug targets. Four distinct transporter proteins have been characterized, most of them expressed on neurons and glial cells. Tiagabine, a clinically used anti-epileptic drug, inhibits GAT-1, and is believed to exert its therapeutic effects by increasing the synaptic concentration of GABA. The pharmacology of the other subtypes, GAT-2, GAT-3, and BGT-1, has not been developed and remains a wide-open field for drug discovery (Soudijn and Wijngaarden, 2000).

The Benzodiazepine Receptor Site on GABA-A Receptors

GABA-A receptors are multimer ligand-gated ion channels, typically composed of two α, two β and at least one additional subunit, often a γ subunit and more rarely a δ, ε, θ, or π subunit (Fig. 4.2). The natural ligand, GABA, binds to a receptor site on the β subunits. Muscimol and bicuculline are direct agonists and antagonists at this binding site, respectively. Barbiturates, benzodiazepines, picrotoxin, and specific steroids called neurosteroids each bind to distinct receptor sites and other subunits. The functionally most

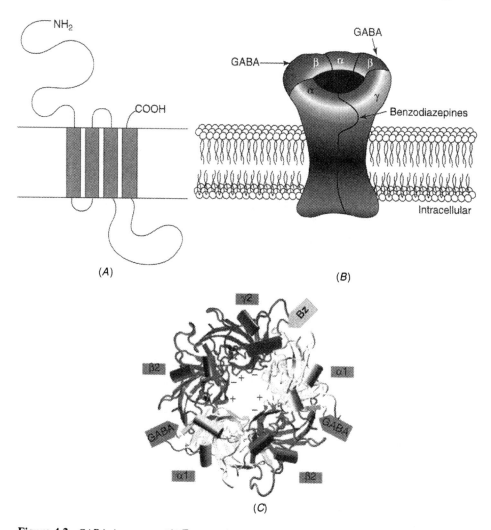

Figure 4.2 GABA-A receptors. (**A**) Transmembrane structure of the GABA-A subunits. (**B**) Assembly of subunits to the functional channel and location of the receptor sites for GABA and drugs. (**C**) Model structure of extracellular domains. (Reprinted with permission, Ernst et al., 2003)

important receptor site, the one mediating the actions of benzodiazepine drugs, is formed by a small number of amino acids at the interface of the α and γ subunits. Those located on the α subunit make the essential contribution to the molecular specificity. It is thus possible to generate benzodiazepine receptor ligands that selectively influence GABA-A receptors containing one of the six α subunits. In the brain different types of GABA-A receptors, with different α subunit compositions, participate in distinct functions and behaviors. The traditional benzodiazepine drugs, such as diazepam, influence most receptor subtypes in similar ways. Their behavioral actions of benzodiazepines include sedation, anxiolysis, and memory dysfunction. Receptors containing the $\alpha1$ subunits mediate the sedative actions. The GABA-A receptors containing $\alpha2$ and $\alpha3$ subunits mediate anxiolysis, whereas the effects on memory are believed to reflect actions on $\alpha5$ containing GABA-A receptors.

The matrix assigning specific receptor subtypes to distinct behaviors is well supported by elegant transgenic animal studies. Since the benzodiazepine receptor does not serve a natural receptor role, it can be mutated without functional consequences, making it possible to generate transgenic animals with mutations of the $\alpha 1$ subunit that do not bind benzodiazepine drugs. In such animals benzodiazepines cause anxiolysis without sedation, supporting the conclusion that $\alpha 1$ containing receptors mediate sedation and other subtypes are responsible for the anxiolytic effects. Several companies have generated subtype-selective benzodiazepine drugs or drug candidates. Zaleplon and zolpidem, two approved sleep-inducing drugs, selectively stimulate the $\alpha 1$ containing GABA-A receptors and thus provide clinical proof for the role of the $\alpha 1$ subtype as the mediator for sedation. Compounds selective for $\alpha 2$ and $\alpha 3$ are anxiolytic in rodents without producing sedation, making these receptors attractive targets for improved future anxiolytic drugs (Mohler et al., 2001).

Studies with transgenic animals and subtype selective compounds link the $\alpha 5$ receptor subunit to the memory disturbances observed with nonselective benzodiazepines. GABA-A receptors are Cl^- channels that serve an inhibitory function in the synaptic cleft. Nonselective benzodiazepines increase opening frequency of these channels and thus decrease the excitability of the postsynaptic neurons. Since these drugs impair memory function, it has been speculated that compounds with opposite effects on the benzodiazepine receptor site, so-called inverse agonists, might improve memory. Early studies with nonselective subtype inverse agonists have provided tantalizing, but very tentative evidence in support of this concept. The selective location of the $\alpha 5$ receptor subunit in the hippocampus, the brain structure with a critical role in memory function, provided the first hint that the effects are mediated by this receptor. Stronger support is provided by $\alpha 5$ knockout mice, which perform better in an animal test for memory function. In the same animal assay, inverse agonists selective for $\alpha 5$-containing receptors also have positive effect, suggesting that such compounds might enhance cognition in humans and be suitable for the treatment of diseases involving memory impairment (Chambers et al., 2002).

The differentiation of benzodiazepine receptor subtypes is perhaps the most elegant example of reverse pharmacology. The selective association of the $\alpha 1$ containing GABA-A receptors with sedation and sleep has been validated by drugs that are effective and commercially successful. While the validation of $\alpha 2$ and $\alpha 3$ containing receptors with anxiety and that of $\alpha 5$ containing receptors with cognition is expected to happen in the future, a cautious remark seems appropriate. Surprises do occur in clinical development, and even the most elegant concepts derived from studies in rodents may not translate into human clinical practice. With regard to the GABA-A receptors, caution is suggested by the experience with pagoclone, a compound with a small degree of selectivity for $\alpha 2$ and $\alpha 3$ containing receptors, which has failed to achieve clinically meaningful anxiolysis in human studies (Bateson, 2003). The clinical efficacy of inverse agonists selective for $\alpha 5$ containing neurons remains to be established. As discussed in Chapter 9, the field of cognitive enhancers has seen many disappointments, and there are no positive control drugs that assure the existence of a sufficient window for enhancing human cognitive function.

GABA-B Receptors

Functional GABA-B receptors are formed by heterodimers of two related subunits, GABA-B_1 and GABA-B_2 (Couve et al., 2000). The former exists in two forms, GABA-B_{1a} and GABA-B_{1b}. The subunits are widely expressed in the central nervous system at pre- and postsynaptic locations in the GABAergic synapse. Baclofen, a drug used for the treatment of spasticity and chronic pain, acts as an agonist at the heterodimeric GABA-B receptors. It is believed to derive its beneficial therapeutic effects from increasing the general inhibition exerted by GABAergic synapses in the spinal cord. The very limited efficacy of baclofen dampens the enthusiasm for a reverse pharmacology approach towards subtype selective GABA-B agonists. However, it is possible that action on one receptor masks potent effects on the other. Subtype selective knockout animal studies will help to address this issue.

GABA-C Receptors

Gene products related to the α subunits of GABA-A receptors, $\rho 1$–$\rho 3$, are able to form functional Cl^- channels that respond to GABA. They are often discussed as a subgroup of the GABA-A receptors. Since these channels are formed by a single subunit alone, do not appear to be heterodimers as the GABA-A receptors, and do not have receptor sites for benzodiazepines or barbiturates, they can be considered a distinct subtype, the GABA-C receptors. These receptors exist at high levels in the retina, but have been detected at lower levels throughout the brain. The functional role remains to be defined as well as their utility as drug targets. Compounds that selectively bind to GABA-C receptors have been identified and serve as tools for the further exploration (Johnston et al., 2003).

4.1.2 Glutamatergic Mechanisms

Glutamate is the dominant excitatory neurotransmitter of the central nervous system. It is the neurotransmitter of the major pathways in the brain and spinal cord. Figure 4.3 shows a diagram of a glutamatergic synapse. Glutamate emerges from the metabolic pathway of the Krebs cycle and can also be formed from glutamine through the catalytic action of glutaminase. Neither of the synthetic pathways involves enzymes selective for the synaptic process, and they do not represent attractive drug targets. Within the synapse glutamate is transported into vesicles by specific vesicular glutamate transporters, VGLT1 and VGLUT2. The two proteins are differentially regulated and expressed. VGLT1 seems to be the dominant transporter in synapses showing plasticity in learning, whereas VGLT2 is the more important transporter in sensory pathways. The pharmacology of the vesicular transporter remains to be explored, and the existence of subtypes may offer opportunities to influence glutamatergic neurotransmission in specific ways.

Ionotropic Glutamate Receptors

Upon release glutamate acts on several types of glutamate receptors (Fig. 4.4). Two highly diverse groups of glutamate receptors have been characterized, the ionotropic receptor group including *N*-methyl-D-aspartate (NMDA) receptors and non-NMDA receptors, and the metabotropic glutamate receptors. Despite the importance of glutamatergic synapse and the high diversity of receptors, only the NMDA receptors can be considered a validated drug target at the glutamatergic synapse. Ketamine, used for anesthesia in children, is an antagonist for them. More recently memantine, a low-affinity NMDA antagonist, has been approved for the treatment of Alzheimer's disease. Similar to the GABA-A receptor, the NMDA receptor is a complex heteromeric assembly of various subunits. It always contains the NMDAR1 subunit that can be associated with one or more of four subunits, called NMDAR2A–2D. Various splicing forms have been described for NMDAR1, and RNA editing has further complicated the molecular analysis. The functional receptors contain several drug receptor sites, including those binding glutamate, Zn^{2+}, glycine, and

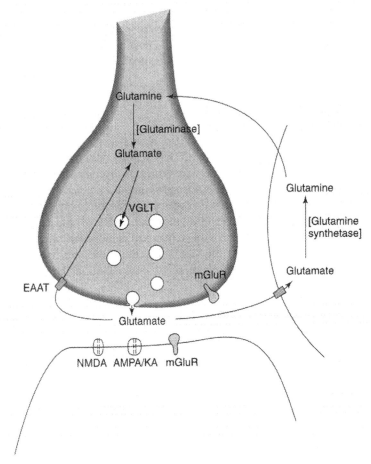

Figure 4.3 Diagram of the glutamatergic synapse. Glutamate emerges from the metabolic pathway of the Krebs cycle and can also be formed from glutamine through the catalytic action of glutaminase. Within the synapse glutamate is transported into vesicles by specific vesicular glutamate transporters (VGLT). The synaptic actions of glutamate are mediated by ion channel NMDA and AMPA/KA receptors and G-protein-coupled (metabotropic) receptors (mGluR). Transmembrane excitatory amino acid transporters (EAAT) terminate the synaptic effects.

polyamines. Binding of glycine is necessary for normal function of the receptor (Marino and Conn, 2002). NMDA antagonists are able to protect neurons from anoxia in vitro and in vivo, suggesting that they may have utility in the treatment of acute injury to the nervous system, ischemic stroke in particular. Several compounds have been tested in clinical trials, as discussed in more detail in Chapter 11.

Non-NMDA glutamate receptors were initially categorized into amino-3-hydroxy-5-methylisozazolepropionic acid (AMPA), kainate (KA), and quisqualate receptors based on binding studies with these ligands. The molecular analysis has not provided a simple molecular correlate to the functional characterization. Non-NMDA glutamate receptors are formed by various subunits of three protein families. These are the GluR1–4 subunits, the GluR5–7 subunits, and KA1 and KA2 subunits. As for the NMDA receptor, various splicing variants and RNA editing complicate the picture. The non-NMDA receptors represent a fertile area for drug discovery. The interest in them as well as in the NMDA receptors

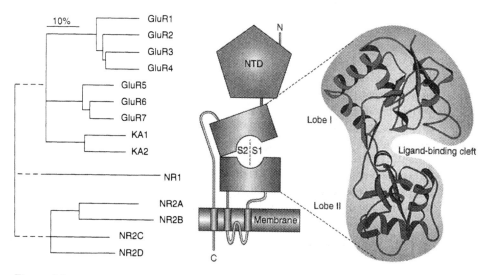

Figure 4.4 Ionotropic glutamate receptors. (**A**) Sequence relationships of ionotropic glutamate receptor proteins. NMDA receptors are formed by heterodimers of NR1 and NR2 subunits. Homo- and heterodimers of GluR and KA receptors form various AMPA and KA receptors. (**B**) The various subunits have a modular structure. The *N*-terminal domain (NTD) is followed by the S1 and S2 domains, which form a cleft for the ligand. Three transmembrane domains participate in the formation of ion channels in homo- and heterodimers. (Reprinted with permission, Ozawa et al., 1998, and Madden, 2002)

is fueled by a wealth of data suggesting utility in schizophrenia, anxiety, Alzheimer's disease, spinal cord injury, and ischemic stroke, and they will remain a very active area for drug discovery in the future (Lerma, 2003).

Metabotropic Glutamate Receptors

Metabotropic glutamate receptors (mGluRs) belong to the large group of G-protein-coupled receptors, making them instantly attractive as putative drug targets. Eight subtypes have been characterized, mGluR1–mGluR8. They are sometimes divided into three groups based on primary coupling mechanisms and pharmacological differences in response to agonists. Group 1 receptors (mGluR1 and mGluR5) stimulate phosphatidyli-nositol hydrolysis, group 2 receptors (mGluR2 and mGluR3), and group 3 receptors (mGluR4, mGluR6, mGluR7, mGluR8) inhibit cAMP formation but show different agonist selectivity. The metabotropic glutamate receptors are modulating the effects of glutamate at the synapse. They occur at locations not typically occupied by the ionotropic receptors, at the presynaptic terminals and in zones immediately surrounding the synaptic cleft. The various subtypes are differentially located throughout the mammalian brain. Besides the receptor site for the neurotransmitter glutamate itself, there are allosteric drug receptor sites. These unusual properties make the mGluRs uniquely attractive as potential targets for drug discovery efforts. Early clinical results suggest that agonists for the mGluR2 receptors in the treatment of anxiety and schizophrenia (Clark et al., 2002). mGluR5 receptors have been linked to reward mechanisms and may represent a novel target to treat addiction (Chiamulera et al., 2001).

Glutamate Transporters

The synaptic action of glutamate is terminated by several transporter molecules that transport glutamate back into the presynaptic terminals or into adjacent glial cells. Five related transporters have been identified, EAAT1–EAAT5. They are structurally related to other neurotransmitter transporter proteins. The EAATs are heterogeneously expressed in various brain regions and with regard to their distribution to neuronal and glial cells. These properties make them attractive targets for drug discovery efforts, in particular, related to schizophrenia, as discussed later in Chapter 6. The diversity of these protein families and their differential expression in many areas of the nervous system offer many appealing target opportunities. While the glutamatergic mechanisms are validated drug targets in their totality, a lot of detailed drug discovery research will be necessary to determine which of the specific target proteins and receptors sites lead to optimal drugs.

4.1.3   Cholinergic Mechanisms

Cholinergic neurons serve various distinct and important functions in the nervous system. The motor neurons that directly control the contractions of the skeletal muscle system use acetylcholine as their transmitter. The parasympathetic neurons and the presynaptic sympathetic neurons of the autonomic nervous system are cholinergic. In the brain the most significant populations are the ascending cholinergic neurons of the pedunculopontine region that play a role in arousal, the ascending cholinergic neurons of the basal forebrain crucial for memory functions, and the cholinergic interneurons of the striatum that form a vital part of the extrapyramidal motor systems. Figure 4.5 shows the diagram of a cholinergic synapse. The transmitter, acetylcholine, is synthesized from choline and acetyl coenzyme A through the catalytic action of choline acetyltransferase (ChAT). Following synthesis, acetylcholine is transported into synaptic storage vesicles by a vesicular transporter (VAChT). No specific inhibitors against ChAT or VAChT have been generated. Their ubiquitous distribution in all cholinergic neurons would predict global disruptive effects on nervous system function, making the two proteins less attractive drug targets than the acetylcholine receptors.

Nicotinic Receptors

The synaptic actions of ACh are mediated by two families of receptors, the nicotinic and the muscarinic receptors. Nicotinic receptors are heterodimers, assemblies of various subunits, α_1–α_9, β_1–β_4, γ, δ, and ε. The best-studied nicotinic receptors of the neuromuscular synapse have the composition $2\alpha_1\beta_1\gamma\delta$. Their composition changes during development. Tubocurarine, succinylcholine, and related neuromuscular blocking agents selectively inhibit their functions. Tubocurarine is one of the ingredients of the toxin "curare" that was used by natives of the Amazon region to cover tips of arrows in combat and hunting, thus paralyzing the victims. Succinylcholine is sometimes used clinically as part of anesthesia for surgical procedures that require complete muscle relaxation. The nicotinic receptors of the central nervous system have various compositions. Dominant forms are $2\alpha_4 3\beta_2$ and $5\alpha_7$ but many other forms appear to exist. Nicotine is an antagonist at the $\alpha_4\beta_2$ receptors but does not bind to the α_7 receptors.

The full potential of nicotinic receptors as drug targets remains yet to be explored. Nicotine is one of the most potent and effective drugs for the human nervous system. It increases the heart rate, causes sweating, alleviates pain, reduces appetite, causes addic-

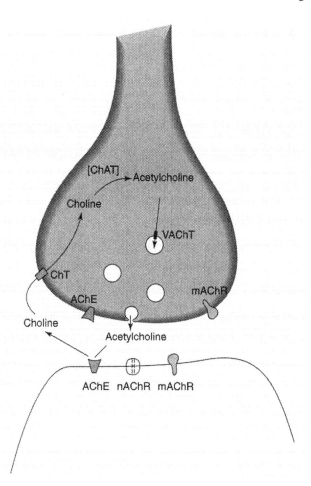

Figure 4.5   Diagram of the cholinergic synapse. Acetylcholine is synthesized from choline and acetyl co-enzyme A through the catalytic action of choline acetyltransferase (ChAT). Following synthesis, acetylcholine is transported into synaptic storage vesicles by a vesicular transporter (VAChT). The synaptic actions of ACh are mediated by two families of receptors, the nicotinic ion channel receptors (nAChR) and the muscarinic G-protein-coupled receptors (mAChR). Acetyl cholinesterase (AChE) inactivates acetylcholine. Choline is taken up again by the presynaptic terminal through a specific transporter (ChT).

tion, and is believed to enhance cognitive functions. Nicotine has too many flaws to be useful for therapeutic purposes. The addictive properties are well known and represent one of the biggest problems of public health. However, if it was possible to separate the undesired effects from desired ones, by ascribing each to specific receptor subtypes, a plethora of highly useful drugs might emerge (Nordberg, 2001).

Muscarinic Receptors

The muscarinic receptors belong to the group of G-protein-coupled receptors. Five subtypes, m1–m5, have been characterized. They are widely distributed in the peripheral and central nervous system, where they serve as postsynaptic mediators of acetylcholine function and as presynaptic receptors regulating acetylcholine synthesis and release. The m2 receptors seem to be specific for the heart. In the brain m1, m3, and m4 are dominant. The muscarinic receptors are very well validated drug targets through atropine, the widely used nonselective antagonist. The actions of atropine are complex and involve most organs. The dominant effects reflect antagonism of the parasympathetic nervous system function. Thus atropine and other nonselective muscarinic blockers stimulate the heart rate, reduce gastrointestinal mobility, induce bladder relaxation, and suppress sweating. Nonselective agonists, including pilocarpine and arecoline, cause central arousal. Arecoline is frequently consumed as ingredient of the betel nut by people in Southeast Asia and serves as a stimulant. Separation of the various effects may lead to clinically useful drugs. The m3 subtype has been linked to urinary incontinence. Selective antagonists for receptors in the bladder would be useful to treat conditions involving bladder hyperreflexia. Selective agonists for the central receptors mediating the stimulatory effects might be useful as cognition enhancers. Several drug discovery research groups have attempted to generate selective m1 agonists for Alzheimer's disease (Beach, 2002).

Acetylcholinesterase

The synaptic action of acetylcholine is terminated by the action of acetyl cholinesterase (AChE), a well-characterized enzyme that cleaves acetylcholine into acetate and choline. Choline is taken up again by the presynaptic terminal through a specific transporter. There appears to be no specific synaptic transporter for acetylcholine itself, making AChE the only player in the termination of acetylcholine actions. In some tissues a related, less specific enzyme, butyrylcholinesterase, can participate in the degradation of acetylcholine. Inhibitors of the cholinesterases have widespread and profound effects on the body by their ability to increase acetylcholine function of all cholinergic synapses. Selective inhibitors of AChE, at small doses, are in clinical use for Alzheimer's disease and Myasthenia gravis, to increase the function of the neuromuscular junction. At higher doses, selective and nonselective cholinesterase inhibitors are invariably toxic, causing convulsions, coma, and death. Following World War II such compounds have been produced in large quantities as weapons of mass destruction that remain a major threat to human welfare (Moretto, 1998).

Botulinum Toxin

While not strictly addressing a medical need, botulinum toxin has found widespread use to locally block neuromuscular transmission for cosmetic purposes and specific forms of local muscle spasms (Simpson, 2004). It is a natural molecule of bacterial origin that preferentially blocks the release of acetylcholine from cholinergic synapses. By cleaving proteins critical for vesicular exocytosis, it shuts down synaptic activity. The unique mechanism of action identifies several proteins involved in neurotransmitter release as putative drug targets. Botulinum toxin requires local injection for clinical utility. Tissue- and cell-specific expression patterns of its target proteins could open an exciting new field for drug discovery.

4.1.4 Dopaminergic Mechanisms

The catecholamines, dopamine, norepinephrine, and epinephrine regulate and influence many functions of the nervous system and of other organs. Dopaminergic neurons are confined to the central nervous system. These neurons and associated molecular mechanisms have been the objects of very intense investigations for many years, because they seem to be particularly attractive from a point of view of drug discovery. Indeed, six molecules associated with dopaminergic mechanisms are clinically validated drug targets, four of them by medically used and approved drugs, and two by illegal drugs of abuse.

The cell bodies of dopaminergic neurons are located in the ventral mesencephalon and in the hypothalamus. The mesencephalic neurons located in the zona compacta of the substantia nigra innervate the corpus striatum and other basal ganglia, forming the nigrostriatal tract, a crucial part of the extrapyramidal motor systems. The adjacent neurons located in the ventral tegmental area project to cortical areas and the nucleus accumbens. They play a significant role in reward and emotional behaviors. The hypothalamic neurons form the tubero-infundibular tract that participates in the regulation of pituitary functions.

Figure 4.6 shows the structure of the dopaminergic synapse and the metabolic pathways. The synthesis of dopamine starts with the hydroxylation of tyrosine by

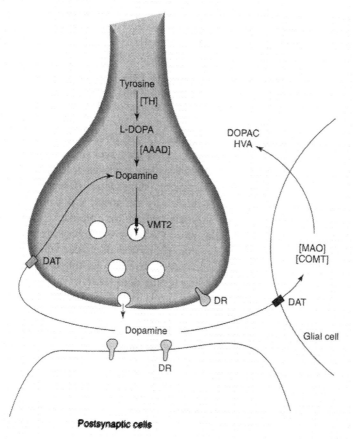

Figure 4.6 Diagram of the dopaminergic synapse. Dopamine synthesis involves hydroxylation of tyrosine by tyrosine hyroxylase (TH), to 3,4-dihydroxyphenylalanine (L-DOPA) and the decarboxylation of L-DOPA to dopamine by aromatic amino acid decarboxylase (AADC). Dopamine is transported into the vesicles by the vesicular monoamine transporter (VMT2). G-protein-coupled receptors (DR) mediate pre- and postsynaptic actions of dopamine. Following release, the synaptic action is terminated by the selective dopamine transporter (DAT) and metabolic degradation catalyzed by monoamine oxidase (MAO), aldehyde dehydrogenase, and catechol-O-methyltransferase (COMT). They generate 3,4-dihydroxyphenylacetic acid (DOPAC) and homovanillic acid (HVA) as principal metabolites.

tyrosine hyroxylase (TH), the rate-limiting enzyme in catecholamine synthesis, to 3,4-dihydroxyphenylalanine (L-DOPA). This intermediate is then decarboxylated to dopamine by aromatic amino acid decarboxylase (AADC). L-DOPA is therapeutically used to treat Parkinson's disease because of its ability to replenish dopamine in the brain. Following synthesis of dopamine in the presynaptic terminals, the transmitter molecules are transported into the vesicles by the vesicular monoamine transporter (VMT2), a molecule related to VMT1, the catecholamine transporter expressed in adrenal cells. Reserpine inhibits VMT2, thus shunting most of the synthesized dopamine directly toward metabolism. Reserpine has been used medically as antipsychotic drug and sedative but has been replaced by more specific drugs in the recent past. Amphetamine, a widely abused stimulant, promotes the release of dopamine and other monoamines through a mechanism that is not fully understood. Their actions are believed to reflect mainly the overstimulation of dopamine receptors in the synaptic cleft.

Five types of dopamine receptors have been identified, DA_1–DA_5 receptors. The D_2 receptor is most widely expressed. It is the target for both antischizophrenia drugs (D_2 antagonists) and drugs for the treatment of Parkinson's disease (D_2 agonists). The D_2 receptors typically are negatively linked to adenylate cyclase. In contrast, the D_1 receptors increase cAMP formation and the phosphorylation of DARPP-32, a protein with multiple effects on metabolic events in postsynaptic cells. The expression pattern of D_1 receptors overlaps in part with that of D_2 receptors, suggesting utility as an alternative drug target to the D_2 receptors. Despite many years of effort, the role of D_1 receptors remains somewhat unclear, and no D_1 selective drugs have entered medical practice as yet. It is very actively pursued as a target for cognition enhancers. D_3 and D_4 receptors have been linked to psychosis and remain under investigation as targets for novel antischizophrenia drugs. D_5 receptors are sparsely expressed only. While widely explored for many decades, the dopamine receptors continue to be attractive putative drug targets (Greengard, 2001).

The synaptic action of dopamine is terminated by the selective dopamine transporter (DAT) and metabolic degradation. Three enzymes catalyze the embolic steps, monoamine oxidase (MAO), aldehyde dehydrogenase, and catechol-O-methyltransferase (COMT). Their sequential actions generate 3,4-dihydroxyphenylacetaldehyde, which is instantly converted by the ubiquitous aldehyde dehydrogenase to 3,4-dihydroxyphenylacetic acid (DOPAC) and further by COMT to homovanillic acid (HVA). The sequence of the steps can vary, generating alternative intermediates; however, DOPAC and HVA are the principal metabolites of dopamine in the brain and serve as readout for dopamine turnover and metabolism. MAO is the target of antidepressant drugs. It exists in two forms, MAO-B and MAO-B. COMT inhibitors are used as adjunct treatment in Parkinson's disease.

4.1.5 Noradrenergic Mechanisms

Norepinephrine (synonymous to noradrenaline) serves as transmitter of distinct populations of central neurons as well as the postsynaptic neurons of the sympathetic nervous system. Given its pronounced effects on many organs, norepinephrine mechanisms have been widely explored in drug discovery, for diseases of the cardiovascular in particular. In the brain norepinephrine is the transmitter of an important modulatory neural system, the ascending noradrenergic pathway emanating from the locus coeruleus. The neurons project to essentially all brain areas, making the system one of the dominant divergent, modulatory systems of the brain.

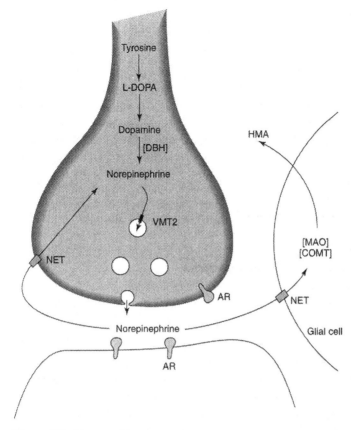

Figure 4.7   Diagram of the noradrenergic synapse. Metabolic pathways and proteins involved are related to those of dopamine. Norepinephrine is synthesized from dopamine by dopamine-β-hydroxylase (DBH). Norepinephrine is transported into the vesicles by the vesicular monoamine transporter (VMT2). Adrenergic G-protein-coupled receptors (AR) mediate pre- and postsynaptic actions. Synaptic effects are terminated by the norepinephrine transporter (NET) and metabolic degradation catalyzed MAO, aldehyde dehydrogenase, and COMT that yield the dominant metabolite 3-methoxy-4-hydroxymandelic acid (HMA).

Figure 4.7 illustrates the noradrenergic synaptic mechanisms. Norepinephrine is synthesized from dopamine by the action of dopamine-β-hydroxylase (DBH). Thus the noradrenergic synapse contains the same enzymatic machinery as the dopaminergic synapse, including TH and AADC, in addition to DBH. Similar to dopamine, norepinephrine is taken up by the transporter VMAT 2 and stored within the synaptic vesicles.

Following synaptic release, the actions of norepinephrine are mediated by three types of G-protein-coupled receptors, the groups of α_1, α_2, and β receptors. The receptors mediate the actions of norepinephrine as well as epinephrine, the hormone secreted by the adrenal medulla. The receptors are therefore typically referred to as adrenergic receptors. Three subtypes exist of each group of the adrenergic receptors, bringing the complete list of adrenergic receptors to α_1A, α_1B, α_1C, α_2A, α_2B, α_2C, β_1, β_2, and β_3. Many of these receptors are targets of drugs used to control blood pressure, reflecting the fact that the sympathetic neurons mediate vessel constriction and increased heart rate. Current medical practice for the treatment of blood pressure includes α as well as β antagonists. Efforts continue to explore subtype selective drugs for this indication area. The α_2 subtype has attracted particular interest since it is located presynaptically, suppressing the release of norepinephrine. None of the adrenergic receptors seems to be located exclusively in the central nervous system. The effects mediated by the peripheral receptors narrow the utility of adrenergic receptors as drug targets for nervous system diseases.

The termination of the synaptic action of norepinephrine is closely similar to that of dopamine. A specific transporter, norepinephrine transporter (NET), mediates the re-uptake of the transmitter into the presynaptic terminals. NET is the target of several antidepressant drugs. Metabolic degradation is mediated by MAO, an aldehyde reductase, and COMT, yielding 3-methoxy-4-hydroxymandelic acid as the principal metabolite.

Noradrenergic mechanisms, as the dopaminergic mechanisms, have been fully explored from a drug discovery perspective. The field has to be considered mature. Nevertheless, there may be further opportunities to make receptor subtype specific drugs for cardiovascular indications. The lack of central nervous system specific receptors limits the utility of these receptors as targets for nervous system diseases.

4.1.6 Serotonergic Mechanisms

The serotonin mechanisms represent the best-explored neurotransmitter system from a drug target point of view, reflecting the unique role of serotoninergic neurons as influential modulators of many functions. Most of the serotoninergic neurons are part of the central nervous system. The central serotonergic neurones form a divergent modulatory system. Their cell bodies are localized in a number of brainstem nuclei from which emerge distinct ascending and descending pathways. Most important are the ascending pathways that originate in the dorsal and medial raphe nuclei and innervate most of the forebrain areas. Serotonergic neurons are part of the innervation of several peripheral organs, including the gastrointestinal system and the bladder, and serotonin is a key mediator of platelet function.

Serotonin is derived from the amino acid tryptophan through two catalytic steps, first by tryptophan hydroxylase (TPH), forming 5-hydroxytryptophan and, second, by AADC, the enzyme also involved in the formation of catecholamines, forming serotonin (5-hydroxytryptamine, 5-HT). Following synthesis, serotonin is taken up by VMAT into the synaptic vesicles and stored for release. Figure 4.8 illustrates the serotonergic synaptic mechanisms.

Four major groups and the total of 13 serotonin receptors have been characterized. The first group, the 5-HT_1 family, contains 5-HT_{1A}, 5-HT_{1B}, 5-HT_{1D}, and 5-HT_{1E}. The second group is formed by 5-HT_{2A}, 5-HT_{2B}, and 5-HT_{2C}. The third group includes 5-HT_4, 5-HT_{5A}, 5-HT_{5B}, 5-HT_6, and 5-HT_7. All these receptors belong to the large group of G-protein-coupled receptors. The fourth group of serotonin receptor, comprising 5-HT_3 alone, is a unique exception in that this receptor is a ligand-gated ion channel related to GABA-A and ionotropic glutamate receptors. 5-HT_{1A} receptors are the target of buspirone, a compound with modest anxiolytic efficacy. $5\text{-HT}_{1B/1D}$ receptors are the targets of the triptans, the antimigraine drugs related to sumatriptan. The 5-HT_{2A} receptors are believed to play an important role in the action of atypical antipsychotic drugs, all of which are mixed $D_2/5\text{-HT}_2$ receptor antagonists. 5-HT_3 antagonists are used to control vomiting. 5-HT4 receptors present only outside the nervous system are the target of cisapride, a 5-HT_4 receptor agonist, used to treat gastrointestinal disorders.

The synaptic action of serotonin is terminated by a selective transporter (SERT), a molecule closely related to the other monoamine transporters (DAT and NET). SERT is

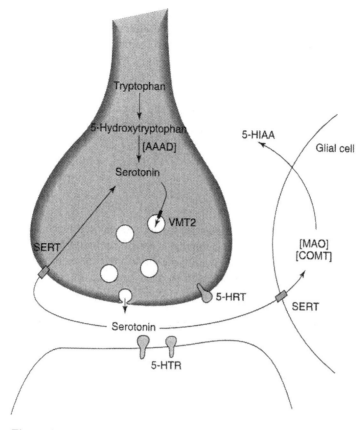

Figure 4.8 Diagram of the serotonergic synapse. Serotonin (5-hydroxytryptophan) is synthesized from tryptophan by tryptophan hydroxylase (TPH) and AADC, and is then taken up by VMAT2 into the synaptic vesicles. Several G-protein-coupled receptors (5-HTR) mediate the actions, which are terminated by the serotonin transporter (SERT). MAO, aldehyde dehydrogenase, and COMT yield the dominant metabolite 5-hydroxyindole acetic acid (5-HIAA).

the target of antidepressant drugs such as fluoxetine. The enzymatic actions of MAO and the aldehyde dehydrogenase form 5-hydroxyindole acetic acid, the principal metabolite of serotonin.

The serotonergic synapse has yielded several highly useful drug targets and has been a favorite area of investigation for drug discovery researchers. The highly divergent nature of the projection system makes it possible to influence most of the brain areas. The high diversity of receptors offers a unique opportunity to refine the current drugs, the uptake inhibitors in particular. Serotonergic receptors are likely to remain one of the most fruitful areas of future drug discovery.

4.1.7 Opiate Receptors

Morphine and its derivatives mimic the action of opioid peptides, enkephalins, and endorphins on opioid receptors. Three receptors have been characterized the μ, δ, and κ receptors by binding studies. Molecular analysis confirmed the existence of three separate genes with various splicing variants. Morphine is a potent agonist for μ receptors and a broad array of findings support the view that the relevant analgesic effects are mediated by the μ receptor alone. Given the broad array of undesired effects of morphine, the addiction, sedation, confusion, gastrointestinal immobility, and respiratory depression, it has been a major goal of pharmacology for more than a century to separate the analgesic from the undesired properties. Despite 100 years of failure these efforts continue and remain exciting.

Opioid peptides belong to the large group of the so-called neuropeptides, meaning peptides active as transmitters or modulators in the nervous system. Substance P, somatostatin, and calcitonin gene-related peptides belong to them. They will be discussed in more detail in the next section of this chapter.

4.1.8 Orphan Drugs

A number of drugs are clinically efficacious and useful, though their mechanism of action is not understood. Several of the earlier compounds found through serendipitous clinical observations fall into this category. They are typically referred to as orphan drugs. The group includes anti-epileptic compounds, such as phenytoin and valproate. Clozapine is a special antipsychotic drug with properties that cannot be explained by its action on dopamine D_2 receptors alone. Modafinil is clinically used for the treatment of narcolepsy, an especially severe form of sleep disorder. Riluzole provides modest improvement in amyotrophic lateral sclerosis. Gabapentin represents the biggest price in the orphan drug group. It is widely used for the treatment of chronic pain. Because of its limited efficacy, the search for mechanisms of action and a more efficacious analogue has become a strong effort in many pharmaceutical companies. NSAIDs can be added to this category because of their ability to prevent Alzheimer's disease. This is a highly intriguing observation believed to hold the key to efficacious preventative treatment for this feared disease. Table 4.2 provides a list of the orphan drugs. For most of them various molecular effects have been described, but these actions have not been decisively linked to the therapeutic effect.

Table 4.2 Orphan drugs (clinically efficacious drugs with unknown primary receptor site)

Therapeutic Use	Drug	Postulated Mechanism of Action
Schizophrenia	Clozapine	DA_4 receptor blockade
Mania	Lithium	Inhibition of kinases and inositol metabolism
Alzheimer's disease	NSAIDs	Inhibition of γ-secretase
Amyotrophic lateral sclerosis	Riluzole	Inhibition of glutamate release
Epilepsy	Carbamazepine Lamotrigine Phenytoin Valproate Felbamate	Inhibition of Na^+ and Ca^{2+} channels, stimulation of GABA mechanisms
Narcolepsy	Modafinil	Stimulation of orexin mechanisms
Pain	Gabapentin	Binding to $\alpha_2\delta$ subunits and inhibition of calcium channels

Establishing the precise mechanism of action of these orphan drugs will identify the drug receptor. Once the receptor has been identified, it is possible to generate a selective and highly potent compound for the clinically validated target, thus providing a direct way to a successful drug. Given this attractive scenario, many pharmaceutical companies have been working on the mechanism of action of orphan drugs. The intriguing and complicated stories of clozapine and gabapentin, to be discussed later, illustrate the difficult nature of this approach. Clozapine binds to a large number of neurotransmitter with high affinity, but it has not been possible to ascribe the clinical benefits to specific receptor types. Gabapentin binds with high affinity to a single subunit of calcium channels, but it has not been possible to conclusively link this binding to the therapeutic benefits. High doses of gabapentin are required for clinical efficacy. At high concentration the compound stimulates several neurotransmitter mechanisms, making it possible that several of these actions combine for the therapeutic benefits.

In the traditional investigations of orphan drugs, the compounds were tested in all the available assays with the hope to make the one revealing observation. In alternative approaches, drugs were modified to cross-link covalently to putative receptor proteins with the hope to then isolate the target protein. Drugs were bound to chromatography columns for affinity chromatography. More recently, array technologies have been explored as a new avenue to explore the mechanism of action of orphan drugs. In one of these approaches, cells on microarray plates are transfected with single cDNAs that represent a large fraction of the genome. Binding of orphan drugs to the entire array of cells will identify the one expressing the drug receptor (Ziauddin and Sabatini, 2001). A further strategy uses the power of *Drosophila* genetics to identify the drug target. The flies are exposed to the orphan drugs to identify any observable phenotype. Genetic mutations reversing this phenotype are then sought. For example, a specific drug may change the feeding behavior of *Drosophila* larvae. Mutations of genes that reverse this effect provide a putative link to the primary mechanism of action of the orphan drug. Yeast genetic techniques offer the possibility to survey drug effects on all proteins of this species (Lum et al., 2004). The methods relying on nonvertebrate species are highly attractive, but they suffer from the fact that small molecules often have unique species selectivity. They may thus lead into an irrelevant direction from the point of view of drug discovery for humans. Genomic or proteomic array technologies may also be employed to compare various drugs that are effective in the same disease but have very different chemical structures and thus bind to different receptor sites. Those genes and proteins affected consistently by all the drugs may lead to the clinically relevant effects.

Orphan drugs and existing drugs with known mechanisms of action continue to provide guidance for the discovery of improved and novel drugs. Neurotransmitter mechanisms, in particular, remain wide open for exploration. The existing drugs identify the synaptic types and neurotransmitters only. There are many choices among the specific molecules that participate in synaptic transmission at each type of synapse. Exploration of validated drug targets and of orphan drug mechanisms thus continues to present an attractive avenue for successful drug discovery.

4.2 EVALUATION OF SPECULATIVE TARGETS

The classical neurotransmitters with their broad functional involvement and general validation remain particularly attractive as future drug targets. However, this approach and any of the reverse pharmacology approaches keep the investigator within the known playing field. They do not capitalize on the vast additional opportunities. As outlined earlier, every gene product, in principle, can serve as drug target, and the number of useful drug targets must be much higher than those currently utilized.

Several general strategies are currently available to broadly evaluate all gene products for suitability as drug targets. Figure 3.3 in the previous chapter shows a general outline of these approaches. In a general gene knockout strategy, genes are deleted randomly and the resulting mice are then evaluated for morphological or behavioral alterations. A putative new drug target is identified if these phenotypic changes are related to the pathophysiology of a nervous system disease. Conditional knockout strategies or knockdown approaches with siRNA provide more useful information in that they distinguish between gene functions relevant for development and those for the function in the adult (Dykxhoorn et al., 2003). While conceptually very attractive, these approaches are unlikely to produce quick results in the neuroscience area because of the complex nature of its diseases. Psychiatric diseases, in particular, tend to be specific for humans, making it very difficult to define a corresponding rodent phenotype. Diseases with severe and easily discernable phenotypes, such as epilepsy, and motoneuron diseases should more easily be replicated and recognized in broad target search efforts.

The probability of success in identifying novel drug targets can be increased if the pool of gene products to be evaluated is narrowed down to include only those proteins with critical physiological roles. For the nervous system these are proteins engaged in functions relating to signal initiation, propagation, and transmission. The key molecules are enzymes and transporters involved in neurotransmitter metabolism and neurotransmitter receptors, the ion channels responsible for the electrical properties of the neurons, and the primary transducers of sensory stimuli. As shown in Table 4.1, most targets of the currently available drugs act on targets in these categories. However, the number of utilized targets is miniscule compared to the total number of relevant enzymes, transporters, receptors, ion channels, and signal transducers, which is likely to exceed 1000. The broad diversity of molecules in these groups offers vast opportunities for drug discovery. Evolution has provided the researcher with a surprisingly large palette of neurotransmitters, neurotransmitter transporters, and neurotransmitter receptors. The classical neurotransmitters and their mechanisms provide just a fraction of the entire group, and even this group has not been fully explored. Beyond the classical neurotransmitter receptors there exist several hundred receptors for neuropeptides awaiting exploration as drug targets. More than 100 diverse ion channels are known that are responsible for signal generation and transmission by neural cells. Many of them may be useful as drug targets. These considerations identify as particularly interesting for drug discovery 1000 to 2000 gene products among the estimated total of 30,000 to 40,000 gene products encoded by human genome. The following section discusses the most attractive groups of putative drug targets.

4.2.1 Classical Neurotransmitter Mechanisms

Most of the classical neurotransmitters and their receptors were discussed in the previous section, based on the fact that at least some of their mechanisms are validated as drug targets. The list of the small-molecules transmitters that includes glutamate, GABA, acetylcholine, catecholamines, and serotonin is completed by glycine, histamine, and the so-called trace amines.

Glycine is an important inhibitory neurotransmitter in the spinal cord and the brain stem that often substitutes for GABA in these areas. It acts on specific receptors with a structure similar to those of the GABA-A receptors. They are pentamers composed of α and β subunits. Four distinct subtypes of α proteins, $\alpha 1$–$\alpha 4$, have been characterized. Strychnine binds to glycine receptors and inhibits their function. Strychnine is a natural alkaloid that has been used for rodent poisoning. It causes fatal convulsions in humans. Strychnine does not inhibit all glycine receptors, providing an opening to explore the entire group. The binding site for glycine on the glycine receptor is distinct from the glycine binding site on NMDA receptors. Nevertheless, the existence of two independent glycine binding sites may complicate the identification of selective drugs. The synaptic action of glycine is terminated by selective transporters, GLYT-1 and GLYT-2. They are expressed in areas not containing glycine receptors and may thus regulate the concentration of glycine at the NMDA synapse. They have potential as drug targets for schizophrenia and other psychiatric conditions (Laube et al., 2002).

Histamine is a principal mediator of the hypersensitivity response, and it regulates many other important organ functions, such as gastric acid secretion. Histamine receptor antagonists are among the most frequently used drugs for the treatment of allergies and stomach ulcers. Histamine serves an additional role as minor neurotransmitter in the brain. The majority of histaminergic cell bodies are located in the hypothalamus and the reticular formation from which they form divergent ascending and descending projections to the many brain areas. Histaminergic neurons thus comprise another important aminergic modulatory system in the brain, in addition to the dopaminergic, catecholaminergic, and serotonergic ones. Early versions of histamine receptor antagonists developed for the treatment of asthma were brain penetrant and induced sedation, confirming a functional role of histamine in the brain.

Histamine is synthesized from the amino acid histidine through AADC or a specific histidine decarboxylase. Following synaptic release, histamine acts on three distinct G-protein-coupled receptors, H_1, H_2, and H_3 receptors that are differentially distributed in the brain. The H_1 receptor mediates the sedative effects of brain-penetrant antihistamine drugs. The H_2 receptor regulates gastric acid secretion. The H_3 receptor occurs in presynaptic locations in the brain, located on catecholaminergic and serotonergic synaptic terminals. Its ability to regulate the release of these modulators makes it an attractive putative drug target. Degradation of histamine follows the pathways of the other amine transporters. Following methylation by histamine methyltransferase, it is converted by MAO and aldehyde dehydrogenase to methyl imidazole acetic acid. Besides the receptors, the specific synthetic and metabolic enzymes deserve consideration as potential drug targets (Phillipu and Prast, 2001).

Additional neurotransmitter substances occur in lower vertebrates and several invertebrate species. They include amines related to the catecholamines that are derived from alternative synthetic pathways, including the examples tyramine and octopamine. These molecules were found to exist at very low concentrations in the mammalian brain and are thus referred to as *trace amines*. Specific receptors have been identified, and they may merit to be evaluated as drug targets.

4.2.2 Neuropeptide Transmitter Mechanisms

Besides the classical neurotransmitters, a large number of diverse peptides serve an important role as transmitters and modulators of synaptic function. Synthetic and metabolic path-

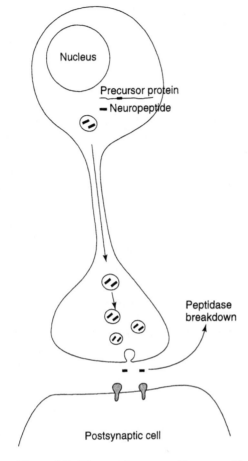

Figure 4.9   Diagram of a neuropeptide synapse. Neuropeptides are cleavage products of larger proteins synthesized in the neuronal cell body. Following cleavage by peptidases, the peptides are packed into secretory (dense-core) vesicles. Following release, they activate specific G-protein-coupled receptors. Synaptic actions are terminated by various peptidases.

ways of neuropeptides are different from those of small molecule transmitters. Figure 4.9 illustrates a generic neuropeptide synapse. Most neuropeptides are cleavage products of larger proteins that are synthesized in the neuronal cell body. Following cleavage by peptidases, the peptides are packed into secretory vesicles that are typically larger than those used by neurons with classical neurotransmitters. In electron microscopy they have electron-dense cores and are thus referred to as dense-core vesicles. Following release the neuropeptide transmitters act on specific postsynaptic receptors. All known neuropeptide receptors belong to the family of G-protein-coupled receptors. No specific transporters are known for neuropeptides. Their synaptic actions are terminated by various peptidases.

Table 4.3 gives on overview of known neuropeptides and their receptors. The existence of a multitude of neuropeptide transmitters, in addition to the already significant number of classical neurotransmitters, has remained an enigma in neuroscience. Just a small number of transmitter substances would seem sufficient from a point of view of information theory. Evolutionary inefficiencies have been invoked to explain the abundance. Whatever the cause, the variety of neurotransmitters and of their receptors provides an astounding opportunity for neuropharmacology. It has been said that the neurotrans-

Table 4.3   Characterized neuropeptides and their receptors

Group	Individual Peptides	Receptors
	Bradykinin	BK$_1$, BK$_2$ receptors
	Calcitonin gene-related peptide (CGRP)	CGRP receptor (associated with receptor-activity-modifying protein-1, RAMP1)
	Cholecystokinin	CCK$_A$, CCK$_B$ receptors
CRF-related peptides	Corticotrophin-releasing factor (CRF)	CRF$_1$, CRF$_2$ receptors
	Urocortin	
	Stresscopin	
	Galanin	GALR1, GALR2, GALR3
	Gastrin releasing-related peptide (GRP)	GRPR
Neurokinins	Substance P	NK$_1$, NK$_2$, NK$_3$ receptors
	Neurokinin A	
	Neurokinin B	
	Neuropeptide Y	Y1, Y2, Y3, Y4, Y5 receptors
	Neurotensin	NTS$_1$, NTS$_2$ receptors
Opioid peptides	Leu-enkephalin	μ, δ, κ opioid receptors
	Met-enkephalin	
	Dynorphin-A	
	Dynorphin-B	
	β-Endorphin	
	Endomorphin-1	
	Endomorphin-2	
Orexins	Orexin A = hypocretin 1	OX$_1$ = hypocretin 1 receptor
	Orexin B = hypocretin 2	OX$_2$ = hypocretin 2 receptor
	OrphaninFQ/nociceptin	ORL1 receptor
	Oxytocin	Oxytocin receptor
	Vasopressin	V$_{1a}$, V$_{1b}$, V$_2$ receptors
	Somatostatin	sst1, sst2, sst3, sst4, sst5 receptors
VIP-related peptides	Vasoactive intestinal peptide (VIP)	VPAC-1, VPAC-2, receptors
	Pituitary adenylate cyclase-activating peptide (PACAP)	PAC(1)-R
	Growth hormone-releasing hormone (GHRH)	

mitter diversity is a gift of the gods to the struggling neuropharmacologists. Indeed, all the current drugs for nervous system diseases are directly or indirectly dependent on their ability to selectively influence a small number of synapses among the highly diverse total synaptic population. The diversity offers ample opportunity for the discovery of novel drugs.

Opiate receptors have been discussed in the previous section as the only example of clinically validated targets among the neuropeptide receptors. Vasopressin and oxytocin can be considered in this group, since they are synthesized by neurons, and since the peptides and ligands for their receptor sites are used clinically for diseases outside of the nervous system. Another group of receptors, the neurokinin receptors that mediate the actions of substance P and related peptides, are the most recent addition to this group. Other neuropeptides of interest include the corticotrophin-releasing factor (CRF), VIP-related peptides, cholecystokinin, neurotensin, calcitonin gene-related peptide (CGRP), bradykinin, somatostatin, and orexin. These peptides together with their receptors and related molecules are presented in more detail below. This will be followed by a discussion of the orphan G-protein-coupled receptors, receptors without known ligands. Given the multitude of peptides and the fact that all known neuropeptide transmitters act on G-protein-coupled receptors strongly suggests that these orphan receptors mediate the actions of peptides.

Neurokinin Receptors

Neurokinin receptors deserve a special place in any textbook of neuropharmacology because one of the ligands, substance P, opened the entire field of neuropeptides. Substance P was purified as acetone powder from brain extracts in 1931 as a pharmacologically active substance. After several decades only was it identified as a peptide (Leeman and Ferguson, 2000) and found to have properties similar to that of the classical neurotransmitters. Most general findings and concepts on neuropeptides were established through research on substance P and its receptor. Substance P serves neurotransmitter functions for primary sensory neurons that mediate pain and, in addition, for distinct populations of brain neurons that control emesis and emotional functions.

Substance P is an undecapeptide derived from the gene product of the neurokinin A gene that gives also raise to the related peptides and neurokinin A. An additional peptide, neurokinin B, is closely related but is derived from a different neurokinin B gene. Receptors mediating the actions of the three peptides are the neurokinin receptors NK_1, NK_2, and NK_3, with partially overlapping selectivity. The actions of substance P are predominantly mediated by the NK_1 receptor.

The location of substance P in primary sensory neurons very early prompted speculations that this neuropeptide is a key mediator of pain. Indeed, many investigators erroneously assumed that the "P" stands for "pain" rather than "powder" as intended by the discoverers. Many companies had strong efforts on substance P mimetics, based on the belief that it would be possible to gradually generate nonpeptidic analogues from neuropeptides. The cloning of the NK receptors drastically changed this approach by making it possible to screen compound libraries on membranes of cells transfected with the human NK_1 gene and expressing this receptor. A publication from the laboratories of Pfizer in 1991 reported the first nonpeptide analogue of substance P and of neuropeptides in general, 60 years after the first characterization of substance P itself. This achievement has radically changed drug discovery in the neurosciences and represents a true landmark in the history of neuropharmacology (Snider et al., 1991).

Several highly potent and selective NK_1 antagonists suitable for human use have been generated in the recent years. As a major negative surprise, the NK_1 antagonists were not effective in alleviating acute or chronic pain (Hill, 2000). This disappointing finding presents a major issue and problem in modern neuropharmacology and will be discussed in more detail in Chapter 15. Besides pain, substance P has been linked to emesis and depression based on indirect evidence and conceptual considerations. Indeed, NK_1 antagonists are highly effective in suppressing emesis in animals and humans (Tattersall et al., 2000). Aprepritant, a selective NK_1 antagonist, was recently approved for the treatment of emesis in humans. Aprepritant is the first example of a clinically effective neuropeptide receptor antagonist and shows the promise of the field. Both NK_2 and NK_3 receptors are expressed in the nervous system and may represent attractive further drug targets.

CRF Receptors

As indicated by the name, corticotrophin-releasing factor, CRF, was purified and identified based on its biological ability to stimulate the release of adrenocorticotrophic hormone (ACTH) from the pituitary. Related to this function, it is heavily expressed in the hypothalamus, but it also occurs in many other parts of the brain, including the cerebral cortex, amygdala, and hippocampus. A related peptide, urocortin, is also expressed in hypothalamic and other brain areas. CRF and urocortin bind with high affinity to the CRF_1 and CRF_2 receptors (Seymour et al., 2003). Both receptors are expressed in the brain and have been linked to the behavioral response to stress. Both receptors are thus attractive putative drug targets for psychiatric indications, anxiety disorders, and depression in particular. Several compounds are in active stages of drug development. A CRF_1 antagonist has been reported to be effective in the treatment of depression. Similar to the NK receptors, the CRF receptors represent an advanced group of putative drug targets. Many pharmacological tools are available and the corresponding knockout mice have been described in detail. Ongoing and planned clinical trials will soon determine their practical utility toward better treatment of human diseases.

Receptors for Other Known Neuropeptides

Several groups of neuropeptides have been characterized over the past few decades, and their receptors have been identified more recently. Many of the neuropeptides occur in the central nervous system and have been tentatively linked to behavioral or physiological functions. Additional roles outside of the nervous system tend to limit the suitability of neuropeptide receptors as targets. Nevertheless, many of them have highly appealing features from a drug discovery point of view. Two peptides, orexin A and B, also called hypocretin-1 and hypocretin-2, and derived from a single gene, prepro-orexin, were first identified in the hypothalamus and were speculatively linked to the regulation of body metabolism. The orexins activate two G-protein-coupled receptors OX_1 and OX_2. These receptors mediate robust effects on feeding behavior as well as the regulation of sleep. Mutations of the OX_2 receptors in animals cause narcolepsy, a sleep disorder characterized by abruptly started episodes of sleep. Narcolepsy in humans is accompanied by changes in orexin levels in the cerebrospinal fluid. The findings make the orexin receptors highly attractive potential targets for drugs to control sleep as well as feeding disorders (Brown, 2003).

Several peptides with homologous sequences, typically referred to as VIP-related peptides, are found in the intestine and related organs, but also in the CNS. They include vasoactive intestinal peptide (VIP), pituitary adenylate cyclase-activating peptide (PACAP), growth hormone-releasing hormone (GHRH), and additional peptides. VIP and PACAP are widely expressed in the nervous system and have been involved in developmental and adult functions, including the control of circadian rhythms. They activate three G-protein-linked receptors, VPAC-1, VPAC-2, and PAC(1)-R with different selectivity (Labourthe et al., 2002).

Other peptides mediate important behavioral as well as physiological functions. Among them are somatostatin, cholecystokinin (CCK), neuropeptide Y (NPY), neurotensin, bradykinin, and calcitonin gene-related peptide (CGRP), which are all products of different genes. Five different receptors have been characterized for somatostatin (sst1–sst5) as well as for NPY (Y_1–Y_5), with differential expression in the nervous system. CCK activates two G-protein-coupled receptors (CCK_A and CCK_B), as do neurotensin (NTR_1 and NTR_2) and bradykinin (BK_1 and BK_2 receptors), whereas CGRP binds to a single receptor whose selectivity is defined by associated protein, receptor-activity-modifying protein-1 (RAMP1).

The peptide ligands and their receptors have been linked to various behavioral functions. Earlier studies with intracerebral injections of the peptides and more recent evaluations of various receptor and peptide knockout mice have revealed a complex array of behavioral and physiological changes in the animals. They speculatively associate various peptide receptors with many indications, including control of feeding behavior, emotional behavior, and pain. The known neuropeptide receptors represent a highly fertile area for drug discovery research (Oliver et al., 2000).

4.2.3 Orphan G-Protein-Coupled Receptors

With very few exceptions, all known neuropeptide receptors, the metabotropic glu and GABA receptors, all catecholamine, serotonin, histamine, and neuropeptide receptors, belong to the G-protein-coupled receptor superfamily. Figure 4.10 provides an overview of G-protein-coupled receptors. There are approximately 1500 in the human genome, the majority of them are odorant receptors that are less interesting from a drug target point of view. About 200 of identified G-protein-coupled receptors have known ligands, about 300 are currently classified as non-odorant, orphan G-protein-coupled receptors. At a rapid rate, ligands are being identified for the orphan receptors. Very likely all of these receptors will be "de-orphanized" within just a few years.

The G-protein-coupled receptors have traditionally been are a fruitful area for drug discovery research. Several of the currently used drugs in the nervous system area and cardiovascular area bind to receptor sites on G-protein-coupled receptors. It is probable that there are many additional and as yet undiscovered drug targets among this class of proteins. The binding pockets of the G-protein-coupled receptors for their natural ligands typically offer suitable drug receptor sites and are favored by the expert medicinal chemists. Thus orphan G-protein-coupled receptors remain the most appealing group of molecules for a guided exploration as drug targets in the neuroscience area.

Two principal approaches are being pursued in the broad evaluation of G-protein-coupled receptors as drug targets. The first approach centers on the identification of the natural ligand. Concentrated peptide extracts from brain or other tissues serve as starting material. Esoteric sources, such as extracts from amphibian skins, are preferred because they contain particularly rich mixtures of unusual peptides. Once a peptidic ligand is identified, the natural ligand in the nervous system is easily found through homology DNA sequence searches. Expression patterns of the ligand and the receptor may lead to specific hypotheses on physiological functions. The hypotheses are tested by injections of the peptides into the brain or organs innervated by peripheral nerves and monitoring of physiological or behavioral parameters that are predicted to respond. A recent example for this approach is provided by the discovery of neuropeptide W as ligand for orphan G-protein-coupled receptors GPR7 and GPR8. The peptide was isolated from the bovine hypothalamus. When injected into the brain, it changed food intake by the animals, leading to the exploration of GPR7 or GPR8 as targets for future drugs to control appetite (Shimomura et al., 2002).

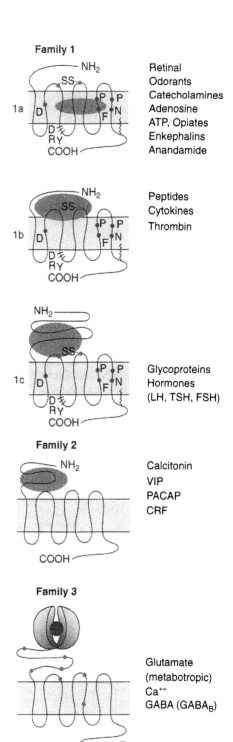

Family 1

Retinal
Odorants
Catecholamines
Adenosine
ATP, Opiates
Enkephalins
Anandamide

Peptides
Cytokines
Thrombin

Glycoproteins
Hormones
(LH, TSH, FSH)

Family 2

Calcitonin
VIP
PACAP
CRF

Family 3

Glutamate
(metabotropic)
Ca^{++}
GABA (GABA$_B$)

Figure 4.10 G-protein-coupled receptors. Sequence homologies determine three main families. The largest, family 1, contains many receptors for neurotransmitters and neuropeptides as well as odorant receptors and glycoprotein hormones. Family 2 includes neuropeptide and hormone receptors. Family 3 contains metabo-tropic glutamate and GABA receptors. The shaded area indicates the ligand binding site. (Reproduced with permission, Bockaert and Pin, 1999)

In the second approach, the ligand is bypassed. Orphan G-protein-coupled receptor functions are prevented through knockout mutations. The phenotype is then analyzed with a broad spectrum of physiological and behavioral tests. It they reveal utility from a therapeutic point of view, a medicinal chemistry program is initiated with the goal to make a small molecule agonist or antagonists as suggested from the functional understanding. If the resulting molecule shows the desired effect in animal models of human disease, a drug candidate has been generated without identification of the natural ligand for the drug receptor. The approach is conceptually very attractive. Indeed, several companies have taken a general approach to deleting all orphan G-protein-coupled receptors for drug target identification. An interesting example is the recent identification of orphan G-protein-coupled receptors believed to be depression targets (Branckek and Blackburn, 2003).

4.2.4 Sodium Channels

Ion channels are responsible for maintaining the resting membrane potential of cells and, in neurons, for the propagation of signals along dendrites and axons as well as for the release of neurotransmitters at the synapse. Many of the ion channels respond to changes in voltage across the membrane rather than to signaling molecules and are called voltage-gated ion channels. Various subtypes exist that are selective for Ca^{2+}, Na^+, or K^+. The functional channels are typically composed of several subunits of related gene products. There is an extremely high degree of heterogeneity among the genes, creating many subforms of functional channels and providing a vast opportunity for drug discovery. Drugs that globally influence an entire class of ion channels are likely to have drastic consequences and will not be therapeutically useful except for local administration. Indeed, nonselective blockers of Na^+ channels, such as lidocaine, are widely used for local anesthesia in clinical and dental practice.

Ten distinct voltage-gated Na^+ channels have been characterized for the mammalian nervous system. Figure 4.11 illustrates the complexity of the Na^+ channel groups.

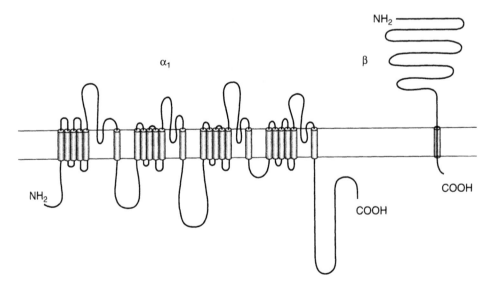

Figure 4.11 Voltage-gated Na^+ channels. The channels are formed by single $\alpha 1$ subunits with 4 repeated 6-transmembrane/1-pore domains. They are associated with two transmembrane β subunits.

Table 4.4 Voltage-gated Na^+ channels

α-Subunit	Other Name	Sensitivity to Tetrodotoxin
$Na_v1.1$	Type I	+
$Na_v1.2$	Type II	+
$Na_v1.3$	Type III	+
$Na_v1.4$	SKM (skeletal muscle)	+
$Na_v1.5$	H1	−
$Na_v1.6$	PN4	+
$Na_v1.7$	PN1, NaS	+
$Na_v1.8$	PN3, SNS	−
$Na_v1.9$	PN5, NaN	−

Overlapping terminologies tend to complicate the picture, however, the terminology $Na_v1.1$–$Na_v1.9$, and Na_v2, has become widely accepted but other terminologies persist in the literature (Table 4.4). The functional channels are formed by a single $\alpha1$ protein with four repeats each containing six transmembrane and one pore domain. They are typically associated with two transmembrane β proteins. Four of the genes, $Na_v1.1$, $Na_v1.2$, $Na_v1.3$, and $Na_v1.6$, are expressed in the central nervous system. Their subcellular location is not uniform. $Na_v1.1$ and $Na_v1.3$ are predominantly located at the soma and dendrites of the neurons, whereas $Na_v1.2$ and $Na_v1.6$ appear to serve axonal functions. Other channels are abundant in the peripheral nervous system, $Na_v1.8$, $Na_v1.9$, and Na_v2. The channel $Na_v1.8$ has attracted particular interest because it is selectively expressed by sensory neurons, making it a highly attractive putative drug target for pain control. Findings that this channel is upregulated in chronic pain states further fuel this enthusiasm. The diversity of Na^+ channels offers an obvious opportunity for drug discovery (Catterall, 2000; Clare et al., 2000).

4.2.5 Potassium Channels

Among the ion channels, the K^+ channels present the most complex picture. More than 200 gene products have been identified that participate in the formation of various functional K^+ channels (Fig. 4.12). Voltage-gated K^+ channels (K_v) are tetramers of α subunits,

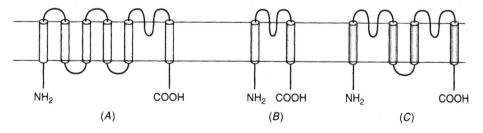

(A) (B) (C)

Figure 4.12 K^+ channels. (**A**) The voltage-gated K^+ channels are composed of 6-transmembrane/1-pore channel proteins, typically tetramers of the α subunits shown, and sometimes associated with cytoplasmic β subunit. More than 40 α subunits are known. (**B**) The inward rectifier K^+ channels (K_{ir}) are tetramers of 2-transmembrane/1-pore channel proteins. (**C**) The K_{2P} channels mediating the resting potential are dimers of 4-transmembrane/2-pore channel proteins.

each with six transmembrane segments and a loop that participates in the formation of the hydrophilic core. Some of the K^+ channels also contain a β subunit (K_vβ) that is located at the cytoplasmic side of the channel complex. More than 40 α subunits have been identified. The K_v1–K_v9 proteins, each with various subforms are the most complex subfamily. hERG and K_vLQT are additional important subfamilies (Coghlan et al., 2001; Shieh et al., 2000).

Nonselective K^+ channel blockers, such as 4-aminopyridine, are available as experimental tools, but they are not suitable for clinical use because of their multiple actions on crucial cellular processes. They bind to a receptor site at the intracellular side of the pore. Several invertebrate venoms, including those from scorpions and sea anemones, contain toxic peptides that block K^+ channels, binding alternative receptor sites. Many of the K_v channels are expressed in the brain and are heterogeneously distributed. Specific mutations of K_vLQT proteins have been discovered that cause epilepsy (Cooper et al., 2000). The existence of various drug-binding sites and the complexity of expression make the K_v channels one of the most open and fertile area for drug discovery.

Since many of the K_v proteins are expressed by neural cells as wells as by cells outside of the nervous system, selectivity is the key issue for drug discovery. The magnitude of this problem is succinctly illustrated by hERG, a voltage-gated K^+ channel that exists in the brain and heart, where it controls the QT interval of the cardiac contraction sequence. The channel is a notorious problem in many drug discovery efforts because it has binding sites with poor selectivity that recognize many small organic molecules. The broad affinity profiles of these binding sites and the critical role of the channel in heart function cause hERG to complicate and delay many medicinal chemistry programs. The pharmaceutical industry is flush with stories of excellent chemical series that had to be abandoned because of insurmountable hERG binding. To overcome this problem, most companies have introduced early hERG counterscreening as a regular feature into their medicinal chemistry programs (Picard and Lacroix, 2003).

Besides the K_v channels there are two additional groups of K^+ channels, the inward rectifier K^+ channels (K_{ir}) and the two-pore channels (K_{2P}). These proteins are structurally quite different and not homologous to the six-transmembrane channel proteins of the Na_v, K_v, and Ca_v channels. The K_{ir} channels are tetramers of proteins with two transmembrane segments and a pore loop between them. They are important for re-establishing the resting membrane potential following an action potential. They are also called G-protein-gated inwardly rectifying K^+ (GIRK) channels because many of them are regulated directly by G-protein-coupled receptors. Their function is furthermore influenced by intracellular gating compounds, including Mg^{2+} and polyamines. Seven protein subfamilies, K_{ir}1–K_{ir}7, have been identified that contain several individual gene products. Many of them are expressed in the nervous system in regionally differential ways. The variety and differential expression makes the K_{ir} receptors interesting to explore as drug targets. The field is wide open for investigation and remains to be explored for drug discovery. The K_{ir} channels tend to fall in the background because it appears easier to explore the G-protein-coupled receptors that regulate them. However, individual members of the two classes of proteins have different distribution patterns in the nervous system. It may be possible to affect selective behavioral functions with K_{ir} ligands, which cannot selectively associated with a G-protein-coupled receptor (Sadja et al., 2003).

The four transmembrane two-pore K_{2P} channels are structurally unrelated to the other two classes of K^+ channels (Bayliss et al., 2003). They exist as dimers of gene products with four transmembrane segments and two pore-forming domains. Fourteen members of this superfamily have been identified. The K_{2P} channels mediate the resting K^+ currents (leak K^+ currents) that maintain the resting membrane potential of neurons and other cells and thus serve a vital biological function. Reflecting this, the K_{2P} channel proteins are expressed widely, within and outside of the nervous system. In the nervous system individual K_{2P} channel proteins have differential expression patterns, creating attractive opportunities for drug discovery. Recent evidence suggests that these channels are one of the molecular targets for the volatile anesthetics such as halothane (Yost, 2003). Subtype selective ligands for the K_{2P} channels may thus affect behavioral functions in much more defined and therapeutically useful ways.

4.2.6 Calcium Channels

Ca^{2+} channels are composed of $\alpha1$ subunits with four repeats of six transmembrane segments and a pore loop in a similar way as the Na_v channels (Fig. 4.13). Three subtypes of Ca^{2+} channels have been characterized, Ca_v1, Ca_v2, and Ca_v3, each of which has 3–4 subforms. Table 4.5 summarizes the existing terminologies. The functional channels typically contain additional proteins, an intracellular β subunit and a transmembrane $\alpha2\delta$ subunit. Four subforms of the β subunit are known, creating further diversity among the channels. An earlier terminology categorizes the channels into L-, N, P/Q, R, and T-type Ca^{2+} based on electrical characteristics of the resulting currents, a terminology that is still frequently used in the pharmacological literature (Ertel et al., 2000). The Ca_v channels are responsible for the Ca^{2+} influx that is triggered by depolarization of the membrane, a central role in many cellular functions. In the nervous system these channels control the transition of axonal signal propagation to synaptic signal transmission. They are activated by the

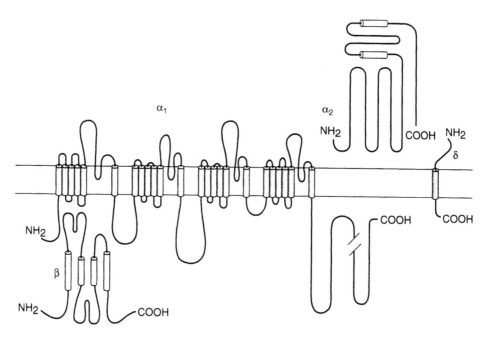

Figure 4.13 Voltage-gated Ca^{2+} channels. The sequence and structure of the pore-forming $\alpha1$ protein is related to that of the voltage-gated Na^+ channels. The transmembrane $\alpha_2\delta$ and the intracellular β-subunits are associated proteins.

Table 4.5   Voltage-gated Ca^{2+} channels

$\alpha 1$-Subunit	Alternative Name for $\alpha 1$ Subunit	Electrophysiological Characterization
$Ca_v 1.1$	$\alpha 1S$	L-type
$Ca_v 1.2$	$\alpha 1C$	L-type
$Ca_v 1.3$	$\alpha 1D$	L-type
$Ca_v 1.4$	$\alpha 1F$	L-type
$Ca_v 2.1$	$\alpha 1A$	P/Q-type
$Ca_v 2.2$	$\alpha 1B$	N-type
$Ca_v 2.3$	$\alpha 1E$	R-type
$Ca_v 3.1$	$\alpha 1G$	T-type
$Ca_v 3.2$	$\alpha 1H$	T-type
$Ca_v 3.3$	$\alpha 1I$	T-type

voltage changes from action potentials and elevate the Ca^{2+} concentrations in the synapse, which then trigger the synaptic neurotransmitter release.

The Ca_v channels are heterogeneously expressed in the nervous system, thus creating many possibilities for the discovery of subtype selective drugs. Disease causing mutations in Ca_v channels further emphasize their suitable as drug targets. For example, familial forms of migraine are linked to a mutation in specific Ca_v channels (Terwindt et al., 2002). The $Ca_v 2.2$ channels are abundant in the dorsal horn of the spinal cord and have been linked to pain mechanisms. They are the target of ziconotide, a peptide that is highly effective in controlling severe pain. However, there are multiple adverse effects of ziconotide mediated by nonneuronal cells. The majority of them can be avoided when ziconotide is administered within the blood-brain barrier. With intrathecal administration, the compound has been used for the control of severe pain in humans. Ziconotide illustrates the enormous potential of the voltage-gated ion channels as drug targets as well as the major hurdle to be encountered, namely the undesired effects mediated by the channels expressed on nonneuronal cells (Penn and Paice, 2000).

4.2.7   Temperature-Gated Ion Channels

The superfamily of transient receptor potential (TRP) ion channels plays a central role in the transduction of many sensory modalities (Fig. 4.14). These proteins are located at the plasma membrane; they contain six putative transmembrane domains and an ankyrin domain that is believed to link them to cytoplasmic proteins. A subgroup of them mediates temperature sensation. They are highly expressed in sensory neurons of the dorsal root ganglia that mediate temperature, touch and pain sensation. The first member of this family discovered was TRPV1, the receptor for capsaicin, the active ingredient of hot peppers. Besides capsaicin, TRPV1 responds to high temperature and H^+ and thus mediates the effects of many noxious stimuli. Its unique pattern of responsiveness, the response to heat as well as "hot" substances contained in peppers and other plants provides a molecular explanation why these molecules are associated with heat in human perception. TRPV1 levels in sensory endings are increased in chronic pain conditions. Capsaicin potently stimulates and then desensitizes TRPV1. The desensitization explains the paradoxical phenomenon that capsaicin, an agonist for TRPV1 is clinically effective against

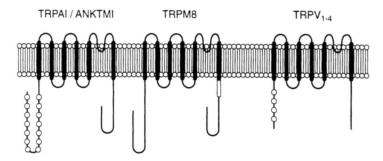

TRPAI / ANKTMI   TRPM8   TRPV$_{1-4}$

Figure 4.14 TRP channels involved in sensory pain transmission. The TRP channels contain six transmembrane elements and different numbers of ankyrin domains at the *N*-terminus, which regulate the location of the proteins to membrane domains. (Adapted from Patapoutian et al., 2003)

Table 4.6 TRP channels involved in thermal and pain sensation

Channel	Temperature Sensitivity	Nonthermal Regulators
TRPV1	>42°C	Capsaicin, H$^+$, anadamide, adenosine
TRPV2	>52°C	
TRPV3	>33°C	
TRPV4	27°–42°C	
TRPM8	<25°C	Menthol
TRPA1/ANKTM1	<17°C	Allyl isothiocyanate

pain. Local administration of capsaicin to the skin has been used experimentally for the treatment of localized chronic pain.

TRPV1 is an obvious and, through the experience with capsaicin, clinically validated drug target for pain therapy. It is very likely that the more recently discovered other temperature sensor will be equally useful drug targets. TRPV2, TRPV3, and TRPV4 all respond differently to temperature, and together, they provide the organism with a remarkably sophisticated biomolecular thermometer. TRPV4 is activated between 27° and 42°C. Temperatures above 33°, 42°, and 52°C activate, in sequence, TRPV3, TRPV1, and TRPV2 (Table 4.6). Pain and heat sensation are closely related. Inflammatory disease states are associated with altered temperature sensation. A battery of drugs able to influence these proteins in selective ways is likely to be useful for the treatment of noxious sensory sensations.

Related molecules are activated by low temperatures and mediate the sensations of cold. TRPM8 responds to temperatures below 25°C. It is also activated by methanol, providing a molecular explanation for the curious cold sensation elicited by this compound. Yet lower temperatures (<18°C) activate TRPA1/ANKTM1, a related channel that also responds to allyl isothiocyanate, the active ingredient of horseradish, wasabi, and mustard. Additional TRP channels are implicated in mechanosensation based on findings in *Drosophila* that they are required for hearing in the flies. The TRP channels represent a highly exciting group of potential drug targets (Patapoutian et al., 2003).

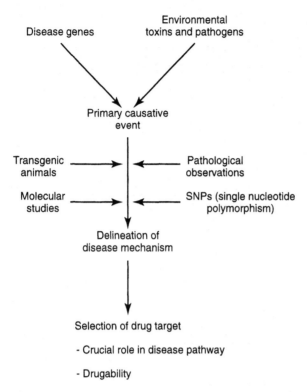

Figure 4.15 Drug target identification based on disease genes and disease mechanisms.

The general approach of exploring protein families with special potential as drug targets continues to be very appealing. While often indirect, time-consuming, and labor intensive, the exploratory efforts are likely to identify many useful targets in the future. The variety of neuropeptide receptors and ion channels provides a vast area of promise and potential. The discovery that the family of temperature sensing proteins, TRPV, contains receptor sites for known drugs illustrates the power of the broad platform approach.

4.3 DISEASE MECHANISMS

Detailed understanding of the specific diseases will directly lead to the most appropriate drug targets. Every disease can be reduced to a single or a small number of causative, initial events. Molecules involved in these first steps will provide targets for drugs to prevent or cure the disease. Molecules participating in downstream events are putative targets for drugs providing symptomatic relief. The road to success may be very difficult and arduous, as illustrated by many examples, but it will ultimately lead there. Trying to identify targets from studies of disease mechanisms is particularly attractive in a field such as neuroscience with its abundance of putative targets and few decisive clues to select among them. The general aspects of this approach.

Pathological and pathophysiological studies of human nervous system tissue may provide observations that directly point to drug targets. In Parkinson's disease, the detection of the dopaminergic neuron degeneration led to the symptomatic dopamine replacement therapy. In Alzheimer's disease, neuropathological studies revealed the loss of basal forebrain cholinergic neurons and provided the justification for the clinical studies with inhibitors of acetylcholinesterase to increase the synaptic concentration of the missing neurotransmitter. In specific conditions of pain, elevated levels of neuropeptides have been detected. They include increases of calcitonin gene-related peptide (CGRP) levels during migraine attacks, and antagonists for the CGRP receptor developed because of these findings are in clinical trials for the treatment migraine pain. Levels of nerve growth factor (NGF) are elevated in painful and inflamed tissue, making a case for NGF antagonists as pain therapeutics.

Pathological studies have been generally disappointing in the area of psychiatric diseases. Despite years of research few reliable postmortem changes have been identified for depression, anxiety, or schizophrenia. The absence of evident pathological alterations suggests that the principal events happen at the level of synaptic activity, processes that can be observed in the living brain only. Modern, functional imaging studies, fMRI (functional magnetic resonance imaging) in particular, may thus be more useful than observations on postmortem tissue. The functional imaging studies are able to link disease states to specific brain areas. If the spacial resolution is sufficient to correlate activity changes with the distribution of specific transmitter systems or structural proteins, they may point to putative drug targets.

The extension of pathological observations to animal models provides a fruitful approach, as illustrated best by the pain area. Pain pathways are anatomically well known in humans and animals. Pain states have been well conserved during evolution and can be relatively easily modeled in animals. Simple injuries cause the release of pain mediators such as substance P, bradykinin, CGRP, and NGF, so their receptors all provide putative pain targets. Many ion channels have been characterized that mediate signal propagation in sensory neurons. Those specific for the pain-mediating sensory neurons are obvious targets for analgesic drugs. Synapses transmitting the sensory signal to spinal cord and brain neurons have been characterized in detail. Those uniquely involved in pain pathway constitute putative drug targets. For example, the NR2B subtype of NMDA receptors is rather selectively expressed by spinal cord neurons of the ascending pain pathways, which cause it to be a highly suitable pain drug target.

Disease genes, if they exist and have been identified, confer a short cut to the understanding of the broader disease mechanism. The recent developments in the Alzheimer field are the best example in support of the view that research on disease genes in combination with pathological studies rapidly accelerates drug target identification. Starting with the purification of amyloid precursor protein from the pathological structures of the brain of Alzheimer victims, a peptide fragment, the Aβ peptide, was identified as a major pathophysiological agent in the disease process. Alzheimer's disease causing mutations were subsequently found in amyloid precursor protein of which Aβ is a fragment. Two enzymes, β- and γ-secretase, were characterized that cleave out Aβ. This was followed by the discovery of disease-causing mutations in γ-secretase, providing strong support for the amyloid cascade as the central event in Alzheimer's disease pathology. The crucial location in the disease process identified the two enzymes as attractive drug targets (Selkoe, 2002). The example offered by the Alzheimer field fuels the enthusiasm for the study of disease mechanisms and the belief that this approach will be the most successful approach. Other diseases of the nervous system are likely to follow the investigational strategy outlined by the research on Alzheimer's disease.

Genomic and proteomic array technologies have only recently been introduced in neurobiology, and their full potential has probably not been realized yet. In a currently explored application, genomic and proteomic profiling is used to identify common pathways of different drugs. In anxiety disorders, benzodiazepine receptor site agonists at GABA-A receptors and agonists to the serotonin 5-HT$_{1A}$ receptors appear to have similar clinical efficacy. Comparison of their genomic or proteomic profiles might be able to identify a common pathway central to the behavioral patterns of anxiety disorders. Understanding these common pathways will likely identify novel drug targets more central to the disease mechanism than those utilized by the current drugs. Gene array and protein array approaches are conceptually very appealing and likely to produce tangible results in the foreseeable future.

While some of the nervous system diseases share common traits, they are all unique. It thus seems appropriate to discuss in detail the drug targets derived from disease mechanisms in the subsequent chapters dealing with individual diseases. The general examples given above hopefully convey the power of using disease mechanisms and disease genes to identify the optimal drug targets.

4.4 CONCLUSIONS

Target selection is the most difficult problem in neuroscience drug discovery. Only a very small number of gene products have been clinically validated as drug targets. Several hundred gene products are attractive putative targets but require further evaluation. Their number vastly exceeds the total drug development capacity of the worldwide biopharmaceutical industry, requiring stringent further selection mechanisms. Three principal approaches are available for successful target selection.

In the first approach, sometimes referred to as reverse pharmacology, target selection relies on existing, clinically validated drugs. Many of the existing drugs act on a small number of related gene products, and they are not absolutely selective for a single receptor site. It is thus possible to improve efficacy and safety of the existing drugs by making them more potent and more selective for the receptor site that mediates the desired action. Most of the existing drugs affect neurotransmitter mechanisms. Expanding the target search to other members of the transmitter machinery yields putative drug targets with a high probability of success. For a small number of drugs, called orphan drugs, the receptor site is not known. Identification of these receptor sites might provide a direct route to a validated drug target.

In the second approach, gene products that appear likely to suit as drug targets are selected for further evaluation. They include proteins involved in neural signaling, namely neurotransmitter receptors and transporters, and the ion channels. Information gained from gene knockout animals is particularly helpful in the further selection among these potential drug targets. In the gene knockout studies developmental gene functions often mask the adult functions that are relevant for drug discovery. Test compounds with agonistic or antagonistic properties are then synthesized to overcome this issue. Conditional gene knockouts and gene knockdown technologies, when generally available, will bypass this labor-intensive path.

The third approach relies on understanding disease mechanisms. Detailed analysis of a specific disease mechanism will identify the crucial events in the process and the gene products mediating them. These gene products have the highest probability of success as drug targets. With the rapid progress in understanding disease mechanisms this approach is likely to become dominant in future years.

REFERENCES

Further Reading

BAYLISS, D.A., SIROIS, J.E., and TALLEY, E.M. The TASK family: Two-pore domain background K⁻ channels. *Mol. Interventions* 3: 205–219, 2003.

BACH, T.G. Muscarinic agonists as preventative therapy for Alzheimer's disease. *Curr. Opin. Investig. Drugs* 3: 1633–1636, 2002.

BOCKART, J., and PIN, J.P. Molecular tinkering of G-protein-coupled receptors: An evolutionary success. *EMBO J.* 18: 17123–1729, 1999.

BROWN, R.E. Involvement of hypocretins/orexins in sleep disorders and narcolepsy. *Drug News Perspect.* 16: 75–79, 2003.

CATTERALL, W.A. From ionic currents to molecular mechanisms: The structure and function of voltage-gated sodium channels. *Neuron* 26: 13–25, 2000.

CLARE, J.J., TATE, S.N., NOBBS, M., and ROMANOS, M.A. Voltage-gated sodium channels as therapeutic targets. *Drug Disc. Today* 5: 506–520, 2000.

COGHLAN, M.J., CARROLL, W.A., and GOPALAKRISHNAN, M. Recent developments in the biology and medicinal chemistry of potassium channel modulators: Update from a decade of progress. *J. Med. Chem.* 44: 1–27, 2001.

COUVE, A., MOSS, S.J., and PANGALOS, M.N. GABA-B receptors: A new paradigm in G protein signaling. *Mol. Cell. Neurosci.* 16: 296–312, 2000.

DYKXHOORN, D.M., NOVINA, C.D., and SHARP, P.A. Killing the messenger: Short RNAs that silence gene expression. *Nature Rev. Mol. Cell Biol.* 4: 457–467, 2003.

GREENGARD, P. The neurobiology of dopamine signaling. *Biosci. Rep.* 21: 247–269, 2001.

JOHNSTON, G.A.R., CHEBIB, M., HANRAHAN, J.R., and MEWETT, K.N. GABA$_C$ receptors as drug targets. *Curr. Drug Targ. CNS Neurol. Disord.* 2: 260–268, 2003.

LABURTHE, M., COUVINEAU, A., and MARIE, J.C. VPAC receptors for VIP and PACAP. *Recept. Channels* 8: 137–153, 2002.

LAUBE, B., MAKSAY, G., SCHEMM, R., and BETZ, H. Modulation of glycine receptor function: a novel approach for therapeutic intervention at inhibitory synapses? *Trends Pharmacol. Sci.* 23: 519–527, 2002.

LEE, D.K., GEORGE, S.R., EVANS, J.F., LYNCH, K.R. and O'DOWD, B.F. Orphan G protein-coupled receptors in the CNS. *Curr. Opin. Pharmacol.* 1: 31–39, 2001.

LEEMAN, S.E., and FERGUSON, S.L. Substance P: An historical perspective. *Neuropeptides* 34: 249–254, 2000.

LERMA, J. Roles and rules of kainite receptors in synaptic transmission. *Nature Rev. Neurosci.* 4: 481–495, 2003.

LUM, P.Y., ARMOUR, C.D., STEPANIANTS, S.B., CAVET, G., WOLF, M.K., BUTLER, J.S., HINSHAW, J.C., GARNI, P., PRESTWICH, G.D., LEONARDSON, A., GARRETT-ENGELE, P., RUSH, C.M., BARD, M., SCHIMMACK, G., PHILLIPS, J.W., ROBERTS, C., and SCHOEMAKER, D.D. Discovering modes of action for therapeutic compounds using a genome-wide screen of yeast heterozygotes. *Cell* 116: 121–137, 2004.

MARINO, M.J., and CONN, P.J. Direct and indirect modulation of the *N*-methyl D-aspartate receptor. *Curr. Drug Targ. CNS Neurol. Disord.* 1: 1–16, 2002.

MOHLER, H.F., CRESTANI, F., and RUDOLPH, U. GABA-A receptor subtypes: A new pharmacology. *Curr. Opin. Pharmacol.* 1: 22–25, 2001.

MORETTO, A. Experimental and clinical toxicology of anticholinesterase agents. *Toxicol. Lett.* 102: 509–513, 1998.

NORDBERG, A. Nicotinic receptor abnormalities of Alzheimer's disease: Therapeutic implications. *Biol. Psychiat.* 49: 200–210, 2001.

OLIVER, K.R., SIRINATSINGHJI, J.S., and HILL, R.G. From basic research on neuropeptide receptors to clinical benefit. *Drug News Perspect.* 13: 530–542, 2000.

PATAPOUTIAN, A., PEIER, A.M., STORY, G.M., and VISHWANATH, V. Thermotrp channels and beyond: Mechanisms of temperature sensation. *Nature Rev. Neurosci.* 4: 529–539, 2003.

PICARD, S., and LACROIX, P. QT interval prolongation and cardiac risk assessment for novel drugs. *Curr. Opin. Investig. Drugs* 4: 303–308, 2003.

SADJA, R., ALAGEM, N., and REUVENY, E. Gating of GIRK channels: Details of an intricate, membrane-delimited signaling complex. *Neuron* 39: 9–12, 2003.

SEYMOUR, P.A., SCHMIDT, A.W., and SCHULZ, D.W. The pharmacology of CP-154,526, a non-peptide antagonist of the CRH1 receptor: A review. *CNS Drug Rev.* 9: 57–96, 2003.

SHIEH, C.C., COGHLAN, M., SULLIVAN, J.P., and GOPALAKRISHNAN, M. Potassium channels: Molecular defects, diseases, and therapeutic opportunities. *Pharmacol. Rev.* 52: 557–593, 2000.

SOUDIJN, W., and VAN WIJNGAARDEN, I. The GABA transporter and its inhibitors. *Curr. Med. Chem.* 7: 1063–1079, 2000.

WISE, A., GEARING, K., and REES, S. Target validation *Drug Disc. Today* 7: 235–246, 2002.

YOST, C.S. Update on tandem pore (2P) domain K⁺ channels. *Curr. Drug Targ.* 4: 347–51, 2003.

Citations

BAILEY, S.N., WU, R.Z., and SABATINI, D.M. Applications of transfected cell microarrays in high-throughput drug discovery. *Drug Disc. Today* 7: S113–118, 2003.

BATESON, A. Pagoclone indevus. *Curr. Opin. Investig. Drugs* 4: 91–95, 2003.

BRANCHEK, T.A., and BLACKBURN, T.P. Trace amine receptors as targets for novel therapeutics: Legend, myth and fact. *Curr. Opin. Pharmacol.* 3: 90–97, 2003.

CHAMBERS, M.S., ATACK, J.R., BROMIDGE, F.A., BROUGHTON, H.B., COOK, S., DAWSON, G.R., HOBBS, S.C., MAUBACH, K.A., REEVE, A.J., SEABROOK, G.R., WAFFORD, K., and MACLEOD, A.M. 6,7-Dihydro-2-benzothiophen-4(5H)-ones: A novel class of GABA-A alpha5 inverse agonists. *J. Med. Chem.* 45: 1176–1179, 2002.

CHIAMULERA, C., EPPING-JORDAN, M.P., ZOCCHI, A., MARCON, C., COTTINY, C., TACCONI, S., CORSI, M., ORZI, F., and CONQUET, F. Reinforcing and locomotor stimulant effects of cocaine are absent in mGluR5 null mutant mice. *Nature Neurosci.* 4: 873–874, 2001.

CLARK, M., JOHNSON, B.G., WRIGHT, R.A., MONN, J.A., and SCHOEPP, D.D. Effects of the mGlu2/3 receptor agonist LY379268 on motor activity in phencyclidine-sensitized rats. *Pharmacol. Biochem. Behav.* 73: 339–346, 2002.

COOPER, E.C., ALDAPE, K.D., ABOSCH, A., BARBARO, N.M., BERGER, M.S., PEACOCK, W.S., JAN, Y.N., and JAN, L.Y. Colocalization and coassembly of two human brain M-type potassium channel subunits that are mutated in epilepsy. *Proc. Natl. Acad. Sci. UAS* 97: 4914–4919, 2000.

ERNST, M., BRAUCHART, D., BORESCH, S., and SIEGHART, W. Comparative modeling of GABA(A) receptors. Limits, insights, future developments. *Neuroscience* 119: 933–943, 2003.

ERTEL, E.A., CAMPBELL, K.P., HARPOLD, M.M., HOFMANN, F., MORI, Y., PEREZ-REYES, E., SCHWARTZ, A., SNUTCH, T.P., TANABE, T., BIRNBAUMER, L., TSIEN, R.W., and CATTERALL, W.A. Nomenclature of voltage-gated calcium channels. *Neuron* 25: 533–535, 2000.

HILL, R. NK1 (substance P) receptor antagonists—Why are they not analgesic in humans? *Trends Pharmacol. Sci.* 21: 244–246, 2000.

OZAWA, S., KAMIYA, H., and TSUZUKI, K. Glutamate receptors in the mammalian central nervous system. *Prog. Neurobiol.* 54: 581–618, 1998.

PENN, R.D., and PAICE, J.A. Adverse effects associated with the intrathecal administration of ziconotide. *Pain* 85: 291–296, 2000.

PHILLIPU, A., and PRAST, H. Importance of histamine in modulatory processes, locomotion and memory. *Behav. Brain. Res.* 124: 151–159, 2001.

SELKOE, D.J. Deciphering the genesis and fate of amyloid beta-protein yields novel therapies for Alzheimer disease. *J. Clin. Invest.* 110: 1375–1381, 2002.

SHIMOMURA, Y., HARADA, M., GOTO, M., SUGO, T., MATSUMOTO, Y., ABE, M., WATANABE, T., ASAMI, T., KITADA, C., MORI, M., ONDA, H., and FUJINO, M. Identification of neuropeptide W as the endogenous ligand for orphan G-protein-coupled receptors GPR7 and GPR8. *J. Biol. Chem.* 277: 35826–35832, 2002.

SIMPSON, L.L. Identification of the major steps in botulinum toxin action. *An. Rev. Pharmacol. Toxicol.* 44: 167–193, 2004.

SNIDER, R.M., CONSTANTINE, J.W., LOWE, J.A. 3rd, LONGO, K.P., LEBEL, W.S., WOODY, H.A., DROZDA, S.E., DESAI, M.C., VINICK, F.J., SPENCER RW, and HESS, H.J. A potent nonpeptide antagonist of the substance P (NK1) receptor. *Science* 251: 435–437, 1991.

TATTERSALL, F.D., RYCROFT, W., CUMBERBATCH, M., MASON, G., TYE, S., WILLIAMSON, D.J., HALE, J.J., MILLS, S.G., FINKE, P.E., MACCOSS, M., SADOWSKI, S., BER, E., CASCIERI, M., HILL, R.G., MACINTYRE, D.E., and HARGREAVES, R.J. The novel NK1 receptor antagonist MK-0869 (L-754,030) and its water soluble phosphoryl prodrug, L-758,298, inhibit acute and delayed cisplatin-induced emesis in ferrets. *Neuropharmacology* 39: 652–663, 2000.

MADDEN, D.R. The structure and function of glutamate receptor ion channels. *Nature Rev. Neurosci.* 3: 91–99, 2002.

TERWINDT, G., KORS, E., HAAN, J., VERMEULEN, F., VAN DEN Maagdenberg, A., FRANTS, R., and FERRARI, M. Mutation analysis of the CACNA1A calcium channel subunit gene in 27 patients with sporadic hemiplegic migraine. *Arch. Neurol.* 59: 1016–1018, 2002.

Chapter 5

From Drug Target to Drug, Neuroscience-Specific Problems

Drug discovery and development are a formidable challenge for all human diseases. Selectivity, efficacy, and appropriate pharmacokinetic properties are difficult to achieve. The safety evaluation often reveals insurmountable issues. Clinical trials require skill and intuition to succeed. The level of difficulty of each of these steps tends to be higher in the neurosciences because of additional complicating factors. For most indications in neurology and psychiatry, compounds have to be able to penetrate the blood-brain barrier to be efficacious. The predictive power of animal models is often poor for nervous system diseases. There are no easy surrogate readouts for efficacy in the clinical trials. Many of the diseases require complex and time-consuming clinical investigations. Results of the clinical trials can be confounded by large placebo effects. The complexity of these issues justifies a special chapter in addition to the preceding description of the general aspects of the drug discovery and development path.

5.1 BRAIN PENETRATION

Most drug targets for psychiatric and neurological diseases are within the blood-brain barrier. Exceptions are the ion channels and receptors on the distal axons of sensory neurons and of motor neurons, as well as those expressed by neurons of the autonomic nervous system. Diseases involving these peripheral systems, for example, pain, can thus be treated with drugs that do not penetrate into the central nervous system. Indeed, it often is an advantage to keep drugs outside of the brain, to minimize undesired effects mediated by receptors within the brain. As discussed in Chapter 15, several important mediators of the initial pain response at the sensory nerve endings have additional functions in the brain that are not related to pain but may mediate adverse effects. Non–brain penetrant ligands for their receptors may thus become ideal drugs for the treatment of pain.

5.1.1 Blood-Brain Barrier

For the majority of the neuroscience drug discovery programs, the need to penetrate into the central nervous system adds a significant hurdle. The term blood-brain barrier encom-

Drug Discovery for Nervous System Diseases, by Franz F. Hefti
ISBN 0-471-46563-1   Copyright © 2005 by John Wiley & Sons, Inc.

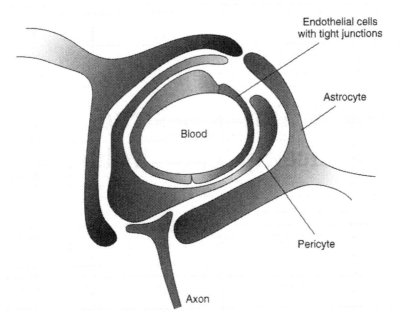

Figure 5.1   Blood-brain barrier. Endothelial cells of the capillary are connected with tight junction. They are surrounded by pericytes and by astrocyte foot processes. Rare axonal processes penetrate innervating the blood vessels penetrate to the surface of the endothelial cells. (Adapted from Pardrige, 2002)

passes several distinct mechanisms that, together, effectively isolate the brain from many chemical influences the body is exposed to (Fig. 5.1). A structural barrier is provided by high-resistance tight junctions between the endothelial cells of the brain capillaries. A biochemical barrier is imposed by endothelial cells and closely located astrocytes that express several ecto-enzymes, which form an enzymatic blood-brain barrier. Among these enzymes are peptidases and esterases that rapidly cleave many bioactive molecules. Various transporter proteins add a third component to the blood-brain barrier. These active efflux transporters rapidly remove many molecules from the extracellular fluid of the brain and spinal cord. p-Glycoprotein is the best known efflux transporter, and it was first recognized as a protein mediating drug resistance because it effectively removed specific drugs from the brain. Many additional transporters have been characterized, including several organic anion transporters (Pardridge, 2002; Sun et al., 2003).

5.1.2   Overcoming the Blood-Brain Barrier

Most small-molecule drugs cross the blood-brain barrier by passive diffusion. Adequate lipophilicity is thus a prerequisite for drugs to be brain penetrant, log P values of 2 to 3 are considered optimal. Small size facilitates the diffusion, making a molecular weight below 500 Da a clear advantage. These prerequisites alone impose well-defined and rather narrow constraints on medicinal chemistry programs. The influence of blood-brain barrier enzymes and efflux transporters set an additional, much less well understood hurdle to these efforts. These enzymes and transporters are only partly known. It is thus currently impossible to address the problem with a complete battery of screening assays for individual enzymes and transporters. Establishing such assays is of high interest for drug discovery, and many academic and industry researchers participate in this activity. It is likely that within a few years the key molecular players regulating drug transport will be identified and predictive tests batteries will be established. In the absence of predictive tests, historical knowledge and intuitive structural thinking by the medicinal chemists provide the principal guidance in medicinal chemistry program. This experience are among the strongest and most intangible assets of established biopharmaceutical companies.

Many researchers have attempted innovative strategies to overcome the blood-brain barrier. The prodrug strategy represents such an approach. For example, carboxylic acid moieties, which impair membrane penetration with their ionic charge at neutral pH, can be masked through ester formation. Following successful penetration into the brain, ubiquitous esterases will release the active molecule in the brain. A further strategy attempts to use existing transporters to carry drugs into the brain. The blood-brain barrier contains several transporters that serve a physiological function. They include transporters for amino acids, glucose, and nucleosides. These transporters can serve as vehicles for the effective transport of drugs into the brain. For example, L-DOPA reaches the brain through transport by the neutral amino acid transporter. However, these transporters are highly selective. Thus attempts to transport drugs by linking them to natural substrates have not been generally successful. A small number of proteins are transported to the brain through selective receptor-mediated transport systems. Insulin, leptin, and other proteins bind to specific receptors that transport the proteins through a sequence of endocytosis and exocytosis through the capillary endothelium cells and into the extracellular space of the brain. The transporter mechanisms might serve as roads for the transport of other molecules coupled to the natural ligands (Banks and Lebel, 2002). However, the overall capacity of the transporters is limited and presents a natural impediment to these innovative approaches.

5.1.3 Measurement of Brain Penetration

In the absence of fully predictive assays for brain penetration, many researchers and companies have attempted to find practical solutions for the complicated problem to predict brain penetration of drug candidates. For a first and quick answer, direct measurements of drug levels in brain homogenates are sometimes carried out. However, the measurement of the overall brain concentrations is not providing a functionally meaningful parameter because it does not distinguish between drug available to the receptor and drug trapped in membranes or other lipophilic cellular compartments. In an attempt to circumvent this issue, microperfusion techniques with push–pull cannulas have been used to assess the concentration in the extracellular fluid. This technique is based on the assumption that there is equilibrium between the drug concentration in the extracellular fluid and the concentration in the pocket perfused by the push–pull cannula. The complex nature of this interaction, however, makes it unlikely that representative levels are being measured. The technique is nevertheless useful for comparing the *relative* levels achieved by various molecules within a specific chemical series. In yet another attempt to obtain information on relevant drug levels in the brain, measurements in the cerebrospinal fluid (CSF) are sometimes used as surrogate measurements for drug concentration in the extracellular fluid of the brain, based on the assumption that the two are in equilibrium. However, this assumption has not been substantiated and specific transporters have been characterized that operate at the interface between brain and CSF. Drug measurements in the CSF can thus not be taken as reliable predictors of brain penetration of drugs (Feng, 2002).

5.1.4 Receptor Occupancy

The direct measurement of receptor occupancy in the brain is indubitably the best solution to the problem of measuring brain penetration. Receptor occupancy provides the pharmacologically relevant parameter and integrates all aspects that regulate brain penetration. Figure 5.2 illustrates a simple receptor occupancy procedure suitable for animals. In essence, a labeled high-affinity ligand for the receptor site is used to occupy the receptor binding sites. This label is then displaced by the test compounds. In animals, ex vivo measurement of the label, typically radioactivity, generates a simple procedure. In humans, an imaging method such as positron emission tomography (PET) or single photon emission

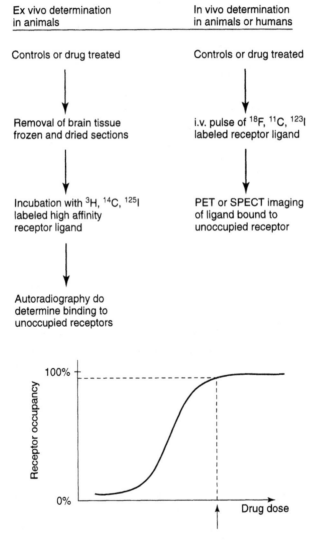

Figure 5.2 Measurement of receptor occupancy in the brain. The drug dose indicated by the arrow results in 99% receptor occupancy. Increasing the dose further will not significantly augment the effects on the drug receptor.

computerized tomography (SPECT) is needed to measure the undisplaced label in the brain. The direct translation of animal measurements to human measurements is an important positive component of this approach. Receptor occupancy measurements have been increasingly accepted as the best readout for brain penetration. For example, in the very active field of neurokinin receptor antagonists they have played a crucial role (Berström et al., 2004; Langlois et al., 2001).

Direct measurement of receptor occupancy is associated with three difficulties. First, a high-affinity label for the receptor site is necessary for these studies to be successful. Generation of such a label is often as difficult as generating the drug candidate itself. The label has to be brain penetrant itself. Its affinity and selectivity must be at least as high as the comparable values for the drug candidate, to avoid that binding to other receptors blurs the signal and generates a high background. Second, receptor occupancy measurements assess the overall brain penetration, integrated over the many molecular components of the blood-brain barrier. This makes it unlikely that in a chemical series of a drug discovery program, a clear structure-activity relationship for brain penetration can be developed. The medicinal chemistry efforts thus operate in the blind, and predictions of successful structures are not possible. Third, many of the efflux transporters show species-specific selectivity. Thus brain penetration studies in animals based on receptor occupancy may generate an erroneous picture and may lead the medicinal chemistry effort in a direction not suitable for drugs to be used in humans. Cell cultures based on human endothelial cells might offer the most attractive solution to this complex problem (Terasaki et al., 2003). Such in vitro blood-brain barrier systems are useful if the cells express the tight junctions, enzymes, and transporters that form the human blood-brain barrier.

5.1.5 Intracerebral Drug Administration

The blood-brain barrier effectively excludes the vast majority of peptides and proteins from the central nervous system. The inability to use biologics, antibodies, and growth factors in particular, represents a major disadvantage for drug discovery of brain diseases. The potential of growth factor and antibody therapy is best illustrated by the experience in immunological diseases, cancer, and disorders of the blood. These approaches are open for diseases of the peripheral nervous system, including motoneuron diseases and pain. For the central nervous system many researchers have pursued alternative administration strategies, including intraventricular and intracerebral infusions by pumps, cell therapy where cells expressing the desired protein are implanted into the brain, and direct gene therapy through injection of appropriate vectors into the brain.

Alternative administration strategies for intracerebral delivery of biologic drugs face many practical and technical hurdles. Infusions into ventricular spaces or within the brain parenchyma require pumping systems that are implanted under the skin. While highly unattractive, because they require invasive surgery and present various risks, infections in particular, they can serve as last resort therapy for difficult diseases. For example, intracerebral and intraparenchymal infusions of glial cell-derived neurotrophic factor (GDNF) are being pursued for patients suffering from advanced Parkinson's disease. Cell therapy with nerve growth factor (NGF) secreting cells is tried as experimental therapy for Alzheimer's disease. Gene therapy would necessitate a single session of invasive surgery only. However, to be successful and safe, intracerebral gene therapy requires vectors that insert the gene into the appropriate cells and convey long-term gene expression. This approach will still require a surgical delivery of the appropriate vector to the targeted brain region. Given the need for surgical intervention, it is unlikely that any of these alternative administration approaches will become mainstream therapy. They may be useful, however, as last resort therapy for severe and life-threatening diseases (Tuszynski, 2003).

5.2 ANIMAL MODELS AND PREDICTABILITY OF EFFECTS IN HUMANS

Drug discovery is greatly facilitated by the availability of animal models for human diseases that predict efficacy of drug candidates. The perfect animal model of a disease replicates the human disease in all its aspects. The cause, the molecular progression, the pathophysiology, and the symptoms are identical. While rare, close to perfect models do exist. For example, tissue damage through injury or burns can be reproduced in animals with a high degree of accuracy. Many tumors that occur regularly in humans have counterparts in animal species, making it possible to optimize in animals the surgical procedures used in humans to excise them. Even in the nervous system there are rare examples of highly suitable animal models. A familial form of ALS that is caused by a mutation in the enzyme superoxide dismutase can be reproduced in transgenic mice that express the mutated human gene. These animals replicate the motoneuron degeneration and the cause of death of the familial form of the human disease. Of course, the emotional aspects of the disease are missing and the time course is accelerated to approximately one year from the typical five years in the human disease (Wong et al., 2002).

The examples also illustrate the difficulties associated with animal models. The absolutely perfect animal model cannot exist, given the many genetic and phenotypic differences that separate species. However, the situation is particularly grave in the nervous system diseases because of evolutionary progress that separates humans from all the animal species. Many other organ systems, for example, the cardiovascular and the reproductive systems, have seen the most significant evolutionary advances at the transition from lower vertebrates to the mammals. In contrast, the major evolutionary steps in brain evolution are those that separate the higher primates, humans in particular, from the lower mammalian species. The cerebral cortex of the human brain is unique. It supports language and all the other aspects of human culture, including artistic and scientific achievements. Higher primate species show abilities of language and comprehension, but it is only the species *Homo sapiens* that has unraveled its genetic code, has developed worldwide instant communication systems, and has found ways to express itself through visual art and music. These abilities reflect the uniqueness of the human cerebral cortex. They illustrate that diseases involving the human brain and the cerebral cortex, in particular, will not be easily modeled in animals.

The difficulty in modeling human nervous system diseases is a function of the evolutionary level of the brain structure involved. The example described above of an excellent animal model for ALS reflects that motor systems are similar throughout the mammalian class. Rodents provide a useful model to study degenerative diseases of the motor nervous system. In a similar way the fundamental behavioral responses to danger, such as fear and anxiety, are believed to have been optimized early in evolution and are thus likely to be a uniform feature of all mammals. It is relatively easy to characterize a fear response in rodents and to define experimental conditions that elicit it in reliable and reproducible ways. In contrast, there currently is no adequate animal model for schizophrenia. The phenotypic picture of the disease is based on verbalization by the patients. They express abnormal thoughts and describe visual and auditory hallucinations. It is not known whether animals can hallucinate, and if they did, they would not be able to express them lacking the ability for verbal communication.

5.2.1 Types of Animal Models

Table 5.1 lists the various types of animal models that are used in nervous system drug discovery research. **Genetic models** appear most attractive, but they are not without limitations. Often they do not replicate the entire disease pattern. In addition they are replications of specific mutations typically running in a small number of families only. Most of the complex diseases are caused by a combination of genetic and environmental influences. The available genetic models for ALS and Alzheimer's disease, discussed in more

Table 5.1   Animal models of nervous system diseases

Genetic Models

Replicate the disease mechanism of familial form of the disease

Examples	APP, γ-secretase mutations	Alzheimer's disease
	α-Synuclein mutations	Parkinson's disease
	Huntingtin mutations	Huntington's disease
	Superoxide dismutase mutation	ALS
	K^+ channel mutations	Epilepsy
	Ca^{2+} channel mutations	Migraine
Advantages	Close to human disease	
Issues	Dependent on genetic background, different life span of humans and animals	

Lesion Models

Microsurgical procedures that lesions of nervous system structures affected in neurological diseases

Examples	Chronic constriction injury	Chronic pain
	Substantia nigra lesions	Parkinson's disease
	Middle cerebral artery occlusion	Ischemic stroke
	Hippocampal lesions	Memory dysfunction
Advantages	Production without breeding delays	
Issues	Acute injury does not replicate disease process	

Behavioral Models

Observation of animals in defined, artificial test situations

Examples	Tail suspension test	Depression
	Open maze test	Anxiety
	Maze performance	Cognitive dysfunction
Advantages	Reproducibility	
Issues	Artificial test environment, anthropomorphic interpretation	

Drug Models

Induction of specific behaviors with known drugs

Examples	Pentylenetetrazole induced seizures	Epilepsy
	Amphetamine-induced hyperactivity	Schizophrenia
	Ketamine-induced head twitch	Schizophrenia
	Atropine-induced memory loss	Cognitive dysfunction
Advantages	Experimental ease	
Issues	Remote from disease process, based on known drug targets	

detail in the respective chapters, are based on rare familial forms of the diseases. The models have become crucial components in the ongoing drug discovery efforts. Clinical studies over the future years will reveal to what extent these models have been good predictors for efficacy in the majority of the patients (Wong et al., 2002).

Lesion models are often used for degenerative diseases of the nervous system, such as Parkinson's disease or Alzheimer's disease. They replicate some of pathological changes and some of the symptoms of disease, but they do not replicate the process of degeneration. The lesion models are thus useful to discover drugs that provide symptomatic relief for a disease, so-called palliative drugs. They are not suitable for the discovery of drugs that prevent the disease process itself.

Behavioral models are specific experimental conditions that induce precisely defined behavioral manifestations and can be easily quantified. Widely used behavioral models are the tail suspension test for depression and the Morris water maze test for cognitive impairment. In the former, rodents are suspended by their tails and the time until the animal stops struggling is used to measure behavioral resilience and to predict the potential as antidepressive drug. The Morris water maze test measures the time an animal needs to find an invisible, submerged platform based on memory from earlier test sessions. Enhanced performance of rodents in this test is interpreted as prediction for improved memory and general cognitive performance in humans. Both models have crucial places in current drug discovery projects. However, their predictive power can only be assessed when many drug candidates chosen by these tests have undergone rigorous clinical testing in humans. Behavioral models put animals in highly artificial situations that would not occur in wild life, and they tend to reflect anthropomorphic interpretations of animal behavior. The tail suspension model for depression vividly illustrates these points. Brain mechanisms are not sufficiently understood to determine whether a rodent struggling to liberate itself from a trap is behaviorally comparable to a human suffering from a depressive episode.

Drug models refer to tests in which drugs are used to create a specific physiological or behavioral state in animals that is believed to be comparable to a human disease. For example, amphetamine stimulates dopamine release in the brain and makes rodents behaviorally hyperactive. Since dopamine antagonists are effective in treating schizophrenia, amphetamine-induced hyperactivity in animals is believed to be a model for human schizophrenia. Amphetamine stimulates dopamine release and dopamine receptor antagonists are used to treat the disease. The animal model thus reflects a circular argument. It allows the investigator to discover other dopamine receptor antagonists, but it is not clear whether the model would be able to detect antischizophrenic drugs acting by a different mechanism. The example illustrates the principal limitation of drug models. They keep drug discovery within the frame of known drugs and drug targets, and they may actually hinder the discovery of new and innovative drugs.

5.2.2 Ethical Aspects of Animal Model Use

In most countries animal research is highly regulated. Ethical aspects of animal research and the potential rights of animals are often debated societal issues. There seems to be a very broad consensus opinion that limited research on animal species, rodents in particular, is justified to find understanding of the human body and mind and to find effective treatment for the human diseases. Researchers are obliged to minimize the number of animals used for research and to avoid procedures that cause severe pain or suffering.

Given the behavioral complexity of the monkey brain, it is imperative from an ethical point of view, that research on monkeys is limited to situations where no rodent model is available. For example, aged monkeys serve as models for the cognitive dysfunction associated with Alzheimer's disease. For many other diseases it is difficult to justify the use of monkeys over that of rodents. Despite the evolutionary proximity between monkeys and humans, there are no suitable monkey models for psychiatric diseases such as depression and schizophrenia. Thus rodent models are dominant in the neuroscience area as for other indication areas. The rapid progress made in genetic models and transgenic technologies will make mouse models yet more dominant in the future and will further reduce the necessity for experimentation with monkeys.

5.3 TRANSLATIONAL MEDICINE, PHARMACOLOGICAL READOUTS

The traditional way of drug development proceeds from animal safety studies, to phase I human safety studies and to the proof-of-concept phase II clinical studies. The outcome of phase II represents the first reliable indication of efficacy. Typically several years of preclinical development work and clinical studies pass before the crucial result is obtained. The high cost and effort associated with drug development provide a strong incentive to the biopharmaceutical companies to seek earlier signs for efficacy. Many months and substantial amounts of money can be saved if drugs that are not efficient are removed from the development path at an earlier time than the end of phase II. Another drawback of the traditional pathway of drug development is the failure to allow the investigators to interpret a negative outcome of a phase II study. Why did the drug fail to produce the expected clinical benefits in phase II? Was the concept wrong or did the drug simply fail to influence the drug target in the desired way? These questions remain unanswered.

In rare situations the problems of the classical development pathway are mitigated by highly visible effects of the drug candidates. Drugs developed for sleep disorders are typically sedative. Sedation is expected to occur in phase I dose escalating studies. If drug candidates fail to induce sedation in phase I, it makes little sense to test them in complex phase II sleep studies where sleep patterns are analyzed with electrophysiological monitoring techniques. The speed of saccadic eye movements represents a particularly sensitive readout of sedation. This parameter is easily measured during phase I studies and this serves as a quantitative endpoint to make a go/no-go decision in the drug development program. Another example is provided by opioid agonists developed for pain. Morphine and related opioid receptor agonists produce a characteristic constriction of the pupil in the eye. While this effect is physiologically unrelated to eventual analgesic properties of the compound, it serves to quickly determine whether a new opioid agonist drug candidate has adequate pharmacological and pharmacokinetic properties to stimulate these receptors in the body. This simple readout can serve to indicate efficacy already in phase I, before the drug candidate is taken into proper phase II pain studies.

Modern drug development puts strong emphasis on pharmacological readouts, surrogate markers, and experimental medicine. The term pharmacological readout is used for any molecular or optical parameter that is affected by a drug candidate and that can be measured in humans. Such readout does not necessarily have to be related to the actual disease process. If such a connection exists, the parameter measured becomes a surrogate marker, standing in for the clinically relevant endpoint. Measurements of surrogate markers are part of experimental medicine, namely medicine in which patients are exper-

Table 5.2   Pharmacological readouts in experimental medicine

---

Imaging Approaches
Receptor Occupancy Determination
Displacement of PET or SPECT labeled ligand with drug candidate
Direct measurement of binding to receptor site

Structural Imaging
Visualization of tumors and infarcts with MRI
Receptor distribution with PET or SPECT
Visualization of pathological structures

Functional Imaging
Visualization of blood flow changes with fMRI
Visualization of cellular morphology with PET/SPECT

Molecular Approaches
Biochemical Measurements in Urine, Blood, and CSF
Enzyme activities, hormone levels, metabolite levels

Genomic Profiling of Epithelial Tissues
mRNA expression profiles in accessible tissues

Proteomic Profiling of Blood and CSF
Protein profiles in accessible body fluids

Metabolomic Profiling of Urine and Blood
Profiles of metabolites in accessible body fluids

Behavioral Approaches
Experimental Human Disease Models
Experimental anxiety, experimental schizophrenia
Experimental pain

---

imental subjects in addition to being patients. Experimental medicine also includes artificial test situations in which humans are exposed to controlled influences that are believed to predict drug effects on the actual disease. Experimental medicine is a rapidly growing part of medicine (Frank and Hargreaves, 2003). Many academic institutions are building up experimental medicine units. Table 5.2 lists the principal approaches of modern experimental medicine.

5.3.1   Imaging Techniques

A direct measurement of receptor occupancy is the most desired approach to demonstrate that a drug candidate binds to its receptor site. Figure 5.2 illustrates the general aspects of this procedure. In animals, receptor occupancy is typically measured by ex vivo binding assays, where an animal is injected with a radiolabeled ligand that binds to the receptor site. The unlabeled test drug is then injected at increasing doses, the animals are killed and the undisplaced radioactivity is measured in the tissue of interest. In humans the labeled ligand is detected by imaging methods, typically PET or SPECT imaging.

Imaging techniques have utility beyond the determination of receptor occupancy. They have made enormous technical progress during the recent years and further rapid advances are expected. Several examples illustrate the elegant ways by which various imaging techniques provide readouts of drug efficacy in humans. Magnetic resonance imaging (MRI) techniques were developed as diagnostic tools, but they also serve as an important tool for drug development. For example, the efficacy of cancer drugs can be directly monitored when the tumor is sufficiently demarcated in imaging, and the drug's ability to shrink the tumor size becomes directly visible. In the brain, MRI allows the detection of infarction and tumor formation. The first notable application in drug discovery has been the use of imaging as surrogate marker for demyelination in MS. Drugs have received regulatory approval based on this marker alone. However, long-term experience revealed a rather complex relationship between the clinical progression of MS and the imaging readouts obtained with MRI (Ingle et al., 2003). Further studies will be needed to firmly establish that MRI provides an accurate surrogate marker for the progression of the disease.

Functional MRI (fMRI) represents the extension of MRI techniques into the study of brain function. MRI readings from the brain reflect the concentration of deoxyhemoglobin and are thus influenced by local blood flow. Neuronal activity and local blood flow are closely related, making it possible to use MRI readings as indicators of regional neuronal activity in the brain. Since MRI readings can be taken in conscious subjects, it is possible to expose humans to various sensory influences and determine the areas of the brain that are activated. For example, showing pictures that induce fear to humans subjects resulted in the activation of neurons in the amygdala. These studies very elegantly confirm the link between the amygdala and emotional processes that was established in animals through various invasive procedures. The impact of fMRI techniques on drug discovery is likely to become substantial. Early experience suggests the possibility to link specific disease states, such as pain, schizophrenia, and anxiety, to fMRI signals, thus providing an opportunity to use them as functional readouts for drug effects (Rauch et al., 2003).

PET, besides determining receptor occupancy of drugs, serves to anatomically locate the drug targets. For example, PET has become the standard technique to assess the survival of dopaminergic neurons in Parkinson's disease. [11]Fluoro-DOPA is administered intravenously and, similar to unlabeled L-DOPA, is taken up by dopaminergic neurons, converted to [11]fluoro-dopamine, and stored in synaptic vesicles. The amount of label thus reflects the density of dopaminergic innervation in the brain. This technique has received excellent validation in transplantation studies in Parkinson's disease (Brooks, 2003). In Alzheimer's disease visualization of pathological structures, the neuritic plaques and neurofibrillary tangles, would provide the best possible surrogate marker for drugs affecting the disease process. The search for suitable PET substrates that accumulate in these structures is the goal of a very active research effort (Kung et al., 2003).

Imaging techniques seem to have unlimited potential in drug discovery and development. Most diseases and drug actions are associated with functional changes in the brain that can be observed with a suitable technical approach. Imaging studies tend to be expensive and experimentally demanding. However, these drawbacks are minimized for indications where clinical studies with large patient populations and of long duration have been needed to obtain meaningful results.

5.3.2 Urological Markers and Metabolomics

For many drugs acting in the brain it is difficult to find appropriate ligands for receptor occupancy determinations, and it is not possible to directly measure their primary effects with imaging techniques in vivo. Most current drugs modify neurotransmitter receptors or ion channels and change biochemical and electrophysiological parameters that do not produce adequately large signals to be detected with imaging techniques and would require complex invasive methodologies for monitoring in vivo. However, some of the drug effects produce downstream events that are reflected by changes in the accessible body fluids, urine, blood, and CSF. For example, L-DOPA administered to Parkinson patients is converted to dopamine in the brain and then to homovanillic acid through the enzymatic conversion by monoamine oxidase and catechol-*O*-methyltransferase. Homovanillic acid is excreted by the kidneys and can be measured in the urine where it provides a reflection of the biochemical efficacy of the drug treatment. Unfortunately, this example is a rare exception, since most other monoamine metabolites found in the urine reflect secretion from the adrenal medulla and neurons of the autonomic nervous system. While popular for many years, measurement of neurotransmitter metabolites in the urine has thus largely been abandoned as irrelevant parameters. These efforts have been jokingly compared to analyzing the composition of the sewage from the Kremlin in an attempt to figure out what its ruler said in the secret chambers. The analogy appears well taken. Similar to the situation with the catecholamines, there are no meaningful metabolite measurements possible in the urine for the other neurotransmitter substances.

Urine analysis to determine drug effects has recently undergone a renaissance because of modern metabolomic techniques. They provide a complete profile of urinary metabolites, without attempting to link individual metabolites to specific biochemical processes in the brain. The metabolite profiles may change under the influence of specific diseases and drugs. Reproducible profile changes could thus serve as pharmacological readout of drug action (Reo, 2002). While highly attractive in principle, metabolomic techniques have not made any practical impact on drug discovery in the neurosciences as yet, and their full potential has to be further explored. The approach is not limited to urine; it can also be applied to blood or CSF samples.

5.3.3 Serological Parameters and Proteomics

Blood components are influenced by brain function and may serve as specific readouts for drug actions. Neurotransmitter metabolites have been discounted as meaningful for similar reasons to those measured in the urine. They reflect peripheral nervous system and adrenal functions predominantly. However, some of the circulating hormones are directly influenced by specific neurotransmitter receptors. For example, dopamine D_2 receptors control the release of prolactin by the pituitary. Activation of D_2 receptors blocks prolactin secretion. Bromocryptine, a dopamine agonist clinically used in the treatment of Parkinson's disease, also serves to stop prolactin secretion and lactation in women after parturition. Conversely, D_2 antagonists, the standard antipsychotic drugs increase prolactin levels, and this parameter can thus serve as a pharmacological readout to monitor efficacy of antagonists (Smith, 2003).

In Alzheimer's disease levels of the $A\beta$ fragment of the amyloid precursor protein are increased in the brain. $A\beta$ has also been detected in the blood, and there appears to be a dynamic relationship between brain and blood levels of $A\beta$. These interactions are not fully understood. Nevertheless, blood levels will be useful for the development of the inhibitors of enzymes that cleave $A\beta$ from its precursor and that are in clinical development. If efficacious in humans, these drugs will reduce $A\beta$ levels in the brain and the blood, making blood $A\beta$ levels an appropriate pharmacological readout for efficacy of the drug (DeMattos et al., 2002).

Proteomic techniques attempt to provide a complete and quantitative picture of the protein content of a specific tissue of body fluid. Proteomic profiling of blood proteins holds enormous promise to make serological markers generally useful as readout for drug actions. Significant disease processes are likely to cause changes in the levels of some of the proteins, generating disease-specific profiles that can be established with proteomic techniques. Modifications of the disease-specific profiles may thus become highly suitable readouts of pharmacologic efficacy. Proteomic methods have become generally available only recently, and their full impact cannot be judged as yet (Petricoin et al., 2002). Technical limitations have made it difficult so far to detect the proteins present at very low levels only. In humans individual variations in life style create variability in the proteomic profiles that might blur more subtle changes induced by drugs.

5.3.4 Cerebrospinal Fluid (CSF)

CSF is an accessible body fluid in humans, though its removal carries a small risk for complications. Infectious agents that have invaded the brain are usually detectable in the CSF. Beyond this diagnostic utility, CSF measurements have had little impact on drug discovery so far. While correlations between disease states and CSF components are often found, the interindividual variability typically precludes their use as surrogate markers. In Alzheimer's disease, for example, the CSF levels of Aβ are generally mildly elevated. However, the correlation is not strong enough to make this marker into a diagnostic tool or a surrogate marker for Alzheimer's disease.

More recently proteomic techniques have been applied to CSF samples from psychiatric patients (Jiang et al., 2003). As for the blood, it may be possible to define disease-specific or drug-specific proteomic or metabolomic profiles in CSF samples. The available experience from human and animal CSF studies raises the concern that the variability of the CSF composition will prevent meaningful results from being obtained.

5.3.5 Tissue Samples and Genomics

Genomic techniques, providing a full picture of gene expression in a tissue, are the most advanced and most promising among the various profiling approaches. They have clear utility for many diseases outside of the nervous system, where tissue samples can be obtained with relative use. In the cancer field, it has been possible to define subtypes of tumors based on their genomic profile (Balmain et al., 2003). In the neuroscience field, genomic techniques are being explored in the study of disease mechanism, using brain tissue samples obtained in postmortem analysis (Mimmack et al., 2002).

Genomic profiles might be useful as disease or drug markers in the neurosciences if they occur in accessible tissues, epithelia in particular. Some of the neuromuscular diseases and the pain area may be directly accessible to genomic approaches, since skin biopsies can be obtained with relative ease. Expression patterns of genes involved in the function of motor and sensory neurons appear attractive as readouts for drug actions.

5.3.6 Behavioral Tests

Several diseases of the brain, psychiatric diseases in particular, are highly heterogeneous and strongly modified by environmental influences. Depression and anxiety disorders are extremely content dependent. Because of these features, clinical trials for new anxiolytic and antidepressant drugs tend to require a very large number of patients to yield statistically meaningful results. Many studies fail, meaning even positive controls do not show a reliable effect. Clinical researchers in biopharmaceutical companies and in academic institutions are thus attempting to test drug candidates in a more controllable environment, in experimental human disease models. The field of anxiety disorders is most advanced and illustrates the possibilities. Several experimental anxiety models have been characterized, including nervousness caused by public speaking and fear of asphyxia caused by brief CO_2 inhalation. Verbal description of the emotions experienced by the patients is used as readouts. While still at an early stage, these human experimental models are highly attractive as early measures of drug efficacy. They have the potential to provide meaningful answers with a small number of patients only (Graeff et al., 2003).

Experimental human disease models will be most useful in depression where clinical trials take many years and the rate of failed trials is particularly high. Unlike anxiety, however, the emotion of depression cannot be created instantly in humans in an ethically acceptable way. The situation is equally complex in schizophrenia. Attempts have been made to induce a schizophrenia-like state with drugs such as cocaine and ketamine that induce hallucinations or exacerbate the symptoms of schizophrenics. However, as discussed earlier for the animal studies, these approaches are linked to known drug targets and thus tend to be limited to the evaluation of drugs acting through the same or a closely related mechanism.

In summary of this section, pharmacological readouts of drug action and surrogate markers are playing an increasingly important role in modern drug discovery and development. Experimental medicine approaches are likely to revolutionize the process from putative drug target to effective drug. The previously well delineated borders between phase I and phase II studies will become more and more blurred. The new approaches will be particularly powerful when it is possible to use the same markers in animal models and human experimental models of the diseases. Direct translation of data from an advanced animal model to a suitable human experimental situation and then to the clinically relevant endpoint delineates the most effective path to new and better drugs.

5.4 PLACEBO EFFECT

Humans respond to a variety of stimuli in real life. At a social dinner, the setting, the composition of the group, the nature of the conversation, all strongly influence our feelings, our emotional and physical status, even the taste of the food. Elderly people who suffer from many age-related ailments tend to feel much better when their children or grandchildren come to visit. In medical practice it is well known that patients tend to feel better and rate their diseases less severe following hospitalization or a visit to the doctor's office. Attention itself has a positive influence. These effects are most obvious at the psychological level. However, they are not restricted to perceptions and have physiological counterparts. The emotional status translates into neural and hormonal differences that influence body function. The body shows how a person feels. Pseudogravity is an extreme version of the influence of psychological status on body function. The strong desire in woman to have a child can produce bodily changes similar to pregnancy, including lactation.

A patient who receives a new medication from the physician expects a beneficial effect. Indeed, the generation of a positive anticipation has therapeutic utility itself and belongs to the repertoire of a successful physician. The effects induced by the anticipation alone are called placebo effects. The literal meaning of placebo in Latin is "I shall please". The placebo effects are real, and they have, as all mental phenomena, a cellular and molecular basis. A study with patients experiencing a placebo effect revealed elevations in dopamine release in the forebrain, tentatively linking the placebo effect to reward mechanisms (de la Fuente-Fernandez et al., 2001). Placebo effects are driven by novelty and tend to be prominent at the beginning of the treatment. They tend to be large for diseases with a large behavioral component, such as depression and anxiety, but play a surprisingly significant role also in diseases such as pain and respiratory allergies. In diseases that involve the nervous system only tangentially, infections and traumatic injuries to limbs for example, the placebo effects are typically not a significant component of the treatment.

When trying to define the benefits of a drug, the placebo effects are a disturbance and have to be separated from the actual drug effects. Double-blinded trial designs are the accepted experimental process to define the drug effects. The effects of a drug are compared with those of a pill or infusion with the same physical properties and appearance except the test compound itself. Neither the physician nor the patient knows which of the two test preparations contains the actual drug. Open label studies where patient and physician know that an active drug is being used are sometimes carried out to get a first subjective impression of the drug effect. The open label trials are fairly predictive for diseases with low placebo effects. In diseases with a high placebo component they do not produce trustworthy results and are often meaningless.

The placebo effects are a severe problem in clinical trials for depression and anxiety disorders, disease of the emotional state itself. Figure 5.3 shows the result of a typical depression trial. The severity of the depression is assessed with the help of a rating scale that is applied in a conversation between the physician and the patients. The attention of the physician has a larger effect than that of the treatment. Many depression trials fail because the drug signal is too small to produce a statistically significant difference over the placebo control group. These trials only succeed if great care is taken to ensure that the double blinding is indeed maintained. Placebo effects are a reality of drug development that requires careful attention.

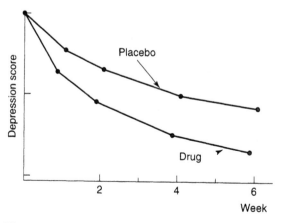

Figure 5.3   Placebo effect. In the example of a depression drug trial, the placebo effect strongly reduces the depression score. The drug results in a further improvement.

5.5 CONCLUSIONS

The development of drugs for diseases of the nervous system is more complex and more demanding than that for other indications. The brain is the most complex organ of the human body. Its evolutionary distance from other mammals is larger than for other organs, and it is specially protected by a blood-brain barrier. The evolutionary uniqueness makes it difficult to identify appropriate animal models for nervous system disease. The existence of the blood-brain barrier imposes an additional hurdle for drug discovery programs. The complexity and diversity of human behavior adds special challenges in the design of clinical trials. Modern translational medicine seeks to identify clinical endpoints that directly reflect the action of the drug and that predict accurately the effects on the clinical parameters relevant for the patients.

The molecular and structural nature of the blood-brain barrier is under active investigation. Detailed knowledge will make it possible to better predict the structural requirements for drug candidates to penetrate into the brain and stimulate the targeted receptor site. Receptor occupancy, measured in vivo, provides the best readout for brain penetration.

The rapidly growing knowledge on disease mechanisms is generating transgenic animal models for human diseases that replicate crucial steps in the disease mechanism. They will gradually replace the lesion models and behavioral models on which the drug discovery researchers have relied so far.

Translational medicine bridges the molecular and cellular knowledge of a drug's mechanism of action and the clinical effects that help the patients. Many new methods, including imaging techniques, proteomics and metabolomics, as well as experimental disease states, provide clinical markers for drug efficacy. These methods will make it possible to establish efficacy of the drug candidates with small groups of patients and to predict the outcome of the large trials demonstrating efficacy that is relevant for the patients.

REFERENCES

Further Reading

BANKS, W.A., and LEBEL, C.R. Strategies for the delivery of leptin to the CNS. *J. Drug Targ.* 10: 297–308, 2002.

FENG, M.R. Assessment of blood-brain barrier penetration: in silico, in vitro and in vivo. *Curr. Drug Metab.* 3: 647–657, 2002.

FRANK, R., and HARGREAVES, R. Clinical biomarkers in drug discovery and development. *Drug Disc. Rev.* 2: 567–580, 2003.

GREAEFF, F.G., PARENTE, A., DEL-BEN, C.M., and GUIMARAES. Pharmacology of human experimental anxiety. *Braz. J. Med. Biol. Res.* 36: 421–432, 2003.

PARDRIGE, W.M. Drug and gene targeting to the brain with molecular Trojan horses. *Nature Rev. Drug Disc.* 1: 131–139, 2002.

PETRICOIN, E.F., ZOON, K.C., KOHN, E.C., BARRETT, J.C., and LIOTTA, L.A. Clinical proteomics: Translating benchside promise into bedside reality. *Nature Rev. Drug Disc.* 1: 683–695, 2002.

REO, N.V. NMR-based metabolomics. *Drug Chem. Toxicol.* 25: 375–382, 2002.

SUN, H., DAI, H., SHAIK, N., and ELMQUIST, W.F. Drug efflux transporters in the CNS. *Adv. Drug Deliv. Rev.* 55: 83–105, 2003.

TUSZYNSKI, M.H. Gene therapy for neurological disease. *Expert Opin. Biol. Ther.* 3: 815–828, 2003.

WONG, P.C., CAI, H., BORCHELT, D.R., and PRICE, D.L. Gene-tically engineered mouse models of neurodegenerative diseases. *Nature Neurosci.* 5: 633–639, 2002.

References

BALMAIN, A., GRAY, J., and PONDER, B. The genetics and genomics of cancer. *Nat. Genet.* 33: 238–244, 2003.

BROOKS, D.J. PET studies on the function of dopamine in health and Parkinson's disease. *Ann. N.Y. Acad. Sci.* 991: 22–35, 2003.

DE LA FUENTE-FERNANDEZ, R., RUTH, T.J., SOSSI, V., SCHULZER, M., CALNE, D.B., and STOESSL, A.J. Expectation and dopamine release: Mechanism of the placebo effect in Parkinson's disease. *Science* 10: 1164–1166, 2001.

DEMATTOS, R.B., BALES, K.R., PARSDANIAN, M., O'DELL, M.A., FOSS, E.M., PAUL, S.M., and HOLTZMAN, D.M. Plaque-associated disruption of CSF and plasma amyloid-beta (Abeta) equilibrium in a mouse model of Alzheimer's disease. *J. Neurochem.* 81: 229–236, 2002.

BERGSTRÖM, M., HARGREAVES, R.J., BURNS, D., GOLDBERG, M.R., SCIBERRAS, D., REINES, S.A., PETTY, K.J., OEGREN, M., ANTONI, G., LANGSTRÖM, B., ESKOLA, O., SCHEININ, M., SOLIN, O., MAJUMDAR, A.K., CONSTANZER, M.L., BATTISTI, W.P., BRADSTREET, T.E., GARGANO, C., and HIETALA, J. Human positron emission tomography studies of brain neurokinin 1 receptor occupancy by aprepitant. *Biol. Psychiat.* 55: 1007–1012, 2004.

JIANG, L., LINDPAINTNER, K., LI, H.F., GU, N.F., LANGEN, H., HE, L., and FOUNTOULAKIS, M. Proteomic analysis of the cerebrospinal fluid of patients with schizophrenia. *Amino Acids* 25: 49–57, 2003.

KUNG, M.P., SKOVRNKSKY, D.M., HOU, C., ZHUANG, Z.P., GUR, T.L., ZHANG, B., TROJANIWSKI, J.Q., LEE, V.M., and KUNG, H.F. Detection of amyloid plaques by radioligands for Abeta40 and Abeta42: Potential imaging agents in Alzheimer patients. *J. Mol. Neurosci.* 20: 15–24, 2003.

INGLE, G.T., STEVENSON, V.L., MILLER, D.H., and THOMPSON, A.J. Primary progressive multiple sclerosis: A 5-year clinical and MR study. *Brain* 126: 2528–2536, 2003.

LANGLOIS, X., TE RIELE, P., WINTMOLDERS, C., LEYSEN, J.E., and JURZAK, M. Use of beta-imager for rapid ex vivo auto-radiography exemplified with central nervous system penetrating neurokinin 3 antagonists. *J. Pharmacol. Exp. Ther.* 299: 712–717, 2001.

MIMMACK, M.L., RYAN, M., BABA, H., NAVARRO-RUIZ, J., IRITANI, S., FAULL, R.L., MCKENNA, P.J., JONES, P.B., ARAI, H., STARKEY, M., EMSON, P.C., and BAHN, S. Gene expression analysis in schizophrenia: Reproducible up-regulation of several members of the apolipoprotein L family located in a high-susceptibility locus for schizophrenia on chromosome 22. *Proc. Natl. Acad. Sci. USA.* 99: 4680–4685, 2005.

RAUCH, S.L., SHIN, L.M., and WRIGHT, C.I. Neuroimaging studies of amygdala function in anxiety disorders. *An. N.Y. Acad. Sci.* 985: 389–410, 2003.

SMITH, S. Effects of antipsychotics on sexual and endocrine implications for clinical practice. *J. Clin. Psychopharmacol.* 23: S27–32, 2003.

TERASAKI, T., OHTSUKI, S., HORI, S., TAKANAGA, H., NAKASHIMA, E., and HOSOYA, K. New approaches to in vitro models of blood-brain barrier drug transport. *Drug Disc. Today* 8: 944–954, 2003.

Chapter 6

Schizophrenia

Among all the diseases of the brain, schizophrenia is perhaps the most cruel one. It affects the very essence of human identity and understanding of the self. There are many well-known victims. The story of Dr. John Forbes Nash, depicted in the movie *A Beautiful Mind* perhaps in an embellished way to make it entertaining, illustrated many of the key features of schizophrenia. They comprise hallucinations, delusions, loss of coherent thinking, and inability to engage in meaningful social contact. The victim, as depicted in the movie, was unable to distinguish between real and imagined people, as if he was living in a gray zone between reality and the perceived veracity of a dream. The story of Dr. Nash also illustrates the limited effectiveness of drug treatment as well as behavioral therapy. A highly supportive family and medical environment could not keep him from leading a bizarre and dysfunctional life. However, the chronicle of Dr. Nash's life and disease also tells the rare possibility of a beautiful resolution of the disease.

Schizophrenia surely played an important role in shaping human history. Many of the visionaries of the antique worlds believed to be the voices of gods were likely to describe their schizophrenic hallucinations, as for example, Cassandra in the tragedy *Agamemnon* by Aeschylus. Cassandra's gripping words, written about 500 years BC, depict the perceived link to the gods, the agony of the hallucinations, and the wish for death to escape the misery, archetypal for schizophrenics:

That is my power—a boon Apollo gave.
—

Woe for me, woe! Again the agony—
Dread pain that sees the future all too well
With ghastly preludes whirls and racks my soul.
—

Grant me one boon—a swift and mortal stroke,
That all unwrung my pain, with ebbing blood
Shed forth in quiet death, I close my eyes.

A most intriguing, well-documented, and even entertaining case of a schizophrenic with historical impact is that of Ludwig II, King of Bavaria from 1864 to 1886. Most visitors to Disneyland or Disney World may not be aware that the wonderful Disney castle, now a symbol of the company, is not a copy of a medieval castle. It is a replication of the castle Neuschwanstein in the German state Bavaria, a neo-historical castle built by Ludwig II less then 150 years ago. Theater artists decorated the castle in medieval style. Ludwig became king as a young man and soon developed features strange for his position. He hid

Drug Discovery for Nervous System Diseases. by Franz F. Hefti
ISBN 0-471-46563-1   Copyright © 2005 by John Wiley & Sons, Inc.

himself, stayed away from governmental functions, abandoned his beautiful fiancée, and gradually withdrew in a dream world of newly built, highly extravagant castles. Lavish parties, sled rides with candle illumination, fantastical discussions with actors filled his world. After many years in formal power, the king was deposed. Despite his disease, he seemed to have understood the events, since he drowned himself three days later in a lake, taking with him the psychiatrist who had justified his deposition. The castles built by Ludwig II are now a major tourist attraction and source of income for the state of Bavaria. From a historical point of view, it is important that Ludwig's extravagant constructions depleted the treasury of the then independent kingdom of Bavaria. He reigned during the foundation of the Second German Empire organized by Bismarck and Prussia. It is believed that Ludwig, whose coffers were empty, accepted money from Bismarck in return for agreeing to merge Bavaria into the new German empire. Without Bavaria, the German Empire would not have gained superiority over the Austrian Empire, and it would have been too small to start World War I. There wouldn't have been World War II with its atrocities and the holocaust. Fantastic psychiatric speculations? Perhaps, but it is captivating to think that the world might look very different now without the schizophrenia of a single man.

6.1 SYMPTOMS AND DISEASE MECHANISM

Most schizophrenia victims receive drug treatment now, making it more difficult for full-blown symptoms to become manifest. Before the advent of antipsychotic drugs in the 1950s patients developed the symptoms in an unhindered way. Detailed descriptions by the physician who coined the term schizophrenia in 1916, Eugen Bleuler, still provide one of the best and most complete picture. Sensory hallucinations are the primary hallmark of the disease. Auditory hallucinations, hearing voices, are often the most disturbing ones, since they can force victims into bizarre or criminal behavior. Delusions, including delusion of grandeur or unjustified paranoia, are a typical part of the disease picture. There were untreated patients who crowned themselves to kings and emperors. Many suffer from messianic illusions; others fear of being followed or persecuted by secret agents. Most patients have difficulties to think coherently and to express reasoned behavioral patterns. Many loose the normal patterns of affective behavior as well as the ability to engage in meaningful social contact. Bleuler coined the term schizophrenia "because the *splitting* of different psychic functions is one its most important characteristics." In the modern medical terminology, thought disturbances, verbal limitations, and reduced affection are referred to as negative symptoms, whereas hallucinations and delusions represent the positive symptoms of schizophrenia.

Schizophrenia affects roughly 1% of individuals during their life span. Its societal consequences and costs are enormous. Many of the patients require long-term care and disability benefits. Schizophrenic adolescents tend to disrupt and even destroy functional families. The suicide rate is high among the disease victims. Before antipsychotic drugs became widely available, schizophrenic patients were typically kept in an insane asylum, where restraint and isolation were the only options to avoid danger for the patients and caregivers. During the recent decades most patients have been moved to outpatient status. Many of the homeless individuals of the modern metropolitan areas suffer from schizophrenia or related psychiatric diseases. During the period of 1960 to 1980, society and the health care community saw environmental factors as the major cause for psychiatric diseases and favored attempts to reintegrate patients into normal life rather than keeping them institutionalized. More recently financial constraints of the health care systems limit the availability of care, institutional care in particular, further limiting the available care. To this day, schizophrenia remains one of the most difficult, devastating, and stigmatized human diseases.

Despite major research efforts we are far away from a coherent picture of the disease mechanisms of schizophrenia. Most often schizophrenia develops during late adolescence, but the onset can occur anytime between late adolescence and early middle age. The earliest time of onset coincides with the late stages of synaptic pruning in mammalian development, so that schizophrenia can be considered a developmental disorder. There are only very few consistent pathological observations. Enlarged cerebral ventricles are most prominent among them, lending support to the view that brain atrophy is a feature of the disease. Atrophic changes have been described for the prefrontal area of the cortex, a brain area associated with higher cognitive functions, decision making, and consciousness. Twin and family studies suggest a strong genetic component of the disease, with a concordance rate of approximately 40% for monozygotic twins. The discoveries of disease-causing genes strongly support this view. In 2000 the research group of David Porteus in Scotland reported the first identification of a disease-causing gene (Millar et al., 2000). They found that a translocation of DISC1 (disrupted-in-schizophrenia 1) co-segregated with schizophrenia. A similar mutation was later found in an independent family in Finland (Ekelund et al., 2001). Carriers of the DISC1 translocation develop schizophrenia, bipolar depression, or major unipolar depression. This highly intriguing observation demonstrates that a single genetic alteration is sufficient to cause schizophrenia and, furthermore, that the genetic environment of this mutations or the cultural environment determine the precise nature of the symptomatology. The new findings support the view that schizophrenia is a multifactorial disease that like diabetes is typically caused by a combination of genetic and environmental influences.

6.2 ANTIPSYCHOTICS AND DOPAMINE D_2 RECEPTORS

The symptoms of schizophrenia, in particular the positive symptoms, are effectively treated with antipsychotic drugs such as chlorpromazine, haloperidol, and thioridazine (Fig. 6.1). Serendipitous observations made at the bedside led to their discovery during the middle of the last century. The mechanism of their antipsychotic action remained unclear for two decades, because neuropharmacology had only few experimental tools available at that time and because these drugs showed effects in many of the existing test systems. This unhappy situation changed dramatically when monoamine receptors were functionally characterized through binding studies, and when a correlation between inhibition of dopamine receptors and clinical potency became evident (Seeman and Lee, 1975). Figure 6.2 reproduces the original graph. The correlation between the in vitro potency and clinical dose in humans is astonishingly robust, when one considers that variability among the compounds in absorbance, liver metabolism, brain penetration, and distribution within the brain could have muddled this picture substantially. In retrospect, the approach to correlate clinical dose to receptor affinities without considering the many steps in between seems naïve and simple, but it certainly led to the correct conclusions. The seminal observations enlightened the schizophrenia field and all of neuropharmacology. They opened the way for the creation of selective dopamine antagonists such as spiperone and raclopride. Later studies on cloned dopamine receptors revealed that the D_2 receptor type is broadly responsible for the antipsychotic actions. Dopamine D_2 receptor antagonists

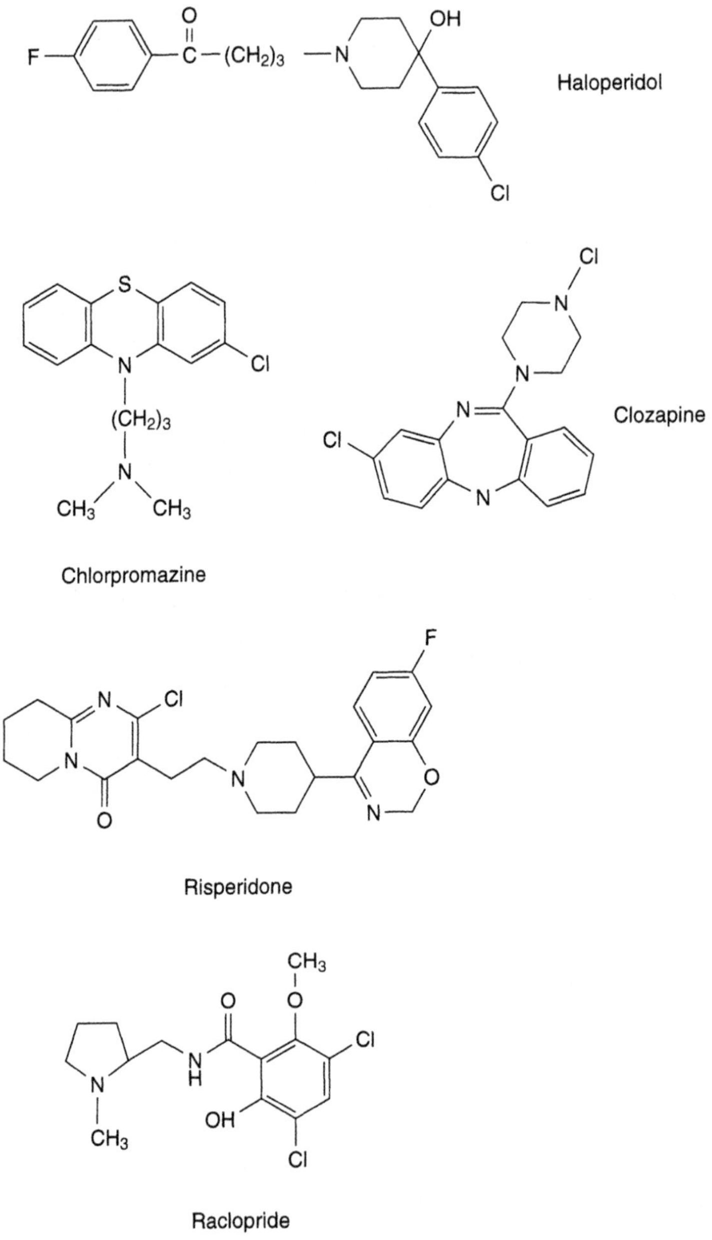

Haloperidol

Chlorpromazine

Clozapine

Risperidone

Raclopride

Figure 6.1 Examples of current antipsychotic drugs.

remain the cornerstone of schizophrenia treatment at the current time (Bennett, 1998; Freedman, 2003).

Additional observations support a link between schizophrenia and dopamine systems. Among the major drugs of addiction, amphetamine and cocaine are able to induce hallucinations, in particular, when used at high doses and chronically. These drugs stimulate the release and block the reuptake of monoamines. They increase the concentration of dopamine, norepinephrine, and serotonin at synaptic locations, resulting in excessive

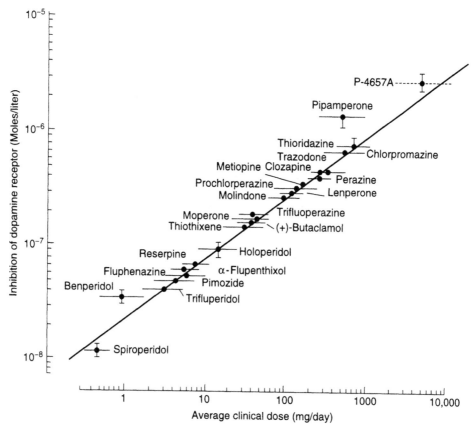

Figure 6.2   The discovery of antipsychotics as dopamine receptor antagonists. Correlation between the therapeutic dose of antipsychotic drugs and the inhibition of a dopamine D₂ receptor mediated effect. (Reproduced with permission, Seeman and Lee, 1975, AAAS)

stimulation of the postsynaptic receptors. Dopamine plays an important part in these behavioral stimulations, since selective dopamine D₂ receptor antagonists can block most of the actions of amphetamine and cocaine. Parkinson's disease, discussed in more detail in Chapter 10, is characterized by the loss dopaminergic neurotransmitter systems in the brain. Most of these patients are treated with L-DOPA, the precursor of dopamine. The doses needed for clinical efficacy massively elevate dopamine levels in the brain. After several years of therapy, many of the patients experience visual hallucinations. There are examples of patients who buy additional groceries for people imagined to live in their house, or patients who call the fire department reporting that there house is on fire when it is not. While these observations strongly suggest a major role for dopamine in schizophrenia, they also illustrate the limited nature of this association. Hallucinations caused by L-DOPA involve the visual sense only; auditory or other sensory hallucinations have not been reported. The patients do not develop a schizoid personality with its incoherence, intellectual and emotional impairments.

The connection between dopamine and schizophrenia represents the basis for animal assays often used to predict antipsychotic actions. Cocaine, amphetamine, L-DOPA, as well as direct dopamine D₂ receptor antagonists (apomorphine) induce locomotor hyperactivity in rodents. Antipsychotic drugs such as chlorpromazine and haloperidol suppress this hyperactivity because they block the D_2 receptors. The models thus keep drug discovery research within the frame of dopamine antagonism. They do not lead to novel drug targets. However, cocaine- or amphetamine-induced hyperactivity is very useful as readouts for brain penetration and receptor occupancy in the brain, in drug discovery programs for antipsychotics where D_2 receptor antagonism is at least a component.

6.3   DOPAMINE D_1, D_3, AND D_4 RECEPTORS

The dopamine D_2 receptor is the most abundant receptor for this neurotransmitter in the brain of rodents, primates, and humans. It is widely expressed in the basal ganglia as well as the cortex and other telencephalic structures. Accordingly, activation or inactivation of these receptors affects behavior in a global and massive way. Mice with deletions of the D_2 receptor gene, D_2 knockouts, are behaviorally inactive, similar as animals treated with high doses of D_2 antagonists. Selective D_2 agonists globally activate animals, alike the indirect activators amphetamine and cocaine. The other members of the dopamine receptor family, the D_1, D_3, and D_4 receptors, are more discreetly expressed and their role is more subtle. Nevertheless, each of them has attracted and continues to attract great interest from schizophrenia researchers. All dopamine receptors belong to the group of G-protein-coupled receptors, making them appealing for drug discovery. The D_2, D_3, and D_4 are closely related and share a long third intracellular loop, which is believed to be a determinant of the interactions with G-proteins and the downstream signaling cascade, whereas D_1 receptors lack this feature defining it as a unique molecule (Missale et al., 1998).

The D_4 receptor is responsible for one of the more intriguing stories of drug discovery. Soon after its cloning and the discovery that the D_4 receptor is expressed in the cortex, the most intriguing observation was published that levels are elevated in the brain of schizophrenics (Seeman et al., 1993). The D_4 receptor became a celebrity drug target, a must for the pharmaceutical industry. Concerns appeared along the way. Awaited confirmatory publications failed to emerge. D_4 antagonists had no behavioral effects in animals. Nevertheless, many pharmaceutical companies moved rapidly ahead, and researchers at Merck & Co. were first in identifying a selective D_4 antagonist that was suitable as drug candidate. The compound swiftly moved through development and was taken into a phase IIa proof-of-concept clinical study. The result was clearly negative, without even a hint of a positive effect, perhaps not entirely surprising given the limited expression of D_4 receptors in the human brain (Kramer et al., 1997). There may be other therapeutic uses for D_4 antagonists, as suggested by the observation that D_4 knockout mice respond differently to cocaine, amphetamine, and also ethanol (Rubenstein et al., 1997). Nevertheless, the D_4/schizophrenia story serves as an educational example for the mercurial and unpredictable nature of neuroscience drug discovery, certainly of the past but perhaps also for the near future.

Many of the antipsychotic D_2 antagonists also inhibit D_1 dopamine receptors, which thus could contribute to their therapeutic actions. In contrast to the situation with the D_2 receptor, deletion of the D_1 gene does not cause massive behavioral changes in the knockout mice. Locomotor behavior is unchanged, perhaps slightly elevated. Interestingly though, the animals no longer respond to cocaine, suggesting a link to addiction or hallucinations. From a point of view of schizophrenia, it is particularly interesting that the D_1 receptors are expressed at relatively high levels in the prefrontal cortex. This brain area has been associated with decision making and higher level thinking in humans, the behaviors most affected in schizophrenia. Blood flow in the prefrontal cortex is increased during intellectual activity. The blood flow changes are less prominent in schizophrenia patients. There is evidence for cytoarchitectonic changes in the prefrontal cortex of schizophrenics. Cells appear more densely packed, most likely because the synaptic network is atrophic and takes up less space. Functional studies in humans suggest that prefrontal cortex alterations lead to pathological elevations in dopaminergic transmission (Meyer-Lindenberg et al., 2002), creating a link to the current pharmacotherapy. The observations can be linked together into a speculative hypothesis predicting that D$_1$ antagonism is a beneficial feature of antipsychotic drugs. A modification of this hypothesis predicts that D$_2$ antagonism exacerbates the cognitive problems in schizophrenia and that D$_1$ agonists might be beneficial in connection with D$_2$ antagonism. Experimental studies on primates support the latter hypothesis. In these studies monkeys were treated with the D$_2$ antagonist haloperidol until their performance declined in memory tests. These deficits were reversed when a D$_1$ agonist was given to the animals (Castner et al., 2000).

The hypothesis that prefrontal cortex dopaminergic functions are altered in schizophrenia has received additional support from rather intriguing findings on the enzyme catechol-O-methyltransferase (COMT) that is part of the inactivation mechanism of dopamine. Two forms of this enzyme are encoded that differ in a single amino acid (valine/methione). The val/val genotype has been tentatively identified as risk factor for schizophrenia. Functional imaging studies with fMRI on humans suggest that people with the val/val genotype respond excessively to dopaminergic stimulation. The genotype is furthermore associated with higher expression of tyrosine hydroxylase (TH) in the human brain (Akil et al., 2003). Postmortem studies on brain tissue from schizophrenia patients revealed alterations in COMT expression patters in the prefrontal cortex (Matsumoto et al., 2003). These findings together with those related to D$_1$ receptors create a tentative but tantalizing picture of dopaminergic dysfunction in the prefrontal cortex of schizophrenic patients, and they support the view that D$_1$ receptors as well as COMT warrant further exploration as putative drug targets.

Dopamine D$_3$ receptors are located in many brain areas outside of the motor systems, at particularly high levels in the nucleus accumbens, a well-defined small area around the anterior commissure of the basal forebrain. Dopaminergic afferents from the medioventral forebrain adjacent to the substantia nigra form the mesolimbic dopaminergic pathway. Together with the adjacent nigrostriatal dopaminergic pathway the mesolimbic pathway constitutes the major ascending dopaminergic projection in the mammalian brain. These pathways have been in the center of attention of neuropharmacologists since the discovery of that dopamine has neurotransmitter function in the brain. Stimulation and lesion studies allowed investigators to distinguish between actions on motor functions and non-motor functions mediated by the nigrostriatal and the mesolimbic pathways, respectively. Reward and addiction appear to require intact mesolimbic systems. While this separation is conceptually very intriguing and helps to formulate testable hypotheses, it has to be kept in mind that the two pathways are not separated in an absolute way. There is a gradual anatomical transition from one to the other. Nevertheless, the projections to the nucleus accumbens are intriguing from a point of view of schizophrenia, since this nucleus is connected to the prefrontal cortex, and the hippocampus, the amygdala, and other nuclei linked to memory and affective mechanisms. It is tempting to speculate that the nucleus accumbens may serve a central function in mediating integration of various behaviors in the brain. Disturbed integrative functions are the key feature of schizophrenia, explaining the research interest in the nucleus accumbens despite its relatively small size. Figure 6.3 shows a diagram of nucleus accumbens afferents and efferents. Many of the antipsychotic drugs, including haloperidol and chlorpromazine, have similar affinities to D$_3$ receptors as

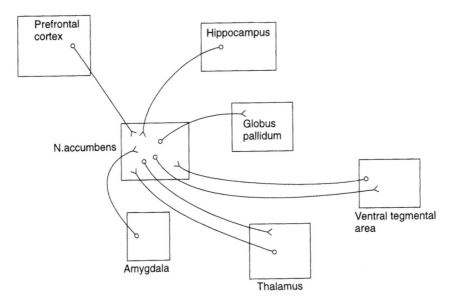

Figure 6.3 Anatomical connections of the nucleus accumbens. The nucleus is connected to many brain areas and neural circuits linked to schizophrenia and other psychiatric disorders.

they have to the D_2 receptors, making it possible that the former may mediate some of the therapeutic effects. However, a minor rather than major role of D_3 receptors is suggested from studies in knockout animals. Mice with deletions of the D_3 receptor gene behave largely normal. They show less inhibition in a novel environment, a feature typically interpreted as suggesting anxiolysis. During recent years several pharmaceutical companies have been engaged in the development of selective D_3 antagonists for schizophrenia and other psychiatric indications.

Understanding of the link between schizophrenia and dopaminergic system and understanding of dopaminergic mechanisms in the brain may lead to improved antipsychotic drugs. However, no specific hypothesis imposes itself as a must and there is no validated drug target beyond the dopamine D_2 receptor. Linkage studies so far have not provided support for a direct and causative role of dopaminergic systems in schizophrenia disease mechanisms. The clinical observations and the scientific knowledge suggest that dopaminergic systems, the D_2 receptors in particular, are essential for the manifestation of schizophrenic symptoms. Reduction of D_2 receptor signal transmission attenuates the disease symptoms but also interferes with normal behaviors, such as motor functions, cognitive and emotional functions. It is likely that D_2 receptor antagonists will always have a role in the treatment of acute psychotic episodes. However, hopefully, more specific drugs can be found that interfere with a more central element of the disease mechanism.

6.4 CLOZAPINE AND THE ATYPICAL ANTIPSYCHOTICS

Clozapine was discovered half a century ago by researchers at a small research department of Wander, the Swiss company who invented Ovaltine. The company later became part of the pharmaceutical company Novartis. The researchers used several simple behavioral rodent models and looked for unusual patterns of behavior that test compounds might elicit. In the ways of the pharmaceutical industry of those days, the test compounds were derivatives of known "psychoactive" compounds. There were few, if any molecular considerations to drive the project. The test compound that became clozapine was an analogue of imipramine, an early antidepressant compound that showed an unusual spectrum of behavioral effects. It was strongly sedating and differed from other imipramine analogues. It was taken into development and proved efficacious in schizophrenia trials. Problems with liver toxicity posed a substantial risk and prevented the company from seeking regulatory approval. However, clinicians who participated in clinical trials with clozapine urged the company to provide more test samples, because they felt that clozapine was superior to the typical antipsychotics and that it worked on some patients who responded poorly to the standard drugs. Clozapine seemed particularly effective in reducing negative symptoms that are typically not corrected by the standard antipsychotic drugs. Reluctantly the company concurred, and was gradually convinced to seek approval for the drug, despite the liver toxicity that strongly curtailed the use. Over many years clozapine found its way into psychiatric practice because of the superior efficacy. The clinical use stimulated drug discovery programs for safe analogues. These newer drugs, together with clozapine, now form the group of atypical antipsychotics.

It is now known that clozapine is a very complex drug that binds to many neurotransmitters with high affinity, including dopamine D_2 and D_4 receptors, α-adrenergic receptors, serotonin 5-HT$_2$ receptors, and histamine H_1 receptors. Possibly the combination of the D_2 antagonism with some of the other affinities is responsible for the improved clinical picture. Despite broad research efforts it has not been possible to ascribe the clinical benefits to specific receptors. The D_4 receptor is unlikely to be a major contributor, given the negative experience with pure D_4 antagonists. Antagonism at the 5-HT$_{2A}$ receptor is believed to be a significant contributor. However, reports that pure 5-HT$_{2A}$ antagonist have antipsychotic activities have not received active confirmation, suggesting that this receptor does not play a major role in the therapeutic effects. Many clozapine-like molecules have entered clinical practice in the past decade. Examples are olanzapine and risperidone. All atypical antipsychotics are D_2 antagonists with additional receptor affinities and lack of liver toxicity that harms clozapine. Cynics claim that all these drugs are just slightly modified dopamine D_2 antagonists and do not represent a significant advantage over the early antipsychotics (Kapur and Remington, 2001). Many psychiatrists maintain the view that the benefits of clozapine are not matched by the newer atypicals. However, at least minor benefits seem to be present for the entire group. For example, tardive dyskinesias, disturbing involuntary movements that occur in a small number of patients chronically treated with typical antipsychotics, are less frequent with the atypical drugs.

Typical and atypical antipsychotic drugs, often also called neuroleptic drugs, represent the backbone of pharmacotherapy for schizophrenia. When titrated carefully and when combined with personal care and behavioral therapy, these drugs can allow a patient to be reasonably functional and to live independently. Patients are often incompliant, however, because they dislike the diminished mental and physical activity produced by the drugs. Many remain trapped in the disabling patterns of the negative symptoms. The current antipsychotics make the disease manageable but do not cure it.

The current clinical and scientific knowledge of the clinically efficacious antipsychotic drugs and dopamine mechanisms does not point to an obvious way toward the discovery of new drugs. For many years drug discovery researchers believed that exploring one receptor affinity after the other of clozapine would ultimately identify a few crucial ones. The negative experiences with highly selective D_4 antagonists and 5-HT$_{2A}$ antagonists have greatly reduced this enthusiasm. Such a sequential trial and error approach takes too much time and is too costly to be attractive. It may not succeed at all, since the beneficial effects of clozapine may reflect the unique combination of actions at several receptors. In absence of credible animal models for schizophrenia, these combinations would have to be evaluated in clinical trials. For each receptor it would be necessary to identify a potent, selective and safe molecule suitable for human use. The molecules would have to be tested alone and in combinations of various doses. Even without referring to statistics, it is obvious that there are too many variables, too high costs, too few patients, to make such a giant experiment even remotely feasible. Progress has to come from new approaches, from other receptor mechanisms, or from better understanding of the disease mechanism.

6.5 NMDA RECEPTORS

Phencyclidine (PCP) and ketamine are drugs initially tested as anesthetics. PCP in particular, but also ketamine, was observed to induce hallucinations in human volunteers. Perhaps because of this property, PCP was never approved as medically useful drug but found an alternative life as drug of abuse, "angel dust." Ketamine is used as anesthetic in children. It does not induce hallucinations or psychosis in children, a very interesting observation given that the onset of detrimental effects coincides with the typical onset of schizophrenia. In schizophrenic patients, ketamine exacerbates the positive symptoms of schizophrenia. Both drugs are antagonists at the glutamate NMDA receptor, and these findings thus provide the basis for the NMDA hypothesis of schizophrenia. The hypothesis predicts that schizophrenic symptoms reflect insufficient stimulation of NMDA receptors and that drugs stimulating these receptors will have a beneficial impact on schizophrenia. In support of this view, psychotic episodes have been observed in clinical trials with new NMDA antagonists tested for efficacy in stroke. These intriguing and provocative observations and speculations have not received support as yet from neuropathological studies. There is no positive evidence for reduced NMDA receptor activity in the brain of schizophrenic patients. However, most beautiful support has been obtained from transgenic mice studies. NMDA receptors are ionotropic receptors composed of at least two subunits, the NR1 subunit together with at least one of the NR2A, NR2B, NR2C, or NR2D subunits. NR1 knockout mice die during intra-uterine development and are not a tool for investigation. However, an incomplete knockout of the NR1 gene has been generated that reaches adulthood. In these NMDA knockdown mice the total number of NMDA receptors is reduced to approximately 10% (Mohn et al., 1999). The knockdown mice exhibit elevated locomotor activity in a similar way as PCP and other NMDA antagonists activate normal mice. Interestingly the NMDA knockdown mice showed deficits in social interactions and sexual functions. Both behaviors were corrected when clozapine was given to them chronically.

Will NMDA agonists be useful for schizophrenia? The answer will be very complex for several reasons. Glutamate and NMDA receptors play a major role in acute neurodegenerative processes, as discussed in detail in Chapter 11. NMDA antagonists reduce neural degeneration in experimental animal models of stroke and traumatic brain injury. These robust findings chip away at the courage to treat humans with general NMDA agonists, since they are likely to worsen neurodegenerative episodes or may induce neurodegenerative events themselves. Glutamatergic synapses are ubiquitous and excitatory in their vast majority, explaining why glutamate agonists can induce seizures, raising an additional concern when considering human use. Nevertheless, highly selective agonists for receptor subtypes may turn out to be useful for schizophrenia. All four of the NR2 subunits are differentially expressed in the brain. During development in rodents, the NR2B subunit is gradually replaced by the NR2A subunit, a process that is influenced by synaptic activity and the environment (Quinlan et al., 1999). These findings encourage the view that NR2A agonists might be effective in schizophrenia. However, the arguments are speculative and may not be sufficient to trigger the substantial efforts of a targeted drug discovery program.

6.6 GLUTAMATERGIC SYNAPSE MODULATORS

NMDA receptors require glycine to be operational. The low-affinity binding site for glycine may provide a safer approach to influence these receptors than direct agonists. It may be possible to stimulate NMDA receptors by increasing the glycine concentration in the brain. The speculation receives tentative support from several small-scale clinical trials in which very high doses of glycine or of its more stable analogue, D-serine, were observed to be beneficial in schizophrenic patients (Heresco-Levy et al., 1999). Specific transporter proteins control the concentration of glycine in the synapse. Two gene products have been characterized, the glycine transporter-1 and transporter-2. The former, GlyT1, is expressed on glial cells surrounding various types of synapses, whereas the latter, GlyT2 appears to regulate the function of glycinergic synapses only. It may thus be possible to influence NMDA receptor function by drugs acting on GlyT1. Indeed, such an influence has been experimentally demonstrated in an oocyte expression system where NMDA receptors were expressed together with GlyT1. Inhibitors of GlyT1 are therefore expected to increase synaptic concentrations of glycine and, in consequence, to increase NMDA receptor function. Such an indirect action on the NMDA receptors might be safer than that of direct activators, since it is more likely to keep receptor function within the physiological range. Based on such considerations, several companies have engaged in drug discovery efforts for specific GlyT1 inhibitors.

The glutamatergic synapse is a complex structure, containing many more receptor molecules than just the NMDA receptors (Fig. 6.4). Kainic acid (KA) receptors and α-amino-3-hydroxy-5-methylisoxazole-4-propionate (AMPA) receptors are further ionotropic glutamate receptors than can occur separately or within the same synapse as NMDA receptors. The family of metabotropic glutamate receptors (mGluR) adds further complexity. The metabotropic glutamate receptors are G-protein-coupled receptors, which makes them particularly attractive from a drug discovery point of view. Several biopharmaceutical companies have engaged in broad research efforts on the mGluR family for these reasons. Researchers at Lilly have identified a drug candidate, LY354740, that is an agonist for both mGluR2 and mGluR3 receptors. This compound counteracts the stimulatory effects of PCP in animals as well as amphetamine.

Transposing this finding to the human situation, one can speculate that LY354740 might counteract PCP-like symptoms, including those of schizophrenia. mGluR2 and mGluR3 receptors are expressed pre-and postsynaptically at glutamatergic synapses, including the NMDA containing synapses of some of the cortical projects. They are often located at the perimeter of the synaptic cleft rather than in the center, and they exist also on glial cells, suggesting a role of modulators rather than central mediators of the synaptic activity. mGluR2/3 agonists such as LY354740 may have beneficial effects in schizophrenia if they elevate the actions of glutamate mediated by the NMDA receptors. mGluR2 and mGluR3 receptors are present in the nucleus accumbens where they can regulate synaptic plasticity, providing an additional speculative link to schizophrenia through this anatomical connection. Drug discovery research on mGluRs is a wide-open, highly attrac-

AMPA Receptor NMDA Receptor   mGlu Receptor

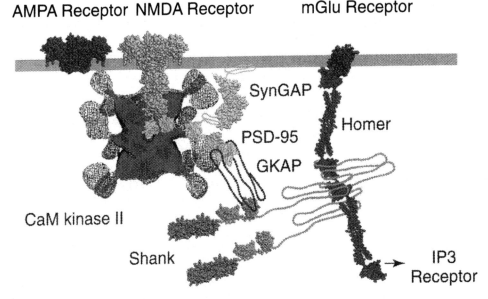

Figure 6.4   Interactions of glutamate receptors in the postsynaptic membrane with several kinase signaling molecules, including Ca^{2+}/calmodulin kinase II (CamKII), guanylate kinase-associated protein (GKAP), synaptic *ras*-GTPase activating protein (SynGAP), and structural proteins of the postsynaptic density, including Homer, Shank, and postsynaptic density-95 (PSD-95). (Reprinted with permission, Kennedy, 2000, AAAS)

tive field, and additional receptors besides mGluR2 and mGluR3 may turn out to be suitable targets for schizophrenia. Several binding sites have been characterized, including novel sites for allosteric potentiators of mGluR receptors (Schoepp and Marek, 2002).

Many glutamatergic synapses contain several types of glutamate receptors. They appear to interact in the signaling process through intracellular proteins that interact with several of the receptors (Kennedy, 2000). Figure 6.4 shows a tentative diagram of proteins involved. They include kinases as well as scaffold proteins that determine the size of the postsynaptic site and the formation of dendritic spines. The components of the postsynaptic signaling mechanism are likely to offer additional opportunities to change the function of glutamatergic synapses in many functional distinct ways.

Transporters of glutamate itself may provide yet another approach to manipulate the activity of glutamatergic synapses. These transporters provide the physiological mechanisms of the termination of glutamate action and play a crucial role in the temporal resolution of synaptic signaling. Five transporters have been characterized, called excitatory amino acid transporters 1–5 (EAAT1–5). The terminology of these molecules remains confusing since other names are frequently used, for example, EAAT1 = GLAST, and EAAT2 = GLT-1. These two transporters are located in glial cells surrounding the synaptic cleft and are thus particularly important in the regulation of synaptic function. Inhibiting them will increase synaptic glutamate concentrations and the activity of glutamatergic synapses.

6.7 FUTURE DRUG TARGETS

The clinical observations with glutamate receptor antagonists and the many possibilities to manipulate it pharmacologically make the glutamatergic synapse a tantalizing area for drug discovery research (Maghaddam, 2003). However, as for the dopaminergic drug targets, glutamatergic targets are identified on the basis of circumstantial evidence and speculations linking clinical and preclinical observations. Only clinical trials will identify the successful drug targets. Preclinical data are too remote from the human disease to give clear guidance for the selection among the various available approaches. Efforts and costs may be just too high to continue such a trial and error approach where clinical studies are needed to choose among many hypothetical drug targets with poor validation.

Real progress and better validated drug targets have to come from better understanding of the disease mechanisms of schizophrenia. Many years of pathological studies on schizophrenic brains have failed to yield a clear picture of the disease process, nor have they led to validated drug targets in a similar way as has happened for Parkinson's disease and Alzheimer's disease. The modern array gene expression technologies may improve the situation by providing a complete overview of gene expression alterations in schizophrenia. Early attempts have generated promising results (Middleton et al., 2002). However, to be successful, the gene array methods require carefully controlled human tissue as a starting point. The limited availability of postmortem material from schizophrenia patients, the fact that tissue has been derived from patients with many years of drug treatment limit the expectations. Real hope for novel targets comes from the recent discoveries of disease-causing genes. In a similar way as early gene discoveries changed Alzheimer's disease research and drug discovery, the schizophrenia genes are the first guideposts for this path. They may not be more than occasional marks for a twisted trail, but they allow the investigators for the first time to set their feet on the trail somewhere. The disease genes are unlikely to be suitable drug targets themselves, but they will lead to specific receptors or enzymes with a crucial role in the disease cascade, as the discovery of mutations in amyloid precursor protein that cause Alzheimer's disease have led to the secretases as suitable drug targets.

DISC1, the first discovered schizophrenia gene, has become an object of intense investigations for the reasons outlined above. It is a complex transmembrane protein whose function remains to be elucidated. In rodents, expression levels in cortex are highest during development. It interacts with proteins such as NudE-like (NUDEL) earlier linked to cortical development. The truncated protein that is associated with the disease is unable to interact with NUDEL. When transfected to neuron-like PC12 cells, truncated but not wild-type DISC1 impairs the outgrowth of neurites from the cells (Ozeki et al., 2003). These findings are compatible with the view that schizophrenia is, at least in part, a disorder of the development of the cortex. The discovery of additional genes causing schizophrenia is likely and is awaited impatiently. Linkage studies have identified neuregulin 1 as a susceptibility gene in Islandic and Scottish populations (Stefansson et al., 2003). Neuregulin is a member of a multigene family of transmembrane proteins (NRG-1–4) that contain an extracellular EGF-like domain necessary for function. They again play an important role in the developmental of neurons and glial cells. A further schizophrenia susceptibility gene identified by linkage studies is dystrobrevin-binding protein 1 (DTNBP1, also called dysbindin). This protein is contained in postsynaptic densities and is believed to have a function in synaptic plasticity (Straub et al., 2002). Several other genes have been tentatively associated with schizophrenia over the recent years. Linkage studies suggest schizophrenia genes on chromosomes 1, 6, 8, and 13, that await discovery and precise description.

In the best of possible worlds, the newly discovered disease genes will lead us to a well-delineated molecular mechanism that causes schizophrenia. Some of the players will be drugable targets such as receptors or enzymes with binding sites amenable for small molecule binding. The disease mechanism will point out the links to dopaminergic and glutamatergic synapses and explain the utility of the current drugs and drug candidates.

Table 6.1 Current and future drug targets for schizophrenia

Current Drugs

Typical neuroleptics (D_2 antagonists)
Atypical neuroleptics (D_2 antagonists with additional receptor affinities)

Future Drugs and Targets

D_1, D_3 dopamine receptor ligands
Modifiers of glutamate receptor mechanisms
   GlyT1 inhibitors
   mGluR ligands
   Glutamate transporter inhibitors
   Ligands to glutamate receptor signaling proteins
Targets identified from disease mechanism

Irrational exuberance? Hopefully not, but there is no guarantee that all of the desired scenario will come into being. The disease may cause aberrant synaptic connections that cannot be rerouted later in development. The essential parts of the disease process may run its course well before the onset of the behavioral symptoms. However, even if the scientific truth follows such a worst-case scenario, the disease mechanism can lead to novel and better drug targets. Downstream mechanisms will be identified that are responsible for the behavioral symptoms, making it possible to improve at least the symptomatic treatment of the disease. Understanding of the disease mechanism may help to identify early markers of schizophrenia, making it perhaps possible to identify future schizophrenia victims during very early development (Table 6.1). Combining neonatal diagnostics with disease-modifying treatment during early years may greatly reduce the number of future victims.

6.8 ANIMAL MODELS AND EXPERIMENTAL MEDICINE

Does schizophrenia occur in animals? Pets, farm, and zoo animals can be hyperactive and lack the social interactions typical for their species. There are many anecdotal reports of difficult cats that are frightful and do not respond at all to other animals or humans. How would we know when an animal is hallucinating? Humans, perhaps just reflecting the vanity of the most successful species, often assume that schizophrenia is a consequence, perhaps the price for massive cerbralization, for the development of our abilities to reason and to speak. However, we just don't know, at least not at this point. The introduction of schizophrenia disease genes into animals may provide an answer in the future. At the present time there are no satisfactory animal models for schizophrenia, because of the lack of observable behavior and the lack of understanding of the disease mechanism.

The animal models currently used in drug discovery programs reflect the existing drugs and drug targets. From the dopamine perspective, amphetamine-, cocaine-, and apomorphine-induced hyperactivity serve this role. Based on the glutamate hypothesis, PCP- and ketamine-induced hyperactivity provide the same utility. Individual researchers tend to use variants of these animal models, some simply scoring locomotor activity and others further distinguishing specific features, for example, those linked to stereotypy. All currently used antipsychotics suppress these behaviors, most likely reflecting their antagonism at the dopamine D_2 receptors. As expected from their mechanism, the experimental drugs acting at the glutamatergic synapse suppress PCP and ketamine hyperactivity. At least some of them also suppress amphetamine and cocaine hyperactivity. These animal assays are linked to the two major groups of current drug targets, the dopaminergic and glutamatergic system. They will not help in the identification of new targets from independent mechanisms.

Many schizophrenic patients show specific changes in behavioral responses that reflect sensory and motor processing. The response to repeated stimulations does not abate in a similar way as in control subjects. Prepulse inhibition (PPI) represents a specific and quantitative measure of this phenomenon. The response to a stimulus (pulse) is inhibited when the same stimulus was given before (prepulse). This phenomenon can be measured in animals and humans using quantitative electrophysiological methods. In animals PPI is disrupted by amphetamine, an effect that is then counteracted by dopamine D_2 antagonist. Genetic disruption of the D_2 but not the D_1 gene also prevents the amphetamine effect, in support of the view that the major effects of the current antipsychotics are mediated by D_2 receptors (Geyer et al., 2002).

The PPI and ketamine hyperactivity animal models may be suitable for translational research that attempts to build direct bridges from animal assays to human experimental studies. For PPI, very similar electrophysiological recordings are possible. For ketamine, subjective descriptions of psychosis-like feelings substitute for the locomotor hyperactivity of the rodents. While the approaches are still linked to their respective mechanistic hypothesis, they will greatly help the clinical investigators in determining the doses to be used in the phase II trials to proof efficacy. So far drug development in schizophrenia has followed the traditional path; the maximally tolerated dose was determined in phase I volunteer studies. The maximal permissible dose was used in the phase IIa proof-of-concept studies. If successful, the dose was then titrated further down in phase IIb studies. Translational research with PPI and ketamine models may allow investigators to establish the optimal dose during small-scale studies and provide an early readout for efficacy. Phase IIa studies in schizophrenia, while still costly and time-consuming, are less cumbersome and mercurial than those in depression and other psychiatric diseases, perhaps limiting the impact of experimental medicine approaches in this disease. However, the saving of even a few months in development has enormous impact on medical practice and commercial aspects of the therapy of schizophrenia.

New, more accurate animal models for schizophrenia are expected to accompany the growing understanding of the disease mechanism. The experience with Alzheimer's disease again provides the guiding example. Insertion of specific combinations of disease-causing mutations produces most, if not all, pathological features of Alzheimer's disease in mice. Disease-causing genes, such as the truncation of DISC-1, can be inserted in transgenic animals. Perhaps it is too high a hope to expect mice with aberrant social behavior or even hallucinations, but such experiments will be the first step in this exciting direction.

6.9 CONCLUSIONS

Schizophrenia is a complex and devastating disease whose mechanism is poorly understood. Only symptomatic treatment is available at the present time. All currently used drugs work primarily through dopamine D_2 receptor antagonism. Relatively pure D_2 antagonists form the group of typical antipsychotics, and drugs with additional effects are grouped into atypical antipsychotics. Despite the saturation of this field with many similar drugs, progress may still be possible through optimized fine-tuning of the various additional activities. More novel, perhaps also more promising, are the many current drug discovery and development programs that are based on the glutamate hypofunction hypothesis of schizophrenia. Modulations of NMDA receptors through metabotropic glutamate receptors appear particularly promising. Neither of these lines of attack is expected to bring a cure for schizophrenia. Novel drug targets for disease-modifying drugs will have to come from the studies of the disease mechanism now launched after the discovery of disease-causing genes.

REFERENCES

Further Reading

BENNETT, M.R. Monoaminergic synapses and schizophrenia: 45 years of neuroleptics. *J. Psychopharmacol.* 12: 289–304, 1998.

CONN, P.J., and PIN, J.P. Pharmacology and functions of metabotropic glutamate receptors. *An. Rev. Pharmacol. Toxicol.* 37: 205–237, 1997.

FREEDMAN, R. Schizophrenia. *N. Eng. J. Med.* 349: 1738–1749, 2003.

GAINETDINOV, R.R., MOHN A.R., and CARON, M.G. Genetic animal models: Focus on schizophrenia. *Trends Neurosci.* 24: 527–533, 2001.

IVERSEN, L. Neurotransmitter transporters: fruitful targets for CNS drug discovery. *Mol. Psych.* 5: 357–362, 2000.

LEWIS, D.A., and LEVITT, P. Schizophrenia as a disorder of neurodevelopment. *An. Rev. Neurosci.* 25: 409–432, 2002.

MOGHADDAM, B. Bringing order to the glutamate chaos in schizophrenia. *Neuron* 40: 881–884, 2003.

MIYAMOTO, S., LaMANTIA, A.S., DUNCAN, G.E., SULLIVAN, P., GILMORE, J.H., and LIEBERMAN, J.A. Recent advances in the neurobiology of schizophrenia. *Mol. Interventi.* 3: 27–39, 2003.

THAKER, G.K., and CARPENTER, W.T. Advances in schizophrenia. *Nature Med.* 7: 667–671, 2001.

Citations

AKIL, M., KOLCHANA, B.S., ROTHMOND, D.A., HYDE, T.M., WEINBERGER, D.R., and KLEINMAN, J.E. Catechol-*O*-methyltransferase genotype and dopamine regulation in the human brain. *J. Neurosci.* 23: 2008–2019, 2003.

BLEULER, E., *Textbook of Psychiatry*. (Transl. from *Lehrbuch der Psychiatrie*, 1916), Ayer Co., Manchester, New Hampshire, 1976.

CARPENTER, W.T., and BUCHANAN, R.W. Schizophrenia. *N. Eng. J. Med.* 330: 681–690, 1994.

CASTNER, S.A., WILLIAMS, G.V., and GOLDMAN-RAKIC, P.S. Reversal of antipsychotic-induced working memory deficits by short-term dopamine D_1 receptor stimulation. *Science* 289: 56–58, 2000.

COYLE, J.T. The glutamatergic dysfunction hypothesis for schizophrenia. *Harv. Rev. Psychiat.* 3: 241–253, 1996.

EKELUND, J., HOVATTA, I., PARKER, A., PAUNIO, T., VARILO, T., MARTIN, R., SUHONEN, J., ELLONEN, P., CHAN, G., SINSHEIMER, J.S., SOBEL, E., JUVONEN, H., ARAJARVI, R., PARTONON, T., SUVISAARI, J., LONNQVIST, J., MEYER, J., and PELTONEN, L. Chromosome 1 loci in Finnish schizophrenia families. *Hum. Mol. Genet.* 10: 1611–1617, 2001.

FARBER, N.B., NOWCOMER, J.W., and OLNEY, J.W. The glutamate synapse in neuropsychiatric disorders: focus on schizophrenia and Alzheimer's disease. *Prog. Brain Res.* 116: 421–437, 1998.

GEYER, M.A., McILWAIN, K.L., and PAYLOR, R. Mouse genetic models for prepulse inhibition: an early review. *Mol. Psych.* 7: 1039–1053, 2002.

GOTO, Y., and O'DONNELL, P. Delayed mesolimbic system alteration in a developmental animal model of schizophrenia. *J. Neurosci.* 22: 9070–9077, 2002.

HERESCO-LEVY, U., JAVITT, D.C., ERMILOV, M., MORDEL, C., SILIPO, G., and LICHTSTEIN, M. Efficacy of high-dose glycine in the treatment of enduring negative symptoms of schizophrenia. *Arch. Gen. Psychiat.* 56: 29–36, 1999.

KAPUR, S., and REMINGTON, G. Dopamine D2 receptors and their role in atypical antipsychotic action: Still necessary and may even be sufficient. *Biol. Psychiat.* 50: 873–883, 2001.

KRAMER, M.S., LAST, B., GETSON, A., and REINES, S.A. The effects of a selective D_4 dopamine receptor antagonist (L-745,870) in acutely psychotic inpatients with schizophrenia: D4 dopamine antagonist group. *Arch. Gen. Psychiat.* 54: 567–572, 1997.

KENNEDY, M.B. Signal-processing machines at the postsynaptic density. *Science* 290: 750–754, 2000.

MATSUMOTO, M., WEICKERT, C.S., BELTAIFA, S., KOLACHANA, B., CHEN, J., HYDE, T.M., HERMAN, M.M.,

WEINBERGER, D.R., and KLEINMAN, J.E. Catechol-*O*-methyltransferase (COMT) mRNA expression in the dorsolateral prefrontal cortex of patients with schizophrenia. *Neuropsychopharmacology* 28: 1521–1530, 2003.

MEYER-LINDENBERG, A., MILETICH, R.S., KOHN, P.D., ESPOSITO, G., CARSON, R.E., QUARANTELLI, M., WEINBERGER, D.R., and BERMAN, K.F. Reduced prefrontal activity predicts exaggerated striatal dopaminergic function in schizophrenia. *Nature Neurosci.* 5: 267–271, 2002.

MIDDLETON, F.A., MIRNICS, K., PIERRI, J.N., LEWIS, D.A., and LEVITT, P. Gene expression profiling reveals alterations of specific metabolic pathways in schizophrenia. *J. Neurosci.* 22: 2718–2729, 2002.

MILLAR, J.K., WILSON-ANNAN, J.C., ANDERSON, S., et al. Disruption of two novel genes by a translocation cosegregating with schizophrenia. *Hum. Mol. Genet.* 9: 1415–1423, 2000.

MISSALE, C., NASH, S.R., ROBINSON, S.W., JABER, M., and CARON, M.G. Dopamine receptors: From structure to function. *Physiol. Revs.* 78: 189–236, 1998.

MOHN, A.R., GAINETDIVINOV, R.R., CARON, M.G., and KOLLER, B.H. Mice with reduced NMDA receptor expression display behaviors related to schizophrenia. *Cell* 98: 427–436, 1999.

OZEKI, Y., TOMODA, T., KLEIDERLEIN, J., KAMIYA, A., BORD, L., FUJII, K., OKAWA, M., YAMADA, N., HATTEN, M.E., SNYDER, S.H., ROSS, C.A., and SAWA, A. Disrupted-in-schizophrenia (DISC-1): Mutant truncation prevents binding to NudE-like (NUDEL) and inhibits neurite outgrowth. *Proc. Natl. Acad. Sci. USA* 100: 289–294, 2003.

PENNARTZ, C.M.A., GROENEWEGEN, H.J., and LOPES DA SILVA, F.H. The nucleus accumbens as a complex of functionally distinct neuronal ensembles: An integration of behavioral, electrophysiological and anatomical data. *Progr. Neurobiol.* 42: 719–761, 1994.

QUINLAN, E.M., PHILPOT, B.D., HUGANIR, R.L., and BEAR, M.F. Rapid, experience-dependent expression of synaptic NMDA receptors in visual cortex in vivo. *Nature Neurosci.* 2: 352–357, 1999.

ROBBE, D., ALONSO, G., CHAUMONT, S., BOCKAERT, J., and MANZONI, O.J. Role of P/Q-Ca^{2+} channels in metabotropic glutamate receptor 2/3-dependent presynaptic long-term depression at nucleus accumbens synapses. *J. Neurosci.* 22: 4346–4356, 2002.

RUBINSTEIN, M. Mice lacking dopamine D$_4$ receptors are supersensitive to ethanol, cocaine, and methamphetamine. *Cell* 90: 991–1001, 1997.

RUBINSTEIN, M., PHILLIPS, T.J., BUNZOW, J.R., FALZONE, T.L., DZIEWCZAPOLSKI, G., ZHANG, G., FANG, Y., LARSON, J.L., MCDOUGALL, J.A., CHESTER, J.A., SAEZ, C., PUGSLEY, T.A., GERSHANIK, O., LOW, M.J., and GRANDY D.K. Mice lacking dopamine D$_4$ receptors are supersensitive to ethanol, cocaine, and methamphetamine. *Cell* 90: 991–1001, 1997.

SCHOEPP, D.D., and MAREK, G. Preclinical pharmacology of mGluR2/3 receptor agonists: Novel agents for schizophrenia? *Curr. Drug Targ. CNS Neurol. Disord.* 1: 215–225, 2002.

SEEMAN, P., GUAN, H.C., and VAN TOL H.H.M. Dopamine D$_4$ receptors elevated in schizophrenia. *Nature* 365: 441–445, 1993.

SEEMAN, P., and LEE, T. Antipsychotic drugs: direct correlation between clinical potency and presynaptic action on dopamine neurons. *Science* 188: 1217–1219, 1975.

SEEMAN, P. Dopamine receptors and the dopamine hypothesis of schizophrenia. Synapse 1: 133–146, 1987.

STEFANSSON, H., SARGINSON, J., KONG, A., YATES, P., STEINTHORDSDOTTIR, V., GUDFINNSSON, E., GUNNARSDOTTIR, S., WALKER, N., PETURSSON, H., CROMBIE, C., INGASON, A., GULCHER, J.R., STEFANSSON, K., and ST. CLAIR, D. Association of neuregulin 1 with schizophrenia confirmed in a Scottish population. *Am. J. Hum. Genet.* 72: 83–87, 2003.

STRAUB, R.E., JIANG, Y., MACLEAN, C.J., MA, Y., WEBB, B.T., MYAKISHEV, M.V., HARRIS-KERR, C., WORMLEY, B., SADEK, H., KADAMBI, B., CESARE, A.J., GIBBERMAN, A., WANG, X., O'NEILL, F.A., WALSH, D., and KENDLER, K.S. Genetic variation in the 6p22.3 gene DTNBP1, the human ortholog of the mouse dysbindin gene, is associated with schizophrenia. *Am. J. Hum. Genet.* 71: 337–348, 2002.

SUPPLISON, S., and BERGMAN, C. Control of NMDA receptor activation by a glycine transporter co-expressed in *Xenopus oocytes*. *J. Neurosci.* 17: 4580–4590, 1997.

Chapter 7

Depression

Human life brings many moments with an emotional value. There are the happy events, some big, such as the birth of a child, the successful completion of an exam, the achievement of professional success and reward, some small, such as a good meal, satisfying sexual activity, or just the victory of the favorite football team. The events create a good mood and generate the feeling of happiness. We all like and wish to be happy. The pursuit of happiness, anchored in the Constitution of the United States, is the dominant driver of human behavior. On the opposite side, sad events, for which there are many examples, generate the feeling of unhappiness, sadness, perhaps gloom, and bring us into a sad or depressed mood. Individual humans differ in the extent these feelings are experienced and expressed. Society tolerates a broad range of individual variations. Every university or company harbors moody, notoriously unhappy, or cranky people we all learn to accept because we see moods as a façade for the underlying real person. Variable moods are a normal feature of human life.

Mood disorders describe conditions where moods become extreme or where there is a clear disconnect between events and the emotional status of a person. Mania refers to a condition of extreme happiness, elation, exuberance, that leads to irrational acts. This chapter is devoted to the opposite condition, depression, the feeling of deep, persistent sadness. Episodes of depression that last several weeks or months are extremely common. Approximately 15% of the human population experience at least one significant depressive episode during the life span. A smaller percentage of people suffer from persistent depression, manifesting itself in multiple, reoccurring depressive episodes or in chronic, constant depression.

Depression is an unpleasant and loathed state. Patients feel weak and tired. Simple actions require a major effort. Self-esteem is low and social contact is avoided. Life seems to have no purpose and to make no sense. Both, the emotional and the intellectual aspects of depression are well documented in historical records and the world literature.

> *I am poured out like water,*
> *And all my bones are out of joint;*
> *My heart is become like wax;*
> *It is melted in mine inmost parts.*
> *My strength is dried up like a potsherd;*
> *And my tongue cleaveth to my throat.*
> *Psalm 22*
>
> *How weary, stale, flat, and unprofitable*
> *Seem to me all the uses of this world.*
> *Shakespeare, Hamlet*

Drug Discovery for Nervous System Diseases, by Franz F. Hefti
ISBN 0-471-46563-1   Copyright © 2005 by John Wiley & Sons, Inc.

Depression must be considered a fatal disease, because it often ends in suicide. The thoughts of worthlessness and lack of purpose prompt patients to contemplate death and self-destruction, and all too often they take suicidal actions. Suicide has been romanticized, as an active and intellectual denial of our limited and often cruel world. Medical investigations, however, make very clear that the vast majority of suicide victims are driven by emotional despair rather than intellectual lucidity. In its mild forms, depression makes people dysfunctional, unproductive, and unhappy. In its extreme form, it destroys them. The currently available drugs make a useful but small contribution to the treatment. Depression remains a giant medical need and field of opportunity for drug discovery research.

7.1 SYMPTOMS AND DISEASE MECHANISM

Depression is the most common disease of the nervous system (Fava and Kendler, 2000). Estimates of prevalence range from 5 to 20% of the general population, when people with mild depressive episodes are included. The prevalence of severe depression has been estimated at 2% of the general population. There are no obvious geographical differences. In all studied areas and countries, females are more likely than males to be diagnosed with depression.

The diagnosis of depression relies on behavioral criteria that are evaluated in a discussion between the patient and a physician. The major determinants are negative mood, feelings of hopelessness, low self-esteem, inability to concentrate, changes in eating and sleeping patterns, decreased interest in pleasurable stimuli (anhedonia), and recurrent thoughts of death and suicide. Several, widely accepted rating scales are utilized that provide a quantitative readout for the severity of the depression. The diagnosis relies strongly on the verbal expression of subjectively felt emotions, explaining why depression ratings tend to be variable and inconsistent. Physician's attention alone can change the emotional status and often has a therapeutic effect on the disease. Behavioral therapy is beneficial for many patients. Clinical trials with antidepressant drugs are difficult because of the therapeutic effect of the enrollment itself (Fig. 5.3). In the clinical trials with the currently approved antidepressant drugs, the quantitative improvement of the depression rating produced by the drugs was only a fractional increment over the benefits achieved by the placebo alone.

Depression is sometimes subdivided based on severity and duration. There is substantial overlap among the various subforms, and they do not represent defined disease entities. Mild episodic depression, often triggered by distinct, negative external factors, is the most common form. Mild or moderate depression symptoms appear over several days and weeks after the triggering event, and the episode resolves over a few or several months. Severe episodic depression is deeper but not necessarily of longer duration. Chronic depression refers to the constant presence of depression symptoms over several years. When mild, the descriptive word dysthymia, from the Greek "bad state of mind," may be used. For severe chronic depression, the term melancholia, introduced by the Greek physician Hippocrates and meaning black bile, becomes the common designation. A small number of patients suffer from cyclic depression, a change of mood state reoccurring at regular frequency. Patients suffering from monopolar cyclic depression experience regularly spaced repetitive depressive episodes. In bipolar depression, also called manic-depressive illness, depressive and manic episodes follow each other over many cycles. Typically the frequency of cycles in cyclic depression is several months. A small number of patients experience much shorter cycles, of several days or even a few hours. The term cyclothymia is used to describe this condition.

Many of the single depression episodes are triggered by severe adverse events of long-lasting consequences, such as a significant professional failure, the rejection by an object of love, or the death of a child or partner. The frequently occurring adolescent and post-partum depressions are set off by drastic changes in reproductive hormones. Numerous medical conditions are accompanied by depression, including several hormonal diseases, diabetes, and Parkinson's disease. Episodic depression frequently follows cardiac stroke and cardiac surgery. Chronic stress, experienced, for example, by caregivers of people with severe illnesses or disabilities or by people with a harsh life in poverty, is believed to be a causative factor for depression. However, people differ in their ability to deal with acute and chronic adverse experiences. An adverse life experience may trigger a severe depressive episode in one person, while leaving another unaffected. Many patients suffer from episodic or chronic depression in absence of a recognized event. These individual differences suggest that there is a significant genetic contribution to depression. Epidemiologic and twin studies estimated the genetic contribution to the risk of depression to be about 50%. Many different genes are likely to contribute, since no familial forms have been defined and no disease-causing genes have been identified as yet. In a similar way as hypertension and diabetes, depression is considered a multi-factorial condition with significant contributions from many genetic risk factors.

The disease mechanism of depression remains to be elucidated (Nestler et al., 2002). Functional imaging studies in patients point to abnormalities in many brain areas including parts of the cerebral cortex. The creation of the subjective feeling of depression is likely to be carried be a multitude of neuronal pathways participate. The mechanism of action of the currently available antidepressant drugs points to a major role of monoaminergic systems in the brain. Studies on the neuronal substrates of stress suggest the participation of neurons located in basal ganglia, amygdala, thalamus, and hypothalamus. Depression is often accompanied by neuroendocrine changes in the hypothalamic-pituitary-adrenal (HPA) axis and its neuropeptide regulators in the brain. These various aspects will be discussed in detail in the sections below on drugs and drug targets. Progress in depression drug discovery has been guiding contributor to the understanding of depression disease mechanisms and is likely to remain so. Depression provides an intriguing example for the benefits of intense interplay between drug discovery and research of disease mechanisms.

7.2 CURRENT ANTIDEPRESSANT DRUGS AND THE MONOAMINE HYPOTHESIS

The currently approved antidepressant drugs all target receptor sites of monoaminergic transmitter mechanisms. They enhance monoaminergic transmission by inhibiting specific steps of the synaptic inactivation machinery. Most of them are blockers of the monoamine transporter proteins, a small number inhibit the enzyme monoamine oxidase (MAO), a critical catabolic step. The introduction of the monoamine antidepressants followed a series of intriguing discoveries around 1960. Reserpine, a drug that induces severe behavioral depression, was discovered to strongly reduce monoamine levels in the brain.

Prompted by the discovery that chlorpromazine, a variant of antihistamine drugs, had antipsychotic effects, a research group at the pharmaceutical company Geigy in Basel, Switzerland, now part of Novartis, synthesized additional homologues for clinical evaluation. One of them, imipramine, failed in the treatment of agitated psychiatric patients but elevated their mood in an unexpected way. Further clinical studies substantiated the mood-elevating effects of imipramine and led to its introduction as antidepressant drug. An independent discovery revealed that iproniazid, a compound developed for the treatment of tuberculosis, had mood-elevating effects, and that this compound inhibited MAO. These parallel and complementing findings created a wave of excitement among neuropharmacologists and psychiatrists of the time. The monoamine hypothesis of affective disorders emerged, the view that dysfunction of monoaminergic neurons are at the root of many psychiatric symptoms. Over the decades the limitations of this concept became apparent. The monoamine antidepressant drugs show incomplete clinical efficacy only, and many other transmitter systems are involved in the disease mechanisms of psychiatric disorders. However, the early discoveries provided an enormous boost to drug discovery in the neurosciences, and up to this day the monoaminergic drugs have remained the only approved and effective antidepressant drugs.

The antidepressant MAO inhibitor iproniazid and the more recently introduced drugs, phenelzine and trancylpromine, inhibit both isoforms of the enzyme, MAO-A and MAO-B. They enhance the actions of all monoamines in the brain, dopamine, norepinephrine, serotonin, and also histamine. Deprenyl, an inhibitor with some selectivity for MAO-B, has been approved for the treatment of Parkinson's disease but is also effective for the treatment of depression. It seems possible that more selective inhibitors of MAO-B or selective MAO-A inhibitors might be clinically effective with differential therapeutic profiles than the existing drugs. Despite the many decades elapsed since the first validation as a drug target, MAO remains a potential opportunity for future drug discovery efforts. However, MAO inhibitors tend to have more serious adverse effects than monoamine uptake blockers and do not differentiate between the various monoamine transmitter systems. For these reasons monoamine transporters have attracted far more interest than MAO as targets for discovery efforts toward new antidepressant drugs.

Imipramine and related first-generation monoamine transport inhibitor antidepressant drugs, for example, amitryptiline and doxepin, have related chemical structures with three chemical ring systems, and are referred to as "tricyclics" (Fig. 7.1). They inhibit the norepinephrine transporter NET and the serotonin transporter SERT, without affecting the dopamine transporter DAT in significant ways. The tricyclics bind to several other receptors sites, including the muscarinic cholinergic receptors for which they are antagonists. Second-generation uptake blockers, the "heterocyclics," including the examples amoxapine and maprotiline, have somewhat higher selectivity for NET and SERT. Their clinical efficacy further strengthens the conclusion that the antidepressant effects of the tricyclics are indeed mediated by the monoamine transporters rather than reflecting one of the off-target activities.

A significant improvement in selectivity of antidepressant drugs was achieved by the researchers at the pharmaceutical company Lilly, in Indianapolis, who showed that inhibition of the serotonin transporter SERT alone is sufficient for antidepressant activity (Fuller et al., 1974). Fluoxetine (Prozac), the first selective serotonin reuptake blocker (SSRI) defined a new class of antidepressant drugs, which now includes paroxetine and sertraline. The SSRIs have become the standard first-line therapy for episodic and chronic depression. Their efficacy has been confirmed in many clinical studies. However, because the maximal efficacy is far less than desired and because of the remaining adverse effects,

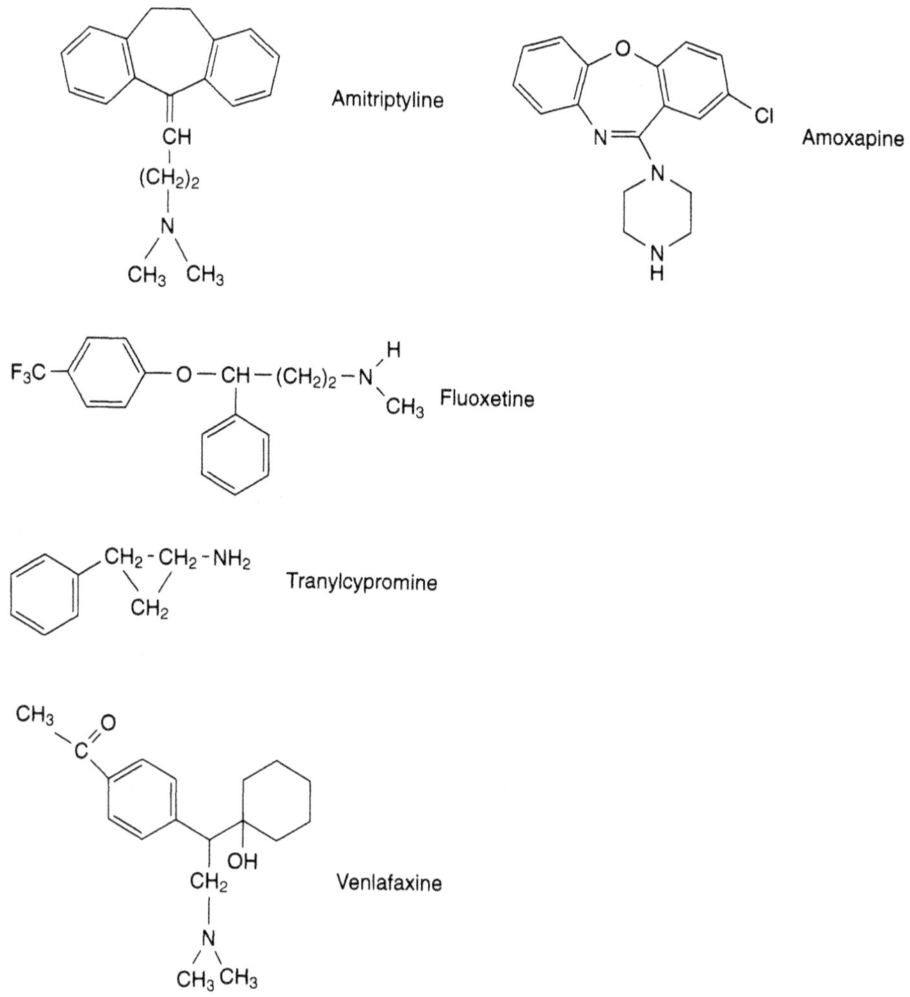

Figure 7.1 Examples of current antidepressant drugs.

the search for improved monoamine uptake inhibitors has been kept alive. More recently the field has shifted back to earlier concepts and favors combined SERT and NET inhibitors such as venlafaxine.

The current psychiatric practitioner has more then ten different monoaminergic anti-depressant drugs to choose from. Their clinical efficacy is comparable, but they differ in their adverse effect profiles. Many of the early tricyclics and heterocyclics produced seda-tion, epithelial dryness and, at high doses, induced seizures and cardiac toxicity. The more recently introduced drugs with improved selectivity lack the more serious adverse effects and are safer, in particular, when considering that some of the patients have suicidal tendencies. Still, even the very selective SSRIs impair sexual function and can reduce alertness. Venlafaxine, the combined SERT and NET inhibitor causes very significant withdrawal symptoms, a serious problem in a patient population with typically poor compliance.

The monoaminergic drugs produce only a small fraction of the desired clinical effect. It takes several days before the antidepressant effects become manifest. In clinical trials where antidepressant drugs are compared with placebos, the drug-induced improvements are discerned after one or two weeks only. Most antidepressant drugs have half-lives of several hours to a few days. Thus the time course of the measurable antidepressant effect bears no relationship to their pharmacokinetic properties. How much of an effect would we expect from a maximally efficacious drug? The maximal effect should bring a person to say "I feel good" without hesitation. The speed of onset should be rapid, reflecting the pharmacokinetic properties of the drug. Most people know from personal experience that unexpected, pleasant events are able to create a feeling of happiness within just a few minutes. These are not unreasonable expectations, when considering the spectrum of everyday human emotions. A unique clinical observation lends support to this optimistic few (Bejjani et al., 1999). A patient implanted with a stimulation electrode in the mesencephalon area to control Parkinson's disease experienced sudden depressive symptoms during stimulation. The patient expressed feelings of sadness and despair, started to cry, and had suicidal thoughts. Cessation of the stimulation immediately returned the normal emotional state. With the consent of the patient, the effect was repeated over several stimulation cycles. This very intriguing clinical observation supports the view that neuronal activities in specific pathways underlie the subjective feeling of mood and that targeting these pathways might lead to highly efficacious antidepressant drugs.

Despite the success of the currently available antidepressant drugs, the quest for safe and efficacious antidepressant drugs remains as important as ever. The monoamine transporters themselves remain targets for the discovery of antidepressant drugs with improved clinical efficacy (Spinks and Spinks, 2002). Attempts have been made to incorporate partial inhibition of DAT into drug candidates, based on the excessive stimulatory effects of selective inhibitors of this transporter and the fear of addiction. Several other putative targets discussed in the following sections have been identified based mechanisms of action of the current drugs and based on neurobiological concepts of depression.

7.3   NEW MONOAMINERGIC DRUG TARGETS

Monoamine uptake blockers and MAO inhibitors delay the removal of serotonin and norepinephrine from the synaptic cleft following release from the presynaptic terminals. They amplify and prolong the stimulation of serotonin and norepinephrine receptors and the downstream events. Direct stimulation of the functionally relevant receptors by selective agonists may be a viable alternative to the existing drugs. This speculation implies that tonic stimulation of postsynaptic neurotransmitter is functionally equivalent to enhancing the neurotransmitter action during each synaptic discharge and maintaining normal patterns of neuronal activity. The success of dopamine agonist therapy in Parkinson's disease lends strong support to the view that this assumption is correct for the modulatory monoaminergic systems. In depression, serotonin and norepinephrine receptor agonists might be effective by themselves, or they might enhance the clinical efficacy of the uptake blockers. The multiple serotonin receptors that are predominantly expressed in the CNS offer a broad field of opportunity for such drug discovery research, more so than the adrenergic receptors, which mediate critical cardiovascular functions that are likely to generate adverse effects.

Among the serotonin receptors, the 5-HT_{1A} subtype has attracted most attention over the recent years. It is widely expressed in the mammalian brain. Postsynaptic 5-HT_{1A}

receptors are abundant in target areas of the serotonergic neurons of the Raphe nuclei. In addition they are expressed by the serotonergic neurons themselves where they function as autoreceptors that provide a regulatory feedback. Stimulation of the 5-HT_{1A} receptors on serotonergic neurons inhibits firing and transmitter release of these cells. Antagonists for 5-HT_{1A} receptors increase serotonin release, and they thus might have antidepressant activity by themselves or they might enhance the effects of reuptake blockers. This concept was explored in clinical trials with pindolol, an antihypertensive drug that inhibits β-adrenoceptors and 5-HT_{1A} receptors, given to patients in combination with SSRIs. The exploratory trials so far failed to provide conclusive support for the view that 5-HT_{1A} antagonists might accelerate and enhance the therapeutic effects of the SSRIs. An opposite speculation was advanced that 5-HT_{1A} agonists rather than antagonists might be effective as adjunct SSRI therapy. Treatment over several days might downregulate the expression of postsynaptic 5-HT receptors and they might be overstimulated during the first few days of treatment. Adding a 5-HT_{1A} agonist, to reduce excessive serotonin release by stimulating the autoreceptors, might prevent this initial overstimulation and may accelerate the onset of the beneficial therapeutic actions. Although marginal, the efficacy of the partial 5-HT_{1A} agonist buspirone in anxiety disorders adds indirect support for the view that agonists might be therapeutically useful. In addition there are tentative findings for a reduction of 5-HT_{1A} receptor levels in the brains of suicide victims. The 5-HT_{1A} receptors represent an intriguing putative target for novel antidepressant drugs. Uncertainty about the precise nature of the ligand necessary for therapeutic effects, however, dampens the enthusiasm. Additional preclinical and clinical studies will be needed to better define this opportunity (Blier and Ward, 2003).

A second serotonin receptor subtype, the 5-HT_{1B} receptors, is located presynaptically and may be attractive as drug target in a similar way as the 5-HT_{1A} subtype. Knockout mice with deletions of the 5-HT_{1B} gene are more aggressive than normal mice, providing support for a role in emotional behavior. The dominant postsynaptic receptor subtypes are the 5-HT_{2A} and 5-HT_{2C} receptors, both of which have attracted interest as putative drug targets (Gingrich, 2002). The phenotype of 5-HT_{2A} knockout mice does not suggest a link to depression, and the clinical trials with a 5-HT_{2A} antagonist in schizophrenic patients has not revealed any effects on mood. The availability of a selective 5-HT_{2A} antagonist and of the atypical antipsychotic $D_2/5\text{-HT}_{2A}$ antagonists makes it possible to explore the utility of this receptor for depression in human studies. Several trials are under way that evaluate the combination of a SSRI with atypical neuroleptics. 5-HT_{2C} receptor knockout mice are obese, an interesting observation from a point of view of depression since the patients often show altered eating habits. Several companies are pursuing 5-HT_{2C} agonists for the treatment of obesity. Compounds acceptable for human studies will surely also be explored in depression trials.

The 5-HT_{5A}, 5-HT_6, and 5-HT_7 subtypes are minor receptors in the brain. Their restricted expression patterns are attractive from a point of view of drug discovery, which favors selective effects over general ones. The 5-HT_{5A} and 5-HT_6 receptors remain to be explored as putative depression targets. The 5-HT_7 subtype is involved in the regulation of circadian rhythms, a tantalizing finding given that the disruption of normal circadian activity patterns is a central aspect of depression. Tentative behavioral studies link the 5-HT_7 receptors to stress and emotional behavior (Pouzet, 2002). Serotonin receptors offer many opportunities for depression drug discovery research. The minor subtypes await detailed exploration. The 5-HT_7 subtype seems particularly attractive for depression research.

7.4   NEUROANATOMICAL PATHWAYS OF DEPRESSION

Serotonergic and noradrenergic pathways are conceptually attractive as regulators of emotions and mood since they are modulatory systems with widespread influence. The serotonergic neurons originate in the Raphe nuclei of the midbrain, and the noradrenergic neurons in the locus coeruleus at the base of the fourth ventricle in the pons. Both nuclei are well defined and harbor only a relative small number of cells, which provide highly divergent innervations to most brain areas and allow them to influence the activity in many neuronal pathways. It is intuitively compelling that such systems, by increasing or decreasing in a coordinated fashion neuronal activity in many systems, might determine the subjective feelings of elation or depression. The current drugs confirm that increased activity of serotonergic and noradrenergic systems is associated with antidepressant effects. While overly simplistic, these concepts may be useful for guiding the search for alternative drug targets for antidepressant medication. They suggest the possibility that modifying the activity of afferents to the Raphe and locus coeruleus neurons might offer a way to activate serotonergic and noradrenergic neurons to generate the desired antidepressant effects.

Figure 7.2 shows a diagram of the Raphe and locus coeruleus nuclei and some of their principal neuroanatomical connections. There is crosstalk between the serotonergic and noradrenergic neurons of the two nuclei, which innervate each other. The noradrenergic neurons provide an excitatory input to the serotonergic neurons that might mediate the beneficial effects of NET blockade. The clinical efficacy of SSRIs makes the point that activation of serotonergic neurons alone is sufficient for an antidepressant response, justifying the further focus on the Raphe nuclei. Major afferent projections to the serotonergic neurons in the Raphe nuclei originate in the prefrontal cortex, the habenula, and the hypothalamus. These projections are likely excitatory, using glutamate as their transmit-

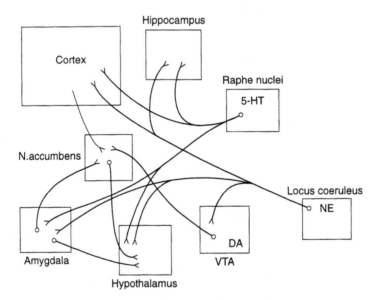

Figure 7.2   Neuronal pathways of depression. Serotonergic neurons of the Raphe nuclei and noradrenergic (NE) of the locus coeruleus provide a modulatory input to many brain areas. Dopaminergic (DA) neurons of the ventral tegmental area (VTA) innervate the nucleus accumbens and cortex. The hypothalamus receives input from many relay nuclei and regulates the hormonal output of the pituitary. The figure only shows part of the connections among these nuclei.

ter. Among the many minor afferents to the Raphe nuclei are a dopaminergic projection from the substantia nigra and several ascending projections from the brainstem. The Raphe nuclei contain several neuropeptides and neuropeptide receptors that may mediate some of these effects. However, there is no precisely defined allocation of neuropeptides to specific pathways that might facilitate drug discovery research. Inhibitory GABAergic interneurons within the Raphe nuclei are able to modify the inputs, further complicating the anatomical picture. The complexity of the afferent pathways offers many opportunities to find targets for drugs to increase serotonergic function. However, without additional knowledge it is impossible to distinguish rationally among the many possibilities.

The various efferent projections from the Raphe nuclei most likely do not make equivalent contributions to the regulation of mood and the mediation of the antidepressant effects of the monoaminergic drugs. It may be possible to define the populations of downstream neurons that are critical for the antidepressant effects and to identify drug targets to selectively influence their activity. Such targets might include serotonin receptor subtypes as discussed above or, alternatively, other neurotransmitter receptors and ion channels selectively expressed by the critical downstream neurons. Interesting projection areas from such a point of view include the nucleus accumbens and the amygdala, since they have been linked to disease processes in schizophrenia and anxiety, respectively. The amygdala contains substance P containing neurons that interact with the serotonergic neurons. The rationale to test substance P NK_1 receptor antagonist in depression is partly based on the speculation that these pathways participate in the regulation of mood. Projections of serotonergic Raphe neurons to cell body and terminal areas of the mesolimbic dopaminergic system suggest an interaction with the reward systems of the brain. Regulating their activity with drugs may generate antidepressant actions. Projections of the Raphe nuclei to the hypothalamus are able to influence many of the peptidergic systems that regulate pituitary and hormonal functions. The connection to the stress response, discussed below, has identified CRF as an important regulatory peptide and drug target opportunity. Other neuropeptides influenced by serotonergic neurons regulate appetite and food intake. Many tantalizing putative drug targets emerge from such speculations, each of which could justify a full-scale drug discovery and development effort. However, the absence of clinical validation, the low probability of success of the speculative targets, together with the high cost and complexity of clinical trials in depression tend to make this approach currently too hazardous. Additional information is required to increase the odds of selecting a successful drug target. Modern molecular biological techniques provide several attractive approaches to this problem. Behavioral analysis of knockout mice of genes identified from neuroanatomical studies may identify those with significant impact. Genomic or proteomic profiling of animals with lesions of specific pathways or treated with antidepressant drugs may reveal profiles relevant for antidepressant activity. The study of gene expression profiles of animals subjected to electroconvulsive treatment, a form of therapy used for extreme forms of chronic severe depression in humans, provides an example for this approach (Altar et al., 2004). The awaited discovery of genes causing depression will provide substantial help in guiding the drug discovery efforts.

7.5 CRF AND THE STRESS RESPONSE

Acute and chronic stress is often a contributing, perhaps even causative factor for episodic and chronic depression. Stressful situations are a normal part of life. Acute physical stress in extreme form occurs during life-threatening emergencies caused by accidents and warfare. Sports and voluntary physical exercise are example of mild physical stress. Chronic psychological stress often reflects difficult situations at the workplace or in the family. Evolution has provided humans and related animals with a mechanism that optimized the body's response to stress and enhances the chance of survival in life-threatening situations. The "stress response" is mediated and coordinated by the hypothalamic-pituitary-adrenal (HPA) hormonal axis (Fig. 7.3). Stressful situations activate hypothalamic neurons that project to the median eminence where they release the neuropeptide CRF (corticotrophin-releasing factor) into the portal vasculature. CRF reaches the anterior pituitary and stimulates CRF_1 receptors on cells that synthesize and release adrenocorticotropic hormone (ACTH). Following release into the general blood stream, ACTH reaches the cortex of the adrenal gland where it stimulates the production and release of glucocorticoids. The steroid hormones influence many organs and processes in a direction that enhances short-term performance and survival of the organism. Energy provision and cardiovascular functions are increased at the expense of functions important for long-term viability such as the immune system. The glucocorticoids penetrate into the brain and provide a negative feedback to CRF-producing cells in the hypothalamus, thus bringing the stress response to conclusion.

The central role of the CRF_1 receptor in the regulation of the HPA axis and the stress response identifies this receptor as an obvious potential drug target (Gutman et al., 2000). Knockout mice with null mutations of the CRF_1 receptor have strongly attenuated responses to stress, in support of this view. Chronic depression is often associated with elevated corticosteroid levels in the blood. Given this strong rationale, several biopharmaceutical companies have generated selective CRF_1 antagonists. In animals they produce behavioral effects considered predictive for antidepressant activity. Several open-label studies have produced tentative evidence for efficacy in human patients suffering from depression.

CRF_1 antagonists are likely to influence functions beyond the classical stress response. CRF is not only expressed in the hypothalamus but also in many other brain areas that can be linked to the regulation of mood and depression. CRF is one among a family of neuropeptides that includes urocortin, stresscopin, and stresscopin-related peptide (Dautzenberg and Hauger, 2002). Similar to CRF, urocortin and stresscopin are widely expressed in the brain, whereas stresscopin-related peptide dominates in peripheral tissue. The four related peptides stimulate CRF_1 and CRF_2 receptors with partially overlapping specificity. CRF_1 receptors exist at high levels in cerebral cortex, hippocampus, cerebellum, anterior pituitary, testis, ovary, and adrenal glands. CRF_1 antagonists in any of these brain areas or peripheral organs may contribute to the antidepressant action but also generate undesired effects. The emerging clinical experience will define the utility of this receptor as drug target. The CRF_2 receptors deserve independent consideration. They are found at highest levels in septum, hippocampus, amygdala, hypothalamus, choroids plexus, skeletal muscle, and the heart. Two different splicing variants with different distribution patterns exist. CRF_2 KO mice show a hypersensitivity to stress independent of the HPA axis. CRF_2 receptors may thus be an interesting drug target in the context of anxiety disorders. Studies in behavioral assays in animals support the view that CRF_2 receptor agonists might have anxiolytic and perhaps also antidepressant properties.

Increased activity of the HPA axis may be contributor to depression rather than just being a consequence on the peripheral functions. Elevated levels of glucocorticoids in the blood may provide a positive feedback to the brain that sustains the depression. These molecules easily pass the blood-brain barrier, and the brain is rich in glucocorticoid receptors. Chronic treatment of rodents with high doses of corticosteroids is able to induce

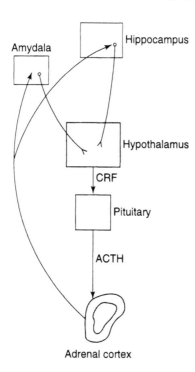

Figure 7.3 Stress response pathway and the central role of CRF. The hypothalamic CRF neurons integrate the stress responses in the brain and stimulate the release of ACTH from the pituitary. ACTH stimulates the release of corticoids from the adrenal medulla, which affect many organs and provide negative feedback control to the brain.

atrophic changes in some of the neuronal populations in the hippocampus. Evidence for small reductions in hippocampal volume have been found in imaging studies on depressed patients (Bremner et al., 2000). These considerations suggest the possibility that glucocorticoid receptors in the brain might be a suitable target for antidepressant therapy. Tentative clinical data in support of this view has been obtained with mifepristone, a glucocorticoid receptor antagonist (Belanoff et al., 2001). Large-scale clinical studies will be necessary to further validate this attractive putative drug target. Together with the CRF receptor, the glucocorticoid receptors represent attractive putative targets that have been identified through studies of the HPA axis and its pathophysiology in depression.

7.6 ANIMAL MODELS AND THEIR USE FOR TARGET IDENTIFICATION

Reliable and predictive animal models of depression would greatly facilitate the study of disease mechanisms and the selection among the many putative drug target opportunities. Unfortunately, animal modeling is a particularly difficult issue in the field of depression research. In humans the feeling of depression represents a subjective sensation that is largely expressed through linguistic communication. It is impossible to obtain adequate linguistic communication from animals. While many dog owners believe to be able to read a depressed mood of their pet, they rely on behavioral associations of human depression, such as absence of spontaneous motor inactivity, lack of response to external stimuli, and perhaps facial expression, which are interpreted in anthropomorphic terms. Rodents, the standard laboratory species, do not have facial expressions, leaving motor activity as the only accessible readout. Perhaps surprisingly, no monkey assay of depression has been generated that might serve as a reliable model for the human disease. The behavioral spectrum of monkeys is far more complex than that of rodents and might offer better opportunities for a differentiated analysis. In lower monkey species behavioral signs reminiscent of human depression, such as social withdrawal, inactivity, huddling, are induced acutely by various drugs. It might be possible to find environmental factors that produce these symptoms as a chronic state, creating a useful model of human depression. Primates might be able to directly communicate feelings of sadness and depression through sign language. However, studies on monkeys tend to be as complex as those on humans, and concerns about animal welfare diminish the willingness to cause depression in the higher species.

Despite the severe limitations, several rodent models have found frequent use in drug discovery research (Table 7.1; Porsolt, 2000). The most frequently used rodent depression assays put the animals in a situation linked to human despair. In the forced swim test they are put in a water tank without any platform or route to escape, and the time interval is measured until the animals remain motionless. The behavior is given the anthropomorphic interpretation of hopelessness. In the tail suspension test, rats or mice are suspended by their tails. They initially struggle but then remain motionless, and the time of active struggle serves as readout of drug efficacy. In the learned helplessness test, the animals are initially exposed to electric shock treatment from which they cannot escape, and in a second session, they tend not to escape when the possibility to escape is given. The time interval until they escape in the second session is measured. In all three models the stop or delay of escape motions is interpreted, in human terms, as loss of hope and despair. The current monoamine antidepressant drugs are effective in all three models, prolonging the time of struggle in the forced swim test and the tail suspension test, and shortening the inactive interval before escape in the learned helplessness assay. The positive effects of clinically efficacious drugs provide a degree of validation of these animal tests as predictive models. However, the example of substance P antagonists discussed below shows the limitations. They cannot be considered reliable predictors for antidepressant action in human patients.

The maternal separation assay takes advantage of a simple behavioral reflex of newborn rodents. When separated from their mothers, newborn pubs vocalize a behavior interpreted as a sign of distress to enforce maternal instincts in the mother. In guinea pig the vocalization is heard as high tone squeaking; in mice it is outside of the audible range for human ears but can be detected by appropriate instruments. Even though the test seems intuitively linked to anxiety rather than depression, it has received validation as depression model because the monoamine antidepressant drugs show a robust effect. In contrast,

Table 7.1 Animal models of depression

Behavioral Despair Assays
Forced swim test
Tail suspension test
Learned helplessness test

Stress Assays
Maternal separation test
Chronic mild stress test

Sensory Deprivation Assays
Olfactory bulbectomy test

---

benzodiazepine drugs that are effective in the treatment of human anxiety do not suppress the vocalization in the test. Similar to the situation of despair tests, substance P antagonists are effective in the rodent maternal separation assay.

The despair tests and the maternal separation test generate situations of acute stress, whereas human depression tends be a consequence of chronic rather than acute stress. The chronic mild stress assay attempts to create a situation similar to a human depression induced by the chronic exposure to adverse events. Animals are exposed to various stressful conditions over a period of several weeks. They include cold exposure, restraint, mild electric shock, disruption of light–dark cycle, and other conditions believed to be unpleasant for rodents. Over time the animals show deficits in hedonistic behaviors, such as sexual activity and consumption of sweets. These pleasure-seeking behaviors are quantified and serve as readout for test compounds with antidepressant potential. Monoamine antidepressant drugs serve as positive controls. The chronic mild stress assay is open to many variations, making it often difficult to compare results of different laboratories.

The rat olfactory bulbectomy model creates a sensory deficit in rodents by surgical removal of the primary neuronal structure mediating the sense of smell. Olfactory sensation serves a primary function in rodents, and the absence of olfactory stimulation is therefore believed to have relevance for human depression, which is associated with the absence of joyful sensory perception. Positive effects of the clinically effective antidepressants in this rat model provide validation for these speculative associations. As for the other models, the predictive power for antidepressant drugs with novel mechanisms is difficult to gage. While the tests are able to reliably predict clinical efficacy of SERT or NET uptake blockers, their usefulness beyond this drug class remains to be established.

The forced swim test, the tail suspension test, and the maternal separation assay are technically simple and have relatively high capacity for evaluating drug candidates. A well-staffed and well-organized research group may be able to evaluate up to perhaps one hundred compounds a year, generating adequate dose–response data for each of them. This high capacity makes it possible to assess many putative drug targets, if suitable pharmacological tools or gene knockout animals are available. Several putative drug targets have been identified with this behavioral screening approach. A few drug candidates arising from this approach have been taken into clinical development. The first example of a compound taken through several phase II and large-scale phase III studies, a substance P antagonist, shows both the promise and the difficulty of this approach.

7.6.1 Substance P Antagonists

Substance P receptors have been pursued as potential new drugs for pain, since the discovery, made several decades ago, that this neuropeptide is a transmitter in pain-mediating sensory neurons. The NK_1 neurokinin receptor, a primary receptor for substance P, is strongly expressed in the spinal cord and participates in mediating the pain sensation to the brain. Both substance P and the NK_1 receptors are also expressed in brain structures mediating the emesis reflex. Indeed, a selective NK_1 antagonist, aprepitant, discovered by research groups at Merck & Co., in New Jersey and the United Kingdom, has recently been approved for the control of emesis that occurs frequently as an adverse event of cancer chemotherapy. The additional expression of substance P and of its NK_1 receptor in brain structures linked to emotional control has given raise to speculation that NK_1

receptors might be a target for drugs to control emotional disturbances, including depression. These speculations received strong support from the demonstration that NK_1 antagonists are effective in the maternal separation test. A proof-of-concept phase II clinical study of aprepritant with a relatively small number of patients provided convincing support for the view that NK_1 antagonists have antidepressant effects in humans (Kramer et al., 1998). These findings were received with high enthusiasm because they identified the first clinically validated depression drug target outside the monoamine systems. NK_1 antagonists were found effective in the tail suspension test for antidepressant activity. Detailed animal studies with NK_1 knockout mice and further functional studies in rodents suggested that substance P provides an indirect inhibition to interneurons of the Raphe nuclei, thus enhancing serotonergic neuron function (Santarelli et al., 2001). Unfortunately, despite the rather convincing preclinical rationale and positive phase II results, the further large-scale phase III studies with aprepritant failed to confirm the clinical efficacy of NK_1 antagonist in human depression.

The experience with substance P antagonists is sobering in several ways. First, it shows the limits of the predictive power of the animal assays. While the widely used rodent assays are able to predict efficacy of monoamine uptake blockers and MAO inhibitors, they are prone to give false positive signals outside of the narrowly defined drug target area. Second, the NK_1 antagonist failed in the clinic despite strong supportive evidence from functional animal studies that linked them to the serotonergic neurons, a key player in the provision of the beneficial effects of the current antidepressant drugs. Third, despite a robust and statistically highly significant effect in a double-blinded phase II study, the larger phase III study did not confirm efficacy. The experience with aprepritant shines an intense beam of cold light onto the major problems of depression drug discovery research, the poor predictive power of animal models, and the difficulty to carry out decisive clinical trials.

7.6.2 Speculative Drug Targets

The simple animal models for depression make it possible to test a large number of receptor antagonists and gene knockout animals, with the expectation to rapidly identify putative targets for antidepressant drugs. For example, an antagonist for the melanin-concentrating hormone-1 receptor, pursued because of its ability to decrease food intake, has also been effective in the rat forced swim test and the guinea-pig maternal separation test (Borowski et al., 2002). Similarly a pentapeptide, nemifitide, has been active in the forced swim test and, based on these data, has been taken into depression studies where tentative evidence for efficacy has emerged (Feighner et al., 2003). Random testing in depression models of drug candidates that have been developed for other indications is likely to identify additional speculative drug targets for depression. Several companies are using industrial-scale efforts to assess all identified genes of the mouse genome as putative depression drug targets. The future years will indubitably bring the publication of many gene deletion studies that produce deficits in depression models. The available experience tentatively suggests that many of the mice with deficits in the depression assays will also show deficits in other behavioral tests. Those with deficits selective for the depression models will be particularly attractive for further studies. The depression assays provide an initial screen only. The experience with substance P antagonist shows very clearly that the currently available animal models do not offer more than a suggestion for further studies.

The current animal models for depression represent a key limiting factor for drug discovery research. It seems unlikely that additional modifications to the existing rodent models will change this picture. Progress may come from generating an appropriate monkey model, by exposing monkeys to chronic low stress and measuring behavioral parameters more relevant to human depression than rodent behaviors. Substantial advances in animal model design will come only from better understanding of disease mechanisms of human depression. Thorough investigations of neuronal pathways mediating the subjective feelings and anticipated discovery of disease genes are expected to generate the necessary breakthroughs. In addition gene and protein array studies in rodents or monkeys exposed to chronic mild stress might identify pathways potentially linked to depression mechanisms to be further explored in studies with human tissue.

7.7 BRAIN-DERIVED NEUROTROPHIC FACTOR (BDNF) AND NEUROGENESIS

There is a good correlation between the clinical efficacy of the antidepressant drugs, both uptake blockers and MAO inhibitors, and their ability to increase monoamine overflow at the synapse, supporting the view that stimulating monoaminergic transmission causes the clinical benefits. However, the delayed onset of therapeutic benefits, misaligned with the neurochemical effects, has kept alive the view that other, yet to be discovered effects might be responsible for the clinical efficacy. Furthermore the findings that depression is sometimes associated with cortical and hippocampal shrinkage suggest that depression might involve more than just a change in activity in existing neuronal pathways. Depression may have a structural component comparable to neurodegenerative diseases such as Alzheimer's or Parkinson's disease. Intriguing discoveries related to neurotrophic factors and neurogenesis have provided a molecular basis for these speculations and point to a bridge between the structural and the transmitter aspects of depression.

Neurotrophic factors regulate neuronal differentiation during development and remain important for synaptic plasticity in the adult nervous system. In the adult brain BDNF appears to play a particularly important role. BDNF and its TrkB receptor are widely expressed in the adult brain, and they participate in the regulation of various forms of synaptic plasticity, including those related to memory formation. Exposure of animals to stress decreases the expression of BDNF. Mice heterozygous for a BDNF null mutation (BDNF$^{+/-}$ mice) and transgenic mice with reduced levels of TrkB activation are resistant to the effects of antidepressants in the forced swim test (Saarelainen et al., 2003). These findings prompt the speculation that depression is associated with a decline in BDNF mechanisms and that antidepressants, through a yet to be established mechanism, stimulate them with a time course in line with the onset of clinical efficacy.

The speculations related to BDNF suggest the TrkB receptor and its downstream signaling molecules as putative drug targets for depression. As discussed in more detail in the chapter on Parkinson's disease, it appears very difficult to identify direct activators or potentiators of TrkB and other transmembrane tyrosine kinase receptors. Thus the focus of drug discovery efforts has shifted to the intracellular signaling pathways. TrkB activation stimulates a number of signaling pathways that mediate diverse cellular functions. Tentative evidence suggests that pathways involving cAMP and the transcriptional regulator CREB (cAMP response element binding protein) are of relevance for depression. Chronic treatment with antidepressants stimulates the cAMP–CREB pathway. These findings provide an attractive link to earlier clinical studies with rolipram, an inhibitor of type 4 phosphodiesterase (PDE4), that controls cAMP levels and CREB activation. Rolipram was efficacious in exploratory depression trials, but because of its poor selectivity, it has many adverse effects and is not suitable for general clinical use. The tentative clinical findings and the related mechanistic concepts provide intriguing support for further trials with selective PDE4 inhibitors in depression (Nestler et al., 2002).

In addition to its role as regulator of synaptic plasticity, BDNF has been identified as a regulator of neurogenesis in the adult brain. In the adult mammalian brain, new neurons are generated in the subventricular zone and in the dentate gyrus of the hippocampus, and this process is accelerated by BDNF. In the dentate gyrus, the newly formed cells differentiate into mature neurons that are integrated into the function of the granule cell layer. Hippocampal neurogenesis is decreased in conditions of stress and increased by treating animals with antidepressants, suggesting the possibility that it contributes to depression and its treatment. Preventing neurogenesis through genetic manipulations or through irradiation blocks the behavioral effects of fluoxetine in an animal test with a time course comparable to that of clinical efficacy in humans (Santarelli et al., 2003).

The discovery that neurogenesis may be a factor in depression and its treatment suggests intriguing new approaches to drug discovery. The regulatory pathways that control neurogenesis remain to be established. Initial findings suggest though the possibility that they might be influenced by neurotransmitter activities and pathways. Chronic treatment of rats with a potentiator of AMPA glutamate receptors has been reported to stimulate hippocampal neurogenesis and to give positive results in the forced swim test and tail suspension test (Bai et al., 2003). The broad search for additional regulators of neurogenesis may identify further novel drug targets for depression outside the currently used monoaminergic drugs.

7.8   BIPOLAR DISORDER AND MOOD STABILIZERS

Manic-depressive disease affects a much smaller number of people than episodic or chronic monopolar depression. Anecdotal reports link bipolar disease to artistic creativity, explaining why it is often erroneously considered a benign, even positive disturbance. In reality bipolar disease is a severe and disturbing illness that often causes accidents during the manic phase and often leads to suicide if left untreated during the depression phase. The genetic contribution to bipolar disease is stronger than that of monopolar depression. Tentative identifications of candidate disease genes have been emerging and, when established, will likely make a significant contribution to understanding disease mechanism of depression. DISC1, one of the genes able to cause schizophrenia, generates the symptomatology of bipolar and unipolar depression in a small number of individuals, pointing out that there must be molecular pathways common to many psychiatric diseases. Any disease gene discovered for bipolar depression will thus make a strong contribution to the understanding of other diseases as well.

The depressive phase of bipolar disease is typically treated with the standard monoamine antidepressant medications. For excessive manic behaviors, antipsychotic dopamine D_2 antagonists or sedative benzodiazepines are helpful. Since its accidental discovery several decades ago, chronic therapy with Li^+ is has been a standard treatment for bipolar disorder. Li^+ dampens the excesses of the emotional phases, the manic one in particular. Drugs initially developed to treat seizure disorders, valproic acid and carbamazepine, have more recently been found to reduce the amplitudes of the mood swings. Together with Li^+ they are now referred to as mood stabilizers. Some patients with extreme bipolar and monopolar disease that does not respond to any of the drugs resort to electroconvulsive therapy. These therapeutic approaches have in common that they do not act on a receptor specifically linked to a neurotransmitter mechanism, in contrast to the monoamine antidepressant drugs.

The mechanism of action of Li^+ and the other mood stabilizers has remained an enigma despite many years of intense search (Coyle and Duman, 2003). Li^+ alters specific steps in a number of signaling pathways, including the phosphoinositol cycle that mediates the action of many extracellular receptor ligands. Li^+ inhibits inositol monophosphatase that converts phosphoinositol to myo-inositol, thereby reducing downstream signaling through diacylclycerol and protein kinase C (PKC), an enzyme controlling several transcriptional regulators. Tentative evidence also links carbamazepine to the phosphoinositol pathways. Li^+ also inhibits glycogen synthase kinase-3β (GSK-3β), an enzyme linked to apoptotic events and to the formation of pathological structures in Alzheimer's disease. Chronic Li^+ treatment affects the expression of the tyrosine kinase Akt, one of the intracellular kinases participating in signaling from the TrkB BDNF receptor (Fig. 7.4). The scientific literature contains descriptions of many additional effects of Li^+ and the mood stabilizers. The plethora of effects will make it difficult to discern the therapeutically relevant ones. It is likely, however, that additional discoveries from disease genes or gene array comparisons of various antidepressant drugs will point out the steps that mediate the effects on mood.

7.9 CLINICAL TRIALS AND EXPERIMENTAL MEDICINE

Clinical trials in depression are difficult to conduct and they have a high failure rate. The high degree of variability among individual patients and the high placebo response illustrated in Figure 5.3 are responsible for this thorny situation. It appears that more than half of the number of double-blinded studies carried out so far have been failed studies. The term "failed study" is used when in the positive control group, an established antidepressant drug such as fluoxetine, does not yield improvement over the placebo preparation. Given the large placebo effect in depression studies, open-label trials without appropriate control groups do not generate interpretable results. The futility of open-label trials in depression cannot be overemphasized. The subtypes of patients selected for the studies influences the outcome. Patients with chronic severe depression represent a relatively uniform population most suitable for clinical studies. At times when several antidepressant drug candidates are being evaluated, clinical research organizations resort to competitive recruitment techniques. Advertisement by Web sites and radio commercials are used to attract more patients. The active enrollment strategies are likely to bring patients to the trials who are not ill enough to seek physician's help and who are driven by a degree of curiosity, thereby confounding the power of the trials. Despite careful considerations applied to the design of depression, the success rate has not increased in recent years. Several phase II and phase III studies are typically necessary to show convincing efficacy of an anti-depressant drug.

The need for repeated studies, for inclusion of large number of patients, and trial durations of several months, make the clinical evaluation of depression drug candidates a very costly and time-consuming enterprise. Many companies shy away from depression pro-

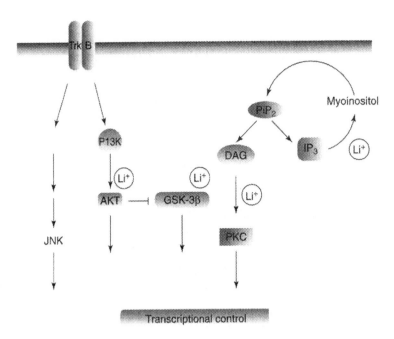

Figure 7.4 Inhibitory effects of Li⁺ and mood stabilizing drugs on intracellular signaling processes of the interlinked inositolphosphate and TrkB receptor pathways. DAG: diacylglycerol; GSK-3β: glycogen synthase kinase-3β; JNK: c-jun-kinase; IP3: inositol-3-posphate; PI3K: phosphatidylinositol-3-kinase; PiP2: phosphatidylinositol-biphosphate; PKC: protein kinase C.

grams because of magnitude of the clinical effort and because the animal models are not able to decisively predict clinical success. Unfortunately, in contrast to other diseases, there has not been any breakthrough progress as yet with alternative approaches of experimental medicine. Accessible biochemical markers, such as blood levels of corticosteroids, show a high degree of variability and do not respond more rapidly than the behavioral readouts. It is unlikely that the morphological changes in the hippocampus and cortex change rapidly. However, imaging studies with functional MRI may be able to identify reliable signals that correlated with the subjective feeling of depression and may have utility as surrogate endpoint. In absence of progress in experimental medicine, depression will lag behind other diseases in drug discovery.

7.10 CONCLUSIONS

Depression is the most prevalent nervous system disease and a salient contributor to human suffering. Its disease mechanism has been slow to emerge and only facets of it are currently understood. Genetic predisposition as well as strong environmental contributions such as chronic stress are causative factors. The genetic basis is likely to include many contributing genes that remain to be identified. Successful therapy most often involves a combination of behavioral and drug therapy. The currently available antidepressant drugs provide a useful therapeutic tool, but they are less efficacious than expected from maximally efficacious compounds expected in the future (Table 7.2).

The currently available antidepressant drugs all increase the synaptic release of the monoamines serotonin and norepinephrine, by blocking mechanisms that terminate their

Table 7.2 Current and future drug targets for depression

Current Targets
Serotonin transporter (SERT)
Norepinephrine transporter (NET)
Monoamine oxidase (MAO)

Future Drugs and Targets
Serotonin receptors
  Postsynaptic: 5-HT_{1A}, 5-HT_{1B}
  Presynaptic: 5-HT_{2A}, 5-HT_{2C}, 5-HT_{5A}, 5-HT_{6}, 5-HT_{7}
CRF1 receptors (antagonists)
CRF2 receptors (agonists)
Glucocorticoid receptors
BDNF mimetics
PDE4 inhibitors

synaptic actions. They inhibit the transporter molecules SERT and NET that are responsible for the reuptake of monoamines after synaptic release or by inhibiting the catalytic enzyme MAO. The action on serotonergic neurons is able to produce effective antidepressant effects alone because selective serotonin uptake blockers are clinically effective. The current drugs identify serotonin receptors as putative novel drug targets. Stimulating postsynaptic serotonin receptors with agonists or inhibiting the negative feedback provided by presynaptic serotonin receptors appear to be attractive strategies. The high diversity in the serotonin receptor family provides a special opportunity. Selective serotonin receptor ligands may be useful by themselves or as adjunct therapy to the uptake blockers.

The central role of serotonergic neurons provides a foothold for the identification of neuronal pathways mediating the subjective feeling of depression. Their cell bodies, located in the Raphe nuclei of the midbrain, have primary afferent and efferent connection areas linked to fear, reward, cognition, and appetite control. While providing a large number of speculative target opportunities, the limited knowledge makes it difficult to select among them. The connection to the hypothalamus is able to influence neuropeptide release involved in the stress response, the stimulation of the HPA hormone axis that stimulates the secretion of corticosteroids by the adrenal gland. Stress is a major contributor to depression, and many patients show elevated corticosteroid levels. The HPA axis is activated by the release of the hypothalamic neuropeptide CRF that stimulates CRF_1 receptors in the pituitary. Corticosteroids penetrate into the brain and may be contributors to the depression. CRF_1 antagonists and glucocorticoid receptor antagonists are being evaluated in clinical trials with depressed patients.

Evidence for shrinkage of cortical and hippocampal structures in chronically depressed patients and the delayed onset of the current drugs points to the possibility that depression involves aspects reminiscent of neurodegenerative disease in addition to the changes in activity of existing neuronal pathways. Tentative evidence suggests that BDNF, a principal neurotrophic factor in the brain, is a player in depression as well as in the action of the current antidepressant drugs. BDNF may be a regulator neurogenesis in the hippocampus and other brain areas, a process that seems to be altered in depression. Mood stabilizers such as Li^+ that are used for the treatment of bipolar depression may derive some of their efficacy from influencing neurogenesis and BDNF signaling processes.

While very vague as yet, the insight in structural processes affected in depression is likely to clarify the disease mechanisms and to identify attractive putative drug targets.

Several rodent models are available that predict efficacy of drugs working by the same mechanisms as the currently approved monoaminergic antidepressants. These models either put animals in a situation of hopelessness or attempt to expose them to situations of stress. The simplicity and high capacity of the animal tests will result in the identification of many putative targets for antidepressant drugs. However, the experience with substance P antagonists that worked reliably in these test but failed to provide robust antidepressant activity in humans emphasizes the limitations of the predictive value of the animal models. This problem together with the difficult nature of clinical trials in depression are a key problem for drug discovery research. Clinical trials have a high failure rate and viable experimental medicine alternatives remain to be developed.

Depression presents one of the most significant needs and challenges for drug discovery. The very limited understanding of the disease mechanism, the poor predictive power of the animal models, the large number of putative drug targets, and the difficult nature of clinical trials create a very problematical situation.

REFERENCES

Further Reading

BLIER, P., and WARD, N.M. Is there a role for 5-HT1A agonists in the treatment of depression? *Biol. Psychiat.* 1: 193–203, 2003.

COYLE, J.T., and DUMAN, R.S. Finding the intracellular signaling pathways affected by mood disorder treatment. *Neuron* 38: 157–160, 2003.

FAVA, M., and KENDLER, K.S. Major depressive disorder. *Neuron* 28: 335–341, 2000.

GINGRICH, J.A. Mutational analysis of the serotonergic system: recent findings using knockout mice. *Curr. Drug Targ. CNS Neurol. Disord.* 1: 449–465, 2002.

GUTMAN, D.A., OWENS, M.J., and NEMEROFF, C.B. Corti-cotropin-releasing factor antagonists as novel psychotherapeutics. *Drugs Fut.* 25: 923–931, 2000.

MULLER-OERLINGSHAUSEN, B., BERGHOFER, A., and BAUER, M. Bipolar disorder. *Lancet* 359: 241–247, 2002.

NESTLER, E.J., BARROT, M., DiLEONE, R.J., EISCH, A.J., GOLD, S.J., and MONTEGGIA, L.M. Neurobiology of depression. *Neuron* 34: 13–25, 2002.

PORSOLT, R.D. Animal models of depression: Utility for transgenic research. *Rev. Neurosci.* 11: 53–58, 2000.

SPINKS, D., and SPINKS, G. Serotonin reuptake inhibition: An update on current research strategies. *Curr. Med. Chem.* 9: 799–810, 2002.

Citations

ALTAR, C.A., LAENG, P., JURATA, L.W., BROCKMAN, J.A., LEMIRE, A., BULLARD, J., BUKHAM, Y.V., YOUNG, T.A., CHARLES, V., and PALFREUMAN, M.G. Electroconvulsive seizures regulate gene expression of distinct neurotrophic signaling pathways. *J. Neurosci.* 24: 2667–2677, 2004.

BAI, F., BERGERON, M., and NELSON, D.L. Chronic AMPA receptor potentiator (LY451646) treatment increases cell proliferation in adult rat hippocampus. *Neuropharmacology* 44: 1013–1021, 2003.

BALDWIN, D., BROICH, K., FRITZE, J., KASPER, S., WESTENBERG, H., and MOLLER, H.J. Placebo-controlled studies in depression: Necessary, ethical and feasible. *Eur. Arch. Psychiat. Clin. Neurosci.* 253: 22–28, 2003.

BELANOFF, J.K., FLORES, B.H., KALEZHAN, M., SUND, B., and SCHATZBERG, A.F. Rapid reversal of psychotic depression using mifepristone. *J. Clin. Psychopharmacol.* 21: 516– 521, 2001.

BEJJANI, B.P., DAMIER, P., ARNULF, I., THIVARD, L., BONNET, A.M., DORMONT, D., CORNU, P., PIDOUX, B., SAMSON, Y., and AGID, Y. Transient acute depression induced by high-frequency deep-brain stimulation. *N. Eng. J. Med.* 340: 1476–1480, 1999.

BOROWSKI, B., DURKIN, M.M., OGOZALEK, K., MARZABADI, M.R., DELEON, J., HEURICH, R., LICHTBLAU, H., SHAPOSHNIK, Z., DANIEWSKY, I., BLACKBURN, T.P., BRANCHEK, T.A., GERALD, C., VAYSSE, P.J., and FORRAY, C. Antide-pressant, anxiolytic and anorectic effects of a melanin-concentrating hormone-1 receptor antagonist. *Nature Med.* 8: 825–834, 2002.

BREMNER, J.D., NARAYAN, M., ANDERSON, E.R., STAIB, L.H., MILLER, H.L., and CHARNEY, D.S. Hippocampal volume reduction in major depression. *Am. J. Psychiat.* 157: 115–118. 2000.

DAUTZENBERG, F.M., and HAUGER, R.L. The CRF peptide family and their receptors: Yet more partners discovered. *Trends Pharmacol. Sci.* 23: 71–77, 2002.

FEIGHNER, J.P., SVERDLOW, L., NICOLAU, G., ABAJIAN, H.B., HLAYKA, J., FREED, J.S., and TONELLI, G., Jr. Clinical effectiveness of nemifitide, a novel pentapeptide antidepressant, in depressed outpatients: Comparison of follow-up re-treatment with initial treatment. *Int. J. Neuropsychopharmacol.* 6: 207–213, 2003.

FULLER, R.W., PERRY, K.W., and MOLLOY, B.B. Effect of Effect of an uptake inhibitor on serotonin metabolism in rat brain: studies with 3-(p-trifluoromethylphenoxy)-N-methyl-3-phenylpropylamine (Lilly 110140). *Life Sci.* 15: 1161–1171. 1974.

POUZET, B. SB-258741: A 5-HT7 receptor antagonist of potential clinical interest. *CNS Drug Rev.* 8: 90–100, 2002.

SAARELAINEN, T., HENDOLIN, P., LUCAS, G., KOPONEN, E., SAIRANEN, M., MACDONALD, E., AGERMAN, K., HAAPASALO, A., NAWA, H., ALOYZ, R., ERNFORS, P., and CASTREN, E. Activation of the TrkB neurotrophin receptor is induced by antidepressant drugs and is required for antidepressant-induced behavioral effects. *J. Neurosci.* 23: 349–357, 2003.

SANTARELLI, L., GOBBI, G., DEBS, P.C., SIBILLE, E.L., BLIER, P., HEN, R., and HEATH, M.J.S. Genetic and pharmacological disruption of neurokinin 1 receptor function decreases anxiety-related behaviors and increases serotonergic function. *Proc. Natl. Acad. Sci. USA.* 98: 1912–1917, 2001.

SANTARELLI, L., SAXE, M., GROSS, C., SURGET, A., BATTAGLIA, F., DULAWA, S., WEISSTAUB, N., LEE, J., DUMAN, R., ARANCIO, O., BELZUNG, C., and HEN, R. Requirement of hippocampal neurogenesis for the behavioral effects of antidepressants. *Science* 301: 805–808, 2003.

Chapter 8

Anxiety Disorders

Anxiety is a natural state and is well within the spectrum of feelings most humans experience every day. We are anxious, or nervous, when sitting through an exam, giving a public lecture, starting a new job, meeting a new date, whenever we encounter a new situation with potentially important consequences. When feeling anxious, we find it difficult to concentrate, to participate in a conversation, and to focus on a single task. We have increased heart rates, feel hot, tend to sweat, and may feel the urge to urinate.

Anxiety disorders represent an exaggeration of the normal anxious response. The term general anxiety disorder is used to describe states where anxiety is present permanently, in absence of situations justifying it. Severe forms of general anxiety disorder interfere with normal activities and often prevent the patients from holding on to a job or from maintaining a satisfactory social life. The term panic attack is used to describe temporary, severe forms of anxiety that last for minutes or hours. In some patients, panic attacks are triggered by specific events or by specific surroundings. In other patients, panic attacks happen in absence of any external triggers. Regular panic attacks tend to incapacitate the patients in a similar way as general anxiety disorders. Patients stay home to avoid the embarrassment of tears and breakdowns in public settings, and they gradually withdraw from professional and social functions.

In addition to the two major subgroups of anxiety disorders, general anxiety disorder and panic attacks, there are various other forms of anxiety that are often considered disease states. The term phobia is used to describe the avoidance of specific situations because patients know or fear that they will trigger a severe anxiety reaction. Social phobia, the avoidance of contact with other people, has been diagnosed with increasing frequency and is considered an exaggeration of natural shyness (Hidalgo et al., 2001). Anxiety adjustment disorder, as the term indicates, describes excessive anxiety in response to a specific, single situation, such as a new neighbor or a new collaborator at work. Post-traumatic stress disorder describes excessive anxiety in response to a significant traumatic event in a patient's life. Obsessive-compulsive disorder, the repetition of ritualized thoughts or behaviors, has been linked to childhood anxiety disorder (Stein, 2002). Finally, premenstrual syndrome can be considered part of this group because of the associated mood changes and neurobiological considerations related to anxiety mechanisms (Sundstrom Poromaa, 2003).

The distinction between normal anxious responses and the pathological exaggerations of anxiety disorders is not precisely defined. Some people worry more and get nervous more easily than others without anybody considering this a disease. An occasional panic response seems normal. Given the gradual change from normal to disease, it is not sur-

Drug Discovery for Nervous System Diseases, by Franz F. Hefti
ISBN 0-471-46563-1   Copyright © 2005 by John Wiley & Sons, Inc.

prising that there are significant cultural differences in the way anxiety is perceived and described. A society where emotional distance and reservation are the norm may call shy a child that stays to itself, whereas the term social phobia may be used in a society that favors easy interpersonal contact and expression of feelings. In many societies there is the tendency to perceive anxiety as weakness and to stigmatize anxiety disorders. Patients tend to present physical complaints, often headaches, chest pain, or breathing difficulties. The term anxiety is avoided and other culturally more acceptable terms are being used, for example, *taijin kyofusho* (fear of losing face and facing situations) in Japanese or *hwa byung* (fire illness) in Korean (Cheng et al., 2002). Anxiety is often paraphrased as excessive activity or excitement. The same benzodiazepine drugs that are prescribed as anxiolytics in the United States are called "calming drugs" (*calmanti, Beruhigungsmittel*) in Italy and Germany.

In addition to the many cultural differences there are philosophical concepts that influence the perception and the expression of anxiety and tend to obscure the recognition of anxiety disorders. Various terms related to anxiety have been given special conceptual meaning. Anxiety and fear are often used as synonyms, but the term fear has been elevated by linking it to the fundamental uncertainty of human life. "Fear of existence" (*angoisse du néant, Existenzangst*) has been used to describe feelings of people who live outside of firm sets of religious beliefs, and these terms are not intended to describe anxiety disorders. The cultural and linguistic differences can make it difficult for the practicing physician to diagnose anxiety. However, these issues should not cloud the fact that anxiety disorders represent distinct medical conditions that require treatment.

In accordance with current medical practice, this volume presents anxiety disorders and depression as different clinical entities and in separate chapters. However, the two diseases are strongly linked and overlap in many aspects. Excessive anxiety is a cardinal feature of depression, and patients suffering from anxiety tend to rate high on depression scales. Monoamine uptake blockers are used in the treatment of both depression and anxiety disorders. The limited knowledge of disease mechanisms shows that similar neuronal pathways are involved in both diseases. It has been argued that the separation between anxiety and depression is artificial and counterproductive, and that they should be bundled together into mood disorders (Shorter and Tyrer, 2003). These considerations are important from the perspective of drug discovery and development, since they show that a drug approved for one of the indications may be beneficial for both.

8.1 SYMPTOMS AND DISEASE MECHANISM

Anxiety disorders affect more than 1% of the population (Kessler and Wittchen, 2002). The unclear separation from normal behavioral states makes it likely that many cases are undiagnosed and that the actual number of affected people is much larger. Anxiety disorders have to be considered a significant and disabling mental illness, for which only inadequate treatment is available today.

Patients suffering from anxiety disorders experience psychological and physiological symptoms. Subjective feelings of apprehension, worries, and fear are common. The thoughts associated with such feelings tend to become dominant in the patients' thinking patterns, and they prevent that proper attention can be given to the normal tasks of life and work. Physiological symptoms include various forms of pain, breathing difficulties, and abdominal discomfort. Patient suffering from general anxiety disorders may initially seek physician's help for headaches and dizziness or for chest pain that is interpreted as weakness of the heart. Abdominal pain or discomfort may reflect digestive problems and bladder hyperreactivity. The diagnosis of general anxiety disorder is reached when other diseases can be ruled out as causes of the typical physiological symptoms and when several psychological and physiological symptoms occur together. Anxiety ratings scales help in the diagnosis and provide a quantitative measure for the severity of the disease.

As for the other major psychiatric diseases, the causes and the diseases mechanism for anxiety disorders are very poorly understood. The majority of the cases cannot be linked to specific traumatic events and must therefore have other environmental or genetic causes. It seems natural to speculate that difficult and stressful episodes during childhood may cause anxiety disorders in the adult, but there is little convincing data in support of this view. No familial forms of anxiety disorders have been described that may help in delineating a disease pathway in a way similar to that emerging for schizophrenia. An interesting potential conduit to disease mechanisms is provided by the studies of fear pathways, and the principally involved brain structure, the amygdala. Lesion studies and functional imaging studies in the human brain clearly demonstrate that activity in this brain structure is linked to feelings of fear and anxiety. The study of the neuronal mechanisms in the amygdala, to be described in more detail below, have the potential to lead to the identification of novel drug targets for anxiety disorders.

8.2 CURRENT TREATMENT OF ANXIETY DISORDERS

As true for all disorders of emotion or mood, anxiety disorders respond best to a combination of behavioral and drug therapy (Gorman, 2003). When specific triggers for the anxiety are known, patients can be helped by providing assistance in avoiding these triggers. Panic attacks triggered by enclosed spaces, such as cars or airlines, are more difficult to avoid because they are often necessary, but patients can be helped by behavioral preparations for these specific situations. It is sometimes possible to teach patients to discern early signs of impending panic attacks and to help them modify the subsequent response. General anxiety disorder and frequent panic attacks respond to several types of drugs, the benzodiazepine-type drugs, antidepressant monoamine uptake blockers, and buspirone (Fig. 8.1). These drugs were discovered based on observations in animals or humans.

8.2.1 Benzodiazepine Drugs

Benzodiazepine drugs have been the mainstay of pharmacotherapy of anxiety disorders since the discovery and introduction of diazepam in the 1960s. These compounds were discovered at the pharmaceutical company Roche, in Basel, Switzerland, because of their unique behavioral effects in animals. Diazepam sedated the animals but, in contrast to other then known sedatives, did not induce anesthesia at high doses. In addition they did not produce any adverse effects such as seizures, cardiac or respiratory depression. While no more efficacious than other known sedatives at that time, the relative benign safety profile helped the benzodiazepines to become the dominant drugs for the treatment of anxiety disorders. They quickly replaced the previously used barbiturates, drugs that are highly toxic at high doses.

By potentiating the action of GABA on the ionotropic GABA-A receptors, the benzodiazepine drugs strengthen inhibitory synaptic transmission throughout the CNS and thus decrease the excitability of most neurons. At low doses, they dampen hyperactivity

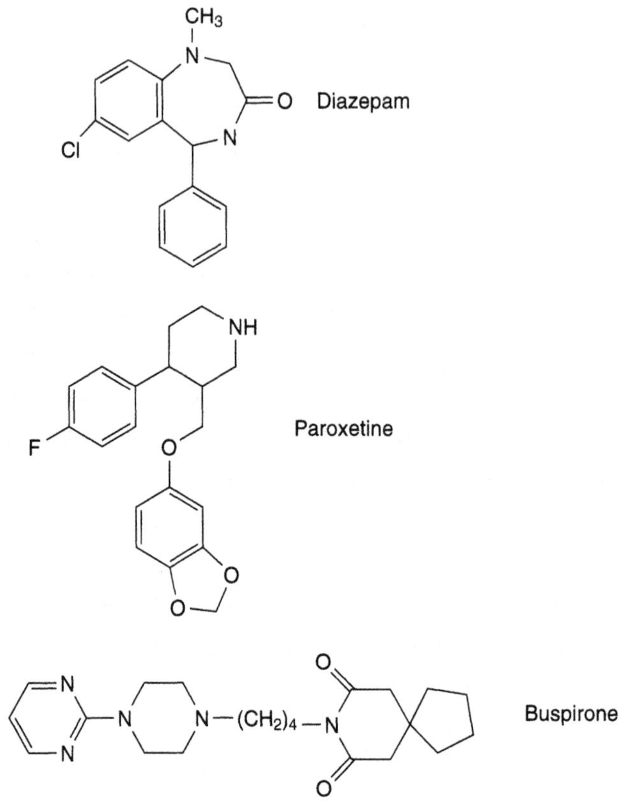

Figure 8.1 Examples of drugs currently used for the treatment of anxiety disorders.

associated with anxiety; at higher doses they are sedative and induce sleep or hypnosis. As described in more detail in Chapter 4, the benzodiazepine drugs bind to a specific benzodiazepine receptor site at the interface of the α and γ subunits of the GABA-A receptors. The anxiolytic benzodiazepines are agonists that increase the frequency of channel opening of the GABA-A ion channels. In consequence more Cl⁻ ions flow through the channels, hyperpolarizing the cells and decreasing the probability that action potentials are generated (Fig. 8.2). Benzodiazepine receptor antagonists prevent the binding of other molecules to this binding site. Since there is no natural ligand, the antagonists are without effects in absence of another active ligand for this receptor site. Flumazenil is an example of a benzodiazepine receptor site antagonist. It serves as important tool in benzodiazepine receptor site drug discovery and can be clinically used to treat benzodiazepine overdosing. Benzodiazepine receptor ligands are found among several classes of chemicals, beyond the original benzodiazepines such as valium. Nevertheless, the term benzodiazepine is firmly anchored in the medical language and textbooks of pharmacology and is used including the molecules from other chemical groups.

The currently available anxiolytic benzodiazepines do not distinguish between the various GABA-A receptor subtypes. They differ in potency and pharmacokinetic properties. Compounds with long half-lives are preferred for the treatment of anxiety disorders, whereas those with short half-lives are preferred for the treatment of sleep disorders. The early benzodiazepines, diazepam and chlordiazepoxide, had long half-lives. Among the

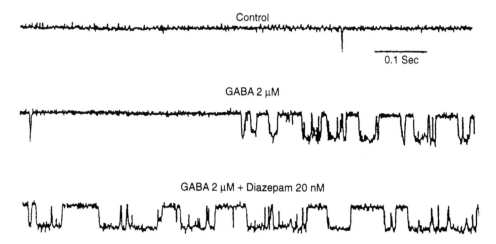

Figure 8.2   Molecular effects of benzodiazepine drugs on GABA-A receptor channel function. Diazepam increases the frequency of channel openings without altering their duration. (Adapted from Twyman et al., 1989)

more recently approved drugs are compounds with very short half-lives, such as triazolam. The approved benzodiazepine drugs are all full agonists at the GABA-A receptors. Partial agonists, compounds that potentiate the actions of GABA to a lesser extend than diazepam, have been described but have not been developed as drugs, since they do not seem to offer significant advantages over the existing fully agonistic drugs.

Benzodiazepines are quite effective in treating anxiety. Their utility is limited by the adverse effects, sedation, addiction, and cognitive impairment. Given the dose-related gradual transition from anxiolytic to sedative effects, it is not surprising that many patients complain of drowsiness. At higher doses benzodiazepines impair motor reflexes, and patients are advised not to drive or to operate machinery when using them. A particular problem derives from the fact that benzodiazepines potentiate the sedative effects of alcohol. A single harmless drink can severely impair motor function when taken by a patient on a benzodiazepine drug. This drug–drug interaction is a particular problem and danger in societies that tolerate low alcohol exposure when driving.

Addiction is frequently mentioned as significant danger associated with benzodiazepine use. However, the addictive potential of benzodiazepines is far less pronounced than that of the powerful addictive drugs like cocaine or heroin. Withdrawal from benzodiazepine used at medically prescribed doses is not associated with significant physiological disturbances. Nevertheless, many patients do cling to their benzodiazepine drugs and find it difficult to abandon them. In absence of robust physiological signs of withdrawal, the desire of the patients to stay on benzodiazepines has been described as psychological dependence rather than physiological addiction. Despite the relatively benign addiction potential, all benzodiazepine drugs carry strong warning labels for addiction. Patients are typically advised not to take them beyond a few months (Salzman, 1998).

Benzodiazepine drugs interfere with memory functions. Anecdotal stories abound of scientists giving poor talks at oversees meetings after having taken benzodiazepine drugs to control jet-lag sleep disturbances. Relatively mild but reproducible deficits in memory have been reliably demonstrated in controlled test settings in animals and humans. They represent a significant disadvantage of the benzodiazepine drugs that can put patients at risk in specific situations. In addition these undesired effects may be used in support of criminal intentions. Some of the benzodiazepines have been added to social drinks to impair the judgment of the victims. The use of benzodiazepines as rape drugs may reflect the combined effects toward sedation and cognitive impairment (Dowd et al., 2002).

Despite their drawbacks benzodiazepines remain medically very useful and are often prescribed. Safety is their key advantage of the benzodiazepines. While high doses are sedative and hypnotic, even highest doses are typically not fatal. Sedation and memory impairment are significant adverse effects that limit their use.

8.2.2 Monoamine Uptake Blockers

All monoamine uptake blockers approved for the treatment of anxiety were initially introduced as antidepressants. These drugs are discussed in detail in Chapter 7. The overlap between depression and anxiety disorders makes it possible to expand the indication territory of a drug into the other group. Several monoamine update blockers have been shown efficacious in randomized and controlled clinical trials. There have been very few conclusive comparative studies so far, leaving it unclear whether selective serotonin or norepinephrine uptake blockers are superior to nonselective uptake blockers or to the benzodiazepines. The side effects of the monoamine uptake blockers limit their usefulness in the treatment of anxiety disorders in a similar way as in depression.

8.2.3 Buspirone

Buspirone represents a class of anxiolytic drug of its own. The compound is an agonist to the 5-HT_{1A} receptors. These receptors mediate some of the postsynaptic actions of serotonin, and they are also located on the serotonergic neurons themselves where they serve as presynaptic sensors of serotonin release. 5-HT_{1A} agonists interfere with this feedback loop and so elevate the amount of serotonin released from the synaptic sites. However, buspirone is only marginally effective in the treatment of human anxiety. The clinical experience with buspirone does not provide strong motivation for the further exploration of the 5-HT_{1A} receptors as drug targets in anxiety.

8.3 FUTURE DRUG TARGETS

Despite the absence of solid knowledge on disease mechanisms of anxiety disorders, there are several promising roads that may lead to the discovery of new anxiolytic drugs. The first approach is an example of reverse pharmacology and attempts to improve the selectivity of the currently used benzodiazepine drugs. Two further approaches are based on the behavioral concept of fear. Animal models of fear and anxiety are used to select effective compounds in random screens or, alternatively, to study the neuronal pathways and neurotransmitter that mediate fear to identify suitable drug targets. These approaches reflect the belief that the mechanism mediating exaggerated anxiety in human disorders are related to those mediating fear and escape in animals. Fear is a subjective feeling that cannot be detected in animals. Escape responses are thus equalized with fear in these tests. Some of the tests have a strong ethological basis. They may use the natural tendency of rodents to seek protection in enclosed spaces or the natural protective responses to a predator. Other tests put the animals in highly artificial conditions that induce fear through the use of unpleasant stimuli. The tests receive validation by the currently used anxiolytics that are effective in the animal models for human anxiety.

8.3.1   Receptor Subtype-Selective Benzodiazepines

The benzodiazepine binding site on GABA-A receptors is a clinically validated drug target. The existence of several GABA-A receptors subunits offers the possibility to improve on existing benzodiazepine drugs through reverse pharmacology approaches, as discussed in more detail in Chapter 4. Briefly, the benzodiazepine receptor site is formed at the interface of the α and γ subunits of the heteromeric GABA-A receptors. Behavioral studies with transgenic animals in which some of the subtypes have been made unresponsive to benzodiazepines suggest that the anxiolytic effects are mediated by receptors containing the $\alpha 2$ or $\alpha 3$ subunits, whereas the sedative actions are mediated by the $\alpha 1$ subunit containing receptors. Animal studies with emerging $\alpha 2$ and $\alpha 3$ selective benzodiazepine receptor ligands support the concept that it is possible to separate the anxiolytic from the sedative properties. In contrast to nonselective benzodiazepine drugs, the subtype selective compounds do not potentiate the sedative actions of ethanol. These compounds not only differ in the affinity to the various subtypes but also in their efficacy. The compound SL651498, for example, binds with high affinity to $\alpha 2$ and $\alpha 1$ containing receptors, and is a full agonist at $\alpha 2$ but only a partial agonist at $\alpha 1$ receptors. This seemingly small difference is sufficient to generate anxiolytic effects in absence of sedation (Griebel et al., 2003). Because compounds can be made with different affinity and different potencies to five different types of GABA-A receptors, it is possible to generate many compounds with subtle differences in their properties. Several compounds with various subtype selectivity are in clinical development. The near future will reveal which ones are useful for human use. If nonsedative benzodiazepines can be obtained for humans, they will likely become highly useful drugs for the treatment of anxiety disorders. While representing a significant improvement for pharmacotherapy of anxiety, these compounds may still have the potential to impair memory functions and to be habit forming.

8.3.2   Target Identification through Animal Model Studies

Many animal models for anxiety are technically simple, and they can be run with reasonably high capacity. It is thus possible to test many available compounds as well as many transgenic animals in these assays. The following putative targets have emerged from studies on animal models of anxiety.

The mGluR5 receptors are expressed in brain areas linked to emotional control. An mGluR5 antagonist, 2-methyl-6-(phenylethynyl)pyridine (MPEP), was synthesized several years ago and found effective in various animal models of anxiety. The efficacy is comparable to that of benzodiazepines and superior to buspirone, suggesting that mGluR5 may be a useful drug target (Brodkin et al., 2002). The interpretations of these findings, however, is made complex by the fact that the test compound MPEP binds to other receptor sites at concentrations only slightly higher than those inhibiting the mGluR5 receptors. These off-target activities may falsely link observed behaviors to mGluR5 receptors or may cloud the effects on mGluR5 receptors. Examinations of mGluR5 knockout mice also provide a complex picture. These animals respond less vigorously to stress, but they differ from control animals in other behavioral aspects too. The availability of an improved mGluR5 antagonist that is devoid of off-target activities (3-[(2-methyl-1,3,-thiazol-4-yl)ethynyl]-pyridine, MTEP) will help resolve the question whether mGluR5 antagonists are useful as therapeutic agents (Cosford et al., 2003).

Other members of the mGluR family have been speculatively linked to anxiety. Similar to mGluR5 receptors, the mGluR2 receptors are widely expressed in the brain, including areas involved in the regulation of emotional behaviors. The mGluR2 agonist LY354740, discussed in Chapter 6 and pursued for the treatment of schizophrenia, has been reported to produce beneficial effects in human experimental anxiety tests (Grillon et al., 2003). Studies with gene knockout mice implicate mGluR7 and mGluR8 in anxiety behaviors. Mice with null mutations of the mGluR7 and mGluR8 receptors exhibit, respectively, decreased and increased activity in animal assays of anxiety (Cryan et al., 2003; Linden et al., 2002). These studies point to both receptors as potential drug targets for anxiety and suggest that mGluR7 antagonists and mGluR8 agonists might have the desired therapeutic activities. Selective compounds will be necessary to further substantiate these hypotheses and to distinguish between developmental and adult functions of the receptors. mGluR2, mGluR5, mGluR7, and mGluR8 are highly attractive putative drug targets for anxiety disorders. The involvement of these receptors in anxiety behaviors strengthens the belief that mGluR receptors in general are especially suitable for drug discovery in the neurosciences.

The peptide vasopressin is predominantly located in the hypothalamus where it plays an important role in the regulation of pituitary hormonal function. In addition vasopressin is expressed in several brain areas outside of the hypothalamus, and it has been functionally linked to memory and emotional processes. Based on these suggestive findings, researchers at the pharmaceutical company Sanofi-Synthelabo, located in Montpellier, France, have synthesized selective antagonists for the receptors mediating the actions of vasopressin. A selective antagonist to the V_{1b} receptor, SSR149415, is highly efficacious in animal models of anxiety, making a strong case for this receptor as putative drug target (Griebel et al., 2002).

A different neuropeptide, orphanin FQ/nociceptin, activates ORL1 receptors, which are homologous to opiate receptors but do not bind morphine or other opioid ligands. Both the peptide and the receptor are widely expressed in the brain. Drug discovery researchers at Roche synthesized a selective agonist for ORL1 receptors, Ro 64-6198. This compound molecule was effective in an anxiety test in rats, thus pointing to the ORL1 receptor as an interesting target opportunity for anxiety (Jenck et al., 2000).

The relative ease and high capacity of behavioral testing in animal anxiety models make it attractive to attempt the identification of drug targets through large-scale, random testing of transgenic animals or test compounds. At the former biotechnology company Deltagen, located in Redwood City, California, knockout mice were generated of many G-protein-coupled receptors and ion channels expressed in the brain. They were then tested in a high-throughput anxiety model. This platform approach rendered a relatively large number of animals with altered performance in the test. Further evaluation of these genes will help to determine their suitability as drug targets. The experience obtained with studies on mGluR and V_{1b} receptors illustrates the difficulties to be encountered. It is not possible to distinguish developmental from adult functions in studies with gene knockout animals. Test compounds that are selective for receptor subtypes and have acceptable pharmacokinetic properties for animal studies have to be generated or, alternatively, approaches to selectively silence gene expression in the adult have to be utilized. Generating test compounds suitable for animal studies remains a difficult and time-consuming effort. Alternative strategies, the siRNA technologies in particular, may be able to bypass the need for small molecules generated with a medical chemistry effort. The experience with mGluR receptors illustrates that effects in anxiety tests discovered with knockout animals or selective receptor ligands often do not occur in isolation. They are frequently accompanied by effects in animal models for other diseases. Many of the knockout mice phenotypes show signals in animal models for anxiety, depression, and schizophrenia. The random approach to identify drug targets by behavioral screening on anxiety models is thus likely to yield a high number of putative targets, requiring many additional studies for further selection. Those receptors that can be linked to selective effects in anxiety models and reflect adult rather than developmental functions will provide the most interesting putative drug targets.

8.3.3 Target Identification from Amygdala Fear Pathways

The amygdala is a small, well-defined neuroanatomical structure located under the lateral cerebral cortex. The name reflects its form, almond-shaped, in Greek. The amygdala is believed to be a phylogenetically old structure that has been preserved through vertebrate evolution. It is not a homogeneous nucleus but comprises several subnuclei with distinct morphology and neuronal connection patterns. Lesion and imaging studies link the amygdala to the emotional feelings of fear and anxiety. Animals with lesions of the amygdala do not exhibit the typical escape responses they display when facing a potentially dangerous situation, such as a predator. Humans with lesions of the amygdala have difficulties recognizing facial expressions. Functional MRI studies show activation of the amygdala when subjects are shown fearful facial expressions. The amygdala is thus considered a crucial brain structure in the perception and expression of fear and anxiety (LeDoux et al., 2000).

A widely studied experimental paradigm called fear conditioning provides further support for a special role of the amygdala. In this paradigm that is a variant of the classical Pavlovian associated learning paradigm, a conditioned stimulus, such as tone or a light flash, is linked to an unpleasant unconditioned stimulus such as an electric shock. Once the association is learned, the conditioned stimulus elicits behavioral and physiologic responses in the animals similar to those experienced by people suffering from chronic anxiety disorders. Animals attempt to escape, or they behaviorally freeze, their heart rate increases and the frequency of urination and defecation is elevated. Fear conditioning is abolished in animals with lesions of the amygdala.

Fear conditioning can be considered a standardized and experimental form of stress-induced learning that occurs in natural life. All humans have stressful and traumatic experiences throughout their lives, and these experiences are typically remembered very vividly. Details of accidents, the precise events, the surroundings, the people affected, are remembered well over many years as if they were carved in stone. Mild stress, for example, in preparation of an exam, affects learning performance, though animal studies suggest significant gender differences in these effects (Shors and Miesegaes, 2002). It seems natural to speculate that the amygdala mechanism related to fear conditioning is altered in patients suffering from anxiety disorders. Hyperactivity in these systems might lead to excessive responses, causing mild stimuli to elicit exaggerated fear and anxiety. Suppressing amygdala fear potentiation might thus lead to better and more specific anxiolytics than the current drugs.

The anatomical connections and synaptic mechanisms of the amygdala that are involved in fear potentiation are fairly well understood (Fig. 8.3). Fear conditioning predominantly involves the basolateral and central nuclei of the amygdala. The basolateral nuclei receive synaptic inputs from neurons in specific thalamic nuclei, which project through the thalamo-amygdala pathway and from neurons in the cortex that are part of the

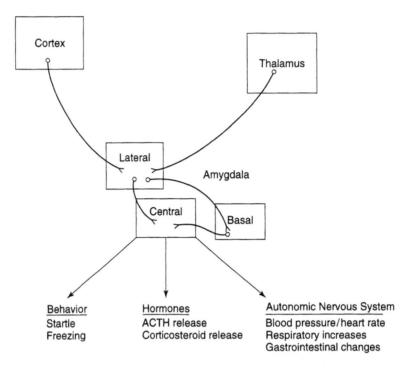

Figure 8.3 Amygdala pathways involved in fear potentiation. Sensory and cognitive inputs from the thalamus and cortex are integrated in the amygdala nuclei. The output regulates behavior, hormonal release, and autonomic functions. (Adapted from Sah et al., 2003)

cortex-amygdala pathway, and transmit sensory inputs from the respective association areas. Long-term potentiation (LTP), an electrophysiological reading that reflects enhancement of synaptic strength through multiple use and is believed to reflect learning, exists at synapses from both pathways. The neurons of the basolateral nuclei project to the central nucleus of the amygdala. A second input to the central nucleus is provided by the accessory basal nucleus that is innervated by the hippocampus, a structure with critical importance for learning. Many modulatory inputs innervate the basolateral or the central nuclei, including dopaminergic, noradrenergic, and serotonergic afferents, as well as cholinergic systems of the basal forebrain. The amygdala is thus able to integrate various sensory and cognitive modalities. The central nucleus provides the efferent output of the structure. Its neurons project to various hypothalamic and brainstem nuclei through which they regulate autonomic and motor functions and thus control the behavioral and physiological signs of fear (Sah et al., 2003).

The synaptic connections of the amygdala and the neurotransmitter mechanisms they use provide a complex picture (Ninan, 1999). As in the cerebral cortex, glutamate and GABA are the principal transmitters of the amygdala. Both the cortico-amygdala and the thalamo-amygdala pathways that innervate the basolateral nuclei use glutamate as their dominant transmitter. NMDA receptors are the most influential component on the postsynaptic side. Nonselective NMDA antagonists inhibit long-term potentiation in the afferent pathways and interfere with fear conditioning. NR2A and NR2B subtypes of the NMDA receptor are expressed in basolateral and central nuclei, and it is not clear whether receptor subtype selective drugs might be able to selectively suppress fear potentiation. The function of the other groups of ionotropic glutamate receptors in the amygdala remains to be explored. Among the metabotropic receptors, the mGluR5 receptors are abundant on dendrites of basolateral nuclei neurons. Long-term potentiation of the thalamo-amygdala pathway is impaired by MPEP, the mGluR5 antagonist discussed above (Rodrigues et al., 2002). The findings further strengthen the case for mGluR5 as an interesting putative drug target for anxiety. The case for mGluR2, made above based on behavioral studies alone, also receives further support from findings on amygdala fear conditioning. The receptor is expressed in the amygdala and direct infusions of the mGluR2 agonist LY354740 impair fear-potentiated startle responses in rats (Walker et al., 2002). Clearly, glutamate receptors are interesting putative drug targets for anxiolytic drugs. The tools provided by the emerging pharmacology of glutamate receptors will be very useful to further explore these possibilities.

GABA receptors that mediate the actions of GABAergic interneurons in the amygdala most likely mediate the anxiolytic actions of benzodiazepines. In support of this view, direct injections of the nonselective GABA-A receptor agonist, muscimol, into the amygdala block fear conditioning. The distribution of GABA-A receptor subunits corroborate that it is the $\alpha 2$ containing receptors that mediate the anxiolytic actions of benzodiazepines. While GABA-A receptors containing $\alpha 1$ or $\alpha 2$ subunits exist in the amygdala, the $\alpha 2$ containing receptors are located at high levels in the central nuclei (Kaufmann et al., 2003).

A particularly intriguing opportunity for drug discovery may be provided by the GABA-A receptors containing $\alpha 4$ subunits. The expression of $\alpha 4$ subunits in the amygdala is regulated by progesterone, providing a potential link to the premenstrual syndrome. In rats subjected to progesterone withdrawal, an animal model of premenstrual syndrome, expression levels of $\alpha 4$ are increased (Gulinello et al., 2003). This seems counterintuitive to a link with premenstrual syndrome, a condition associated with increased anxiety. However, the $\alpha 4$ containing receptors are influenced by so-called neurosteroids, metabolites of progesterone that are decreased following the drop in progesterone and that normally enhance the GABA-A receptor functions. Selective activators of $\alpha 4$ containing GABA-A receptors thus represent a potentially attractive approach for the treatment of premenstrual syndrome. Molecules other than benzodiazepine receptor ligands have to be identified, since this receptor type has very low affinity to standard ligands. The link of $\alpha 4$ to premenstrual syndrome remains speculative at this point, but it seems intriguing enough to deserve further exploration.

Cannabinoid receptors provide an opportunity to indirectly modulate GABAergic synapses in the amygdala. Cannabinoid CB1 receptors are abundantly expressed in the lateral but not central nucleus of the amygdala. They appear to be located on GABAergic interneurons that co-express the neuropeptide cholecystokinin. Electrophysiological studies show that CB1 receptor agonists influence the postsynaptic action of GABA. These actions may represent part of the mechanisms by which cannabis exerts its psychological influences that are perceived as beneficial (Katona et al., 2001).

The amygdala receives several monoaminergic inputs, from serotonergic neurons of the Raphe nuclei, noradrenergic neurons of the locus coeruleus, and dopaminergic cells of the substantia nigra. Enhancement of the serotonergic and noradrenergic inputs to the amygdala may explain the anxiolytic actions of the antidepressant uptake blockers. However, the existing scientific literature provides a complex picture. Infusions of norepinephrine into the amygdala potentiate rather than reduce fear conditioning (LaLumiere et al., 2003). It is tempting to speculate that some the effects may be linked to dopaminergic systems since dopamine enhances long-term potentiation in the lateral nucleus of the amygdala (Bissiere et al., 2003). Several of the subtypes of 5-HT receptors are expressed in the amygdala, including 5-HT_{1A}, 5-HT_{1B}, 5-HT_{2A}, 5-HT_{2C}, 5-HT_3, 5-HT_4, and 5-HT_7 receptors. The 5-HT_{1A} receptor is linked to anxiety through the actions of buspirone. The other subtypes, the 5-HT$_7$ receptor in particular, continue to be worth exploring, since they might be able to modify the synaptic mechanisms of the amygdala in a much more selective way than serotonin uptake blockers.

Many neuropeptides and neuropeptide receptors exist in the amygdala. Very often they co-exist with the primary transmitters, glutamate and GABA, in specific subpopulations of neurons. The neuropeptide receptors may thus provide drug targets with much higher selectivity than the ubiquitous glutamate and GABA receptors. Substance P and its NK$_1$ receptor occur in the amygdala and may mediate some of the antidepressant activities discussed in the previous chapter. Animals with selective ablation of neurons that express NK$_1$ KO mice respond differentially in anxiety tests (Gadd et al., 2003). Neuropeptide Y (NPY) and some of its receptors exist in the amygdala, and this peptide has been linked to anxiety through functional studies. NPY-Y2 receptor knockout mice show reduced anxiety in the animal test (Tschenett et al., 2003). CRF receptors have been discussed in the previous chapter as potential drug targets for depression. A similar argument can be made for anxiety. The lateral amygdala has a high level of expression of CRF$_1$ receptors and injections of a peptidic nonselective CRF receptor antagonist into the amygdala reduced fear-associated learning (Roozendaal et al., 2002). These findings support the view that CRF$_1$ antagonists might be useful for the treatment of depression as well as anxiety.

The receptor for gastrin-releasing peptide (GRPR) was identified as putative drug target in the search for amygdala specific gene expression. Single cells were isolated from the amygdala and their patterns of gene expression compared with those of the hippocampus, in a differential expression screen. Gastrin-releasing peptide was among the genes selectively expressed in the amygdala and was subsequently shown to be expressed at high levels in the basolateral nuclei. The corresponding receptor, GRPR, is located on GABAergic neurons in the amygdala and thus represents an attractive putative drug target to modulate these cells in a similar way as the benzodiazepines. The blockage of GRPRs may reduce the excitatory influence of gastrin-releasing peptide on GABAergic interneurons, thus the inhibitory feedback of the GABAergic interneurons in the amygdala, and so increase the efficacy of fear-potentiation pathways. In support of this view, GRPR knockout mice show enhanced long-term potentiation in the cortico-amygdala pathway and enhanced fear conditioning. This effect is remarkably selective since other forms of learning, in particular the spatial learning that requires hippocampal circuits, are not affected. GRPR knockout mice behave normally in the elevated plus maze test, the standard model used in anxiety testing (Shumyatsky et al., 2002). GRPRs thus represent highly selective and unique putative drug target for anxiety. It remains to be seen whether the limited effects in animals predict efficacy in humans and whether the expression of the receptors outside of the amygdala lead to significant adverse effects. GRPRs appear to also be involved in the control of feeding behavior and circadian rhythms.

Several other neuropeptides and receptors have been detected in the amygdala, including somatostatin, enkephalins, cholecystokinin, and orphanin FQ/nociceptin. The sst(2A) somatostatin receptor is expressed in the basolateral nuclei as well as in regions innervated by amygdala efferent pathways and is thus likely to play a part in fear-related mechanisms. The receptor for orphanin FQ/nociception has been identified as putative anxiety drug target based on animal model studies, as described above. Given the large number of neuropeptides and their G-protein-coupled receptors, the list of putative neuropeptide receptor drug targets is likely to grow yet further. The selective existence in subpopulations of glutamatergic and GABAergic neurons of the amygdala may create special opportunities to very selectively regulate fear pathways.

Table 8.1 Current and future drug targets for anxiety disorders

Current Drugs
GABA-A receptor ligands
Monoamine transporter inhibitors
Buspirone (5-HT$_{1A}$ agonist)

Future Drugs and Targets
GABA-A α2, GABA-A α4 receptors
mGluR2, mGluR7 receptors
V$_{1b}$ vasopressin receptor
ORL1 orphanin FQ/nociception receptor
CB$_1$ cannabinoid receptor
5-HT$_{1B}$, 5-HT$_{2A}$, 5-HT$_{2C}$, 5-HT$_3$, 5-HT$_4$, and 5-HT$_7$ receptors
NPY-Y2 receptor
CRF1 receptors
GRPR (gastrin-related peptide receptor)
sst(2A) somatostatin receptor

The amygdala and its pathways are an integral part of the stress response mechanisms discussed in the previous chapter on depression. The separation between mechanisms of fear potentiation and those of the stress response is somewhat artificial. The division reflects different subfields of neuroscience and the fact that separate groups of scientists embraced and evolved these concepts. The fields overlap by necessity because of the clinical similarities between depression and anxiety disorders. Many patients show symptoms belonging to both diseases, many drugs will be useful for both indications.

The putative drug targets discussed above and listed in Table 8.1 make it appear likely that studies of amygdala fear potentiation mechanisms and the random evaluation of test compounds and transgenic animals in behavioral models will identify a significant number of putative drug targets for anxiety and depression. If future studies corroborate this conjecture, the drug discovery in anxiety and depression will face a difficult capacity problem. In absence of better understanding of disease pathways, it will be very difficult to define selection criteria to identify the most promising ones. There will be the tendency to "just do it" and to push various receptor antagonists and agonist into clinical trials to test for efficacy. However, the number of putative drug targets with a reasonably compelling rationale will vastly exceed the capacity of the biopharmaceutical industry to identify and develop selective and safe drug candidates and to test them in clinical trials. Further studies on the disease mechanism of anxiety are thus urgently needed to identify the targets with the highest likelihood of clinical success. Experimental human anxiety tests will help to increase the capacity of clinical trials and to rapidly establish proof-of-principle for a putative drug target.

8.4 ANIMAL MODELS AND EXPERIMENTAL MEDICINE

Many animal models of anxiety have been developed, and they are widely used in drug discovery (Table 8.2). They broadly tend to fall into two categories. In some models, the animals are exposed to situations that reflect natural conditions they associate with increased danger. In other models, artificial conditions are created that put the animals in a conflict situation because a desired stimulus is coupled to an undesired event, and they have to overcome the associated fear.

8.4.1 Experimental Animal Anxiety

The elevated plus maze for mice and rats is the most widely used animal assay for testing anxiolytic effects. The test apparatus consists of an elevated cross-shaped platform with two covered arms and two open arms. Mice and rats have the natural tendency to hide in covered spaces in situations of danger and to explore open spaces under safe conditions. Since the elevated plus maze is based on naturally occurring behavior of the animals, it can be considered an ethological model of anxiety. An increase in time the animals spend in the open arms is interpreted as anxiolytic effects. Benzodiazepines prolong the time spent in the open space. They validate the model and provide a positive control in the testing of novel compounds. The simplicity of the model, its relatively high capacity, and the broad historical database have made the elevated plus maze model the favorite test system for anxiolytic drugs. However, monoamine uptake blockers that are effective in the treatment of human anxiety disorders do not produce a consistent effect in this model.

Several other ethological animal models make use of the rodent's preference for dark space. In simple versions the animals are given the choice between open, illuminated space and a dark secure compartment. The light–dark box test represents a simple version of this assay. Two boxes are connected by a tunnel, one of them is dark and the other is brightly lit. The ratio of time an animal spends in the two boxes is measured as a readout for anxiety. Various stressors, including mild electric shock, are sometimes added to the open space to increase the magnitude of the difference between secure and dangerous space. These light–dark tests respond well to benzodiazepines and antidepressant monoamine uptake blockers (Hascoet et al., 2001).

In the marble-burying test single rodents are put in a cage with bedding and a number of marbles. The animals have the natural tendency to bury the marbles. Under stress or dangerous conditions this behavior is abolished. Benzodiazepine drugs increase the number of marbles buried. The marble-burying test is technically very simple and serves well those investigators, who are not equipped for complex behavioral assays, to quickly assess the anxiolytic potential of a compound. Stress-induced hyperthermia is another very simple test that does not require special equipment. A group of animals is put into a common cage. The animals are removed, one after the other, and their rectal temperature is measured. The temperature of the animals taken at the end is slightly higher than those taken at the beginning. The difference of the two mean temperatures serves as readout of stress or anxiety. The test responds well to benzodiazepine drugs that serve as positive controls.

The social exploration test focuses on fear-related aspects of social interactions. A rodent that has been kept in isolation is moved to a cage with another animal. The intruder animal has tendency to approach and explore the resident rat by sniffing, grooming, licking, and other species-specific social behaviors. Benzodiazepines increase the amount of time spent in social interactions. The test exists in many variations and is often used to predict anxiolytic effects of drugs, in particular, for their ability to counteract social phobia.

Defensive behavior assays attempt to measure reactions of the animals to dangerous stimuli. Intruder animals, predators, serve as natural stimuli. In many tests they are replaced by artificial substitutes such as electric shock coupled to a light flash. The defensive behaviors include defensive burying, believed to be an escape reaction of the animals, and "freezing," an immobility reaction that is used by many wild animals to avoid predators (De Boer and Koolhaas, 2003).

Fear conditioning, discussed earlier in the context of amygdala function, is based on the freezing reaction in the defensive behavior repertoire. In the traditional fear-conditioning paradigm, the behavioral freezing of mice or rats is measured in response to a conditioned stimulus that has been associated with shock or danger. The fear-potentiated startle assay represents a more elaborate version of the same assay. If a loud tone rather than light is used as conditioned stimulus, the animals show a startle response, they typically jump up. This whole body startling response can be quantified by measuring the force the animals apply to the floor during the jump.

The Geller-Seifert test creates a situation of conflict for the animals that may be related to anxiety states. Rodents are put in a box that provides access to food and allows the experimenter to apply mild food shocks. Access to the food pellets is indicated by lights. When a white light flashes, there is direct food access; when the light is red, the food access is paired with shock. The number of times an animal goes to the food following the red light is measured as "punished response". Benzodiazepines increase the punished response rate, in support of the view that the model can serve to predict anxiolytic effects. The Vogel conflict test is very similar to the Geller-Seifert test. Access to water rather than food is being used as unconditional stimulus. Animals are kept slightly thirsty. The number of times they overcome the fear of the shock and exhibit the punished response serves as readout in this test.

These tests all measure different facets of animal behavior related to fear and anxiety. Many variants of these tests have been described in the scientific literature, and the list of those mentioned above cannot be considered complete. All assays listed are responsive to benzodiazepine drugs that validate them as anxiety assays. The effects of monoamine uptake blockers, including those approved for the clinical use to treat anxiety, are less robust. In same of the assays they produce the opposite, anxiogenic response. There is therefore no perfect or uniformly accepted animal model for anxiety. Furthermore, as is often the case for behavioral assays, variations in animal strains used or minor experimental details can affect the outcome of the studies in anxiety models. Animal behavioral experimentation in support of drug discovery programs for anxiety disorders remains a difficult and complex field.

Table 8.2   Animal models of anxiety

Elevated plus maze
Light–dark box test
Marble-burying test
Stress-induced hyperthermia
Social exploration test
Defensive behavior to intruder or predator
Fear conditioning
Fear-potentiated startle
Geller-Seifert conflict test
Vogel conflict test

8.4.2 Correlating Animal Models with Human Experimental Anxiety

Clinical trials in general anxiety disorders are difficult, similar to the situation in depression. Placebo effects are massive and typically larger than those produced by the drugs themselves. The patient population is heterogeneous in general anxiety disorder. Related conditions, such as social phobia, obsessive-compulsive disorder, and premenstrual syndrome, pose yet additional complexities for clinical trials. Several experimental anxiety models in humans have been investigated for their ability to predict success in studies on patients.

The abundance of available animal assays that are used as models of human anxiety begs the question of the most suitable or most useful one. A lot of time and effort can be spent during the preclinical evaluation of drug candidates, testing them in all the existing animal assays, although such broad testing does not increase the probability of clinical success. Priority needs to be given to the models that directly relate to human conditions. Are there animal models that directly correlate to human experimental conditions and, furthermore, to specific subforms of human anxiety disorders? Successful identification of such direct pathways from animal to human studies will increase the probability of success of the compounds in clinical studies with patients suffering from anxiety disorders (Fig. 8.4).

Simulated public speaking is the mildest currently used experimental human model of anxiety (Graeff et al., 2001). Volunteers are put into a situation that mimics the situation of a speaker addressing a large, potentially critical audience at a scientific or political meeting. Heart rate and blood pressure are measured as parameters reflecting functions of the autonomic nervous. A questionnaire and rating scale serve to evaluate the subjective feeling of anxiety of the subject after the trial. Benzodiazepines have been reported to reduce these parameters. However, the results tend not to be very robust and the model requires further work before it can be considered established. Simulated public speaking

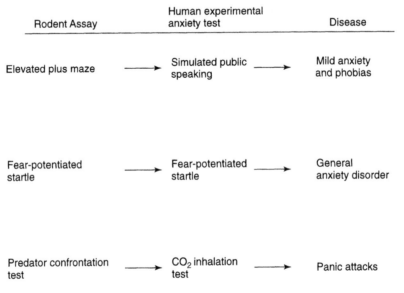

Figure 8.4 Pathways from animal models to human experimental conditions to human disease trials in anxiety disorders.

is a relatively mild condition that reflects a naturally occurring situation. Among the animal models, those reflecting natural situations represent the best analogues. The path from testing a drug candidate in the elevated plus maze in rodents, to testing it in humans in the simulated public speaking model, to clinical studies in mild forms of anxiety, seems intuitively correct. Many additional studies will be needed to properly validate it.

In the CO_2 inhalation test, human subjects are briefly exposed to elevated concentrations of CO_2 that generate the transient feeling of asphyxia or drowning (Shipherd et al., 2001). While transient and relatively mild, these sensations are perceived as unpleasant, stressful, and they generate the feeling of fear and anxiety. Benzodiazepines have been reported to blunt these responses. There is no directly comparable animal model at the present time. Defensive behavior and predator confrontation models perhaps represent suitable comparator models, since they also feature the instant exposure to potentially a life-threatening situation. Therefore the sequential evaluation of test compounds in predator confrontation assays in rodents, the experimental human CO_2 inhalation test, and the clinical trials in patients suffering from panic attacks may represent an effective pathway of drug discovery and development.

Fear-potentiation assays can be done on humans as well as on animals. Volunteers are given a mild electric shock to the skin, of just sufficient strength to make it slightly unpleasant. Lights of different colors indicate time intervals during which a shock stimulus may occur, or that are safe. The actual shock is preceded by a loud noise that elicits eye blinking, a startling response reflex. This reflex is triggered by the noise alone, but the magnitude of the startling response is greater during time periods the shock may occur. The difference in the magnitude of the startling response serves as readout of anxiety. In the practical test situation, the shock is applied only very rarely, since the anticipation of a shock is sufficient to increase the eye blink reflex. In the corresponding fear-potentiated startle animal assay, the whole body startling response is measured rather than the eye blink reflex. Otherwise, the two test situations are very similar. Therefore the sequential evaluation of compounds in an animal fear-potentiated startle assay, a human fear-potentiated startle test, and in clinical trials with patients suffering from general anxiety disorder presents itself as an attractive pathway for drug development.

Research on human experimental anxiety models is still at an early stage. Public speaking tests, CO_2 inhalation assays, and fear-potentiated startle tests remain to be fully validated by drugs that are clinically used. If successful, these studies bring significant progress to the evaluation of drug candidates in anxiety disorders because they will make it possible to pick early the most promising candidates from an increasingly large field of contenders.

8.5 CONCLUSIONS

Anxiety disorders encompass general anxiety disorder, panic attacks, post-traumatic stress disorder, and many additional conditions with an anxiety component, such as obsessive-compulsive disorder and premenstrual syndrome. Since anxiety is a natural part of human behavior, the border between normal and pathological anxiety is blurred and strongly dependent on cultural norms and values. Many anxiety disorders have depression as a component, and the symptomatology of depression often includes excessive anxiety. The separation between anxiety and depression is thus somewhat artificial, although it is generally accepted in modern medical science. Anxiety disorders are frequent and represent a substantial medical need.

Anxiety is linked to the feeling of fear, a subjective feeling believed to be present in animals and to be primitive from an evolutionary point of view. In animals, fear manifests itself in escape and defense responses, behavioral phenomena that are open to neurobiological investigations. The studies of fear mechanisms in the brain have delineated functional fear pathway that give a central role to the amygdala, a subcortical nucleus in the forebrain. No disease genes associated with anxiety have been described as yet.

The current treatment of anxiety disorders uses benzodiazepine drugs, antidepressant monoamine uptake blockers, and buspirone. Benzodiazepines are effective, but their use is limited by the associated sedation and the concerns about their addictive potential. Antidepressants have been proved to be effective in subgroups of anxiety disorders in clinical trials. Buspirone, an agonist to the 5-HT_{1A} serotonin receptor subtype, is an approved but marginally effective drug.

Drug discovery for anxiety disorders is a very active field that is generating an interesting stream of novel drug candidates. Subtype selective benzodiazepine receptor site ligands have been generated that selectively act on those GABA-A receptors mediating the anxiolytic response. Many other putative drug targets have been identified through tests in animal models of anxiety. They include mGluR2, mGluR5, mGluR7, and mGluR8 metabotropic glutamate receptors, V_{1b} vasopressin receptors, and the ORL1 neuropeptide receptor. Functional studies of amygdala fear pathways have identified the receptors for gastrin-releasing peptide (GRPR), NPY-Y2 receptors, sst(2A) somatostatin, as well as CRF_1 receptors as putative drug targets. They also provide a neurobiological basis for the anxiolytic activity of cannabinoid CB_1 receptor ligands.

Clinical trials in anxiety disorders are difficult because of patient heterogeneity and large placebo effects. The number of emerging drug candidates with novel, not clinically validated targets may soon exceed the financial and organizational capacity of the biomedical industry, making it necessary to establish selection criteria before large-scale clinical trials. A coordinated approach linking animal anxiety models to human experimental anxiety and specific anxiety disorders appears most attractive for this purpose.

REFERENCES

Further Reading

DE BOER, S.F., and KOOLHAAS, J.M. Defensive burying in rodents: Ethology, neurobiology and psychopharmacology. *Eur. J. Pharmacol.* 463: 145–161, 2003.

GORMAN, J.M. Treating generalized anxiety disorder. *J. Clin. Psych.* 64 (suppl. 2): 24–29, 2003.

HASCOET, M., BOURIN, M., and DHONNCHADHA, B.A. The mouse light-dark paradigm: A review. *Prog. Neuropsychopharmacol. Biol. Psych.* 25: 141–166, 2001.

HIDALGO, R.B., BARNETT, S.D., and DAVIDSON, R.T. Social anxiety disorder in review: Two decades of progress. *Int. J. Neuropsychopharm.* 4: 279–298, 2001.

LEDOUX, J.E. Emotion circuits in the brain. *An. Rev. Neurosci.* 23: 155–184, 2000.

NINAN, P.T. The functional anatomy, neurochemistry, and pharmacology of anxiety. *J. Clin. Psych.* 60 (suppl. 22): 12–17, 1999.

SAH, P., FABER, E.S., LOPEZ DE ARMENTIA, M., and POWER, J. The amygdaloid complex: Anatomy and physiology. *Physiol. Rev.* 83: 803–834, 2003.

SUNDSTROM POROMAA, I., SMITH, S., and GULINELLO, M. GABA receptors, progesterone and premenstrual dysphoric disorder. *Arch. Women Ment. Health* 6: 23–41, 2003.

STEIN, D.J. Obsessive-compulsive disorder. *Lancet* 360: 397–405, 2002.

Citations

BISSIERE, S., HUMEAU, Y., and LUTHI, A. Dopamine gates LTP induction in lateral amygdala by suppressing feed-forward inhibition. *Nature Neurosci.* 6: 587–591, 2003.

BRODKIN, J., BRADBURY, M., BUSSE, C., WARREN, N., BRISTOW, L.J., and VARNEY, M.A. Reduced stress-induced hyperthermia in mGluR5 knockout mice. *Eur. J. Neurosci.* 16: 2241–2244, 2003.

CHENG, J.P., REICH, L., and CHUNG, H. Anxiety disorders. *West J. Med.* 176: 249–253, 2002.

COSFORD, N.D., TEHRANI, L., ROPPE, J., SCHWEIGER, E., SMITH, N.D., ANDERSON, J., BRISTOW, L., BRODKIN, J., JIANG, X., MCDONALD, I., RAO, S., WASHBURN, M., and VARNEY, M.A. 3[(2-Methyl-1,3-thiazol-4-yl)ethynyl]-pyridine: A potent and highly selective metabotropic glutamate subtype 5 receptor antagonist with anxiolytic activity. *J. Med. Chem.* 46: 204–206, 2003.

CRYAN, J.F., KELLY, P.H., NEIJT, H.C., SANSIG, G., FLOR, P.J., and VAN DER PUTTEN, H. Antidepressant and anxiolytic-like effects in mice lacking the group III metabotropic glutamate receptor mGluR7. *Eur. J. Neurosci.* 17: 2409–2417, 2003.

DOWD, S.M., STRONG, M.J., JANICAK, P.G., and NEGRUSZ, A. The behavioral and cognitive effects of two benzodiazepines associated with drug-facilitated sexual assault. *J. Forensic. Sci.* 47: 1101–1007, 2002.

GADD, C.A., MURTRA, P., DE FELIPE, C., and HUNT, S.P. Neurokinin-1 receptor-expressing neurons in the amygdala modulate morphine reward and anxiety behaviors in the mouse. *J. Neurosci.* 23: 8271–8280, 2003.

GRAEFF, F.G., SILVA, M., DEL BEN, C.M., ZUARDI, A.W., HETEM, L.A., and GUIMARAES, F.S. Comparison between two models of experimental anxiety in healthy volunteers and panic disorder patients. *Neurosci. Biobehav. Rev.* 25: 753–759, 2001.

GRIEBEL, G., SIMIAND, J., SERRADEIL-LE GAL, C., WAGNON, J., PASCAL, M., SCATTON, B., MAFFRAND, J.P., and SOUBRIE, P. Anxiolytic- and antidepressant-like effects of the non-peptide vasopressin V1b receptor antagonists, SSR149415, suggest an innovative approach for the treatment of stress-related disorders. *Proc. Natl. Acad. Sci. USA* 99: 6370–6375, 2002.

GRIEBEL, G., PERRAULT, G., SIMIAND, J., COHEN, C., GRANGER, P., DEPOORTERE, H., FRANCON, D., AVENET, P., SCHOEMAKER, H., EVANNO, Y., SEVRIN, M., GEORGE, P., and SCATTON, B. SL651498, a GABA-A receptor agonist with subtype-selective efficacy, as a potential treatment for generalized anxiety disorder and muscle spasms. *CNS Drug Rev.* 9: 3–20, 2003.

GRILLON, C., CORDOVA, J., LEVINE, L.R., and MORGAN, C.A. Anxiolytic effects of a novel group II metabotropic glutamate receptor agonist (LY354740) in the fear-potentiated startle paradigm in humans. Psychopharmacology 168: 446–454, 2003.

GULINELLO, M., ORMAN, R., and SMITH, S.S. Sex differences in anxiety, sensorimotor gating and expression of the α4 subunit of the GABA-A receptor in the amygdala after progesterone withdrawal. *Eur. J. Neurosci.* 17: 641–648, 2003.

JENCK, F., WICHMANN, J., DAUTZENBERG, F.M., MOREAU, J.L., OUAGAZZAL, A.M., MARTIN, J.R., LUNDSTROM, K., CESURA, A.M., POLI, S.M., ROEVER, S., KOLCZEWSKI, S., ADAM, G., and KILPATRICK, G. A synthetic agonist at the orphanin FQ/nociception receptor ORL1: Anxiolytic profile in the rat. *Proc. Natl. Acad. Sci. USA* 97: 4983–4943, 2000.

KATONA, I., RANCZ, E.A., ACSADY, L., LEDENT, C., MACKIE, K., HAJOS, N., and FREUND, T.F. Distribution of CB1 cannabinoid receptors in the amygdala and their role in the control of GABAergic transmission. *J. Neurosci.* 21: 9506–9518, 2001.

KAUFMANN, W.A., HUMPEL, C., ALHEID, G.F., and MARKSTEINER, J. Compartmentation of alpha 1 and alpha 2 GABA(A) receptor subunits with rat extended amygdala: implications for benzodiazepine action. *Brain Res.* 964: 91–99, 2003.

KESSLER, R.C., and WITTCHEN, H.U. Patterns and correlates of generalized anxiety disorders in community samples. *J. Clin. Psych.* 63 (suppl. 8): 4–10, 2002.

LALUMIERE, R.T., BUEN, T.V., and MCGAUGH, J.L. Post-training intra-basolateral amygdala infusions of norepinephrine enhance consolidation of memory for contextual fear conditioning. *J. Neurosci.* 23: 6754–6758, 2003.

LINDEN, A.M., JOHNSON, B.G., PETERS, S.C., SHANNON, H.E., TIAN, M., WANG, Y., YU, J.L., KOSTER, A., BAEZ, M., and SCHOEPP, D.D. Increased anxiety-related behavior in mice deficient for metabotropic glutamate 8 (mGlu8) receptor. *Neuropharmacology* 43: 251–259, 2002.

RODRIGUES, S.M., BAUER, E.P., FARB, C.R., SCHAFE, G.E., and LEDOUX, J.E. The group I metabotropic glutamate receptor mGluR5 is required for fear memory formation and long-term potentiation in the lateral amygdala. *J. Neurosci.* 22: 5219–5229, 2002.

ROOZENDAAL, B., BRUNSON, K.L., HOLLOWAY, B.L., MCGAUGH, J.L., and BARAM, T.Z. Involvement of stress-released corticotrophin-releasing hormone in the basolateral amygdala in regulating memory consolidation. *Proc. Natl. Acad. Sci. USA* 99: 13908–13913, 2002.

SALZMAN, C. Addiction to benzodiazepines. *Psychiatr. Q.* 69: 251–161, 1998.

SHIPHERD, J.C., BECK, J.G., and OHTAKE, P.J. Relationships between the anxiety sensitivity index, the suffocation fear scale, and responses to CO_2 inhalation. *J. Anxiety Disord.* 15: 247–258, 2001.

SHORS, T.J., and MIESEGAES, G. Testosterone in utero and at birth dictates how stressful experience will affect learning in adulthood. *Proc. Natl. Acad. Sci. USA* 99: 13955–13960, 2002.

SHORTER, E., and TYRER, P. Separation of anxiety and depressive disorders: blind alley in psychopharmacology and classification of disease. *Br. Med. J.* 327: 158–160, 2003.

SHUMYATSKY, G.P., TSEVETKOV, E., MALLERET, G., VRONSKAYA, S., HATTON, M., HAMPTON, L., BATTEY, J.F., DULAC, C., KANDEL, E.R., and BOLSHAKOV, V.Y. Identification of a signaling network in lateral nucleus of amygdala important for inhibiting memory specifically related to learned fear. *Cell* 111: 905–918, 2002.

TSCHENETT, A., SINGEWALD, N., CARLI, M., BALDUCCI, C., SALCHNER, P., VEZZANI, A., HERZOG, H., and SPERK, G. Reduced anxiety and improved stress coping ability in mice lacking NPY-Y2 receptors. *Eur. J. Neurosci.* 18: 143–148, 2003.

TWYMAN, R.E., ROGERS, C.J., and MACDONALD, R.L. Differential regulation of gamma-aminobutyric acid receptor channels by diazepam and phenobarbital. *An. Neurol.* 25: 213–220, 1989.

WALKER, D.L., RATTINER, L.M., and DAVIS, M. Group II metabotropic glutamate receptors within the amygdala regulate fear as assessed with potentiated startle in rats. *Behav. Neurosci.* 116: 1075–1083, 2002.

Chapter 9

Alzheimer's Disease

Loss of memory and cognitive abilities during the course of aging has been considered normal and inevitable for most of human history.

> *A good old man, sir; he will be talking: as they say,*
> *When the age is in the wit is out.*
>   *Shakespeare, Much Ado About Nothing*

The quotation from Shakespeare's play must have been common language, and it reflects common thinking to modern times. Only recently, because of the massive increase in the population of the elderly, has it become evident that people differ enormously in the rate of intellectual decline during aging. Some humans retain high abilities for reasoning and memory into their advanced years. Others go through a relatively rapid process of memory loss, decline of cognitive abilities, to a final stage without speech and recognition. The former president of the United States of America, Ronald Reagan, was believed to have mild memory problems during the final years in office; a decade later he had no recollection of his political past.

Today Alzheimer's disease is recognized as an illness that affects a high percentage of the elderly and that destroys brain matter and function. The name of the disease honors Dr. Alois Alzheimer, a neuropathologist who worked in Munich, Germany, at the beginning of the twentieth century, and who first recognized the correlation between pathological features in the brain and the behavioral consequences. The disease he discovered is a cruel one. It affects and gradually destroys the brain, the essence of human life. At the beginning of the disease, people become less able to remember new events, their ability to make judgmental decisions gets eroded, and they find it difficult to orient themselves in their surroundings. In the advanced stages, they loose their ability to recognize relatives, including their own children or spouses. At the very end, a vegetative state remains where people have no cogniscence of the self and the world.

Alzheimer's disease has become one of the most significant medical and societal problems. Emotional and financial costs are enormous. Caregivers are particularly severely affected. The opposite of helping a child to gain increasing abilities during education, giving care to an Alzheimer patient means assisting a person through progressing and irreversible decline. At advanced stages patients require constant supervision and care, which is very costly in a private or nursing home setting. Alzheimer's disease creates fear of aging in many people. Patients regret their own fate as well as the fact that they are a burden to others. The current therapy makes a marginal difference only. Finding treatment that effectively slows down or blocks the progression of Alzheimer's disease is one of the most important goals of modern drug discovery.

Drug Discovery for Nervous System Diseases. by Franz F. Hefti
ISBN 0-471-46563-1   Copyright © 2005 by John Wiley & Sons, Inc.

9.1 SYMPTOMS AND DISEASE MECHANISM

Alzheimer's disease affects 1 to 2% of the human population. Its prevalence increases with age. At the age of 65, approximately 10% of the population suffers from Alzheimer's disease. At 85, the prevalence increases to 40 to 50%. The correlation between age and prevalence seems to be linear or even exponential, suggesting that if it was possible to extend the human life span beyond the current maximum of 125 years, everybody would come down with Alzheimer's disease. Mild reductions of memory and cognition are a normal feature of aging. Since the severe impairments of Alzheimer's disease seem inevitable given enough time, the illness is sometimes considered an accelerated form of brain aging.

Alzheimer's disease is considered a multifactorial disease with genetic and environmental contributions to the causative factors. A small number of familial forms have been discovered in which a single dominant genetic mutation is sufficient to cause Alzheimer's disease. The discovery of the disease genes had enormous impact for the understanding of the disease mechanisms, but the vast majority of the cases are not caused by such mutations. A protein involved in cholesterol transport, apolipoprotein E (ApoE), has been identified as genetic susceptibility factor. Three alleles of this protein exist (ϵ2, ϵ3, and ϵ4). People carrying the ApoEϵ4 allele have a gene dosage-dependent increase in the risk to be diagnosed with Alzheimer's disease. No material environmental risk factor has been identified. Education seems to reduce the risk.

Alzheimer's disease is a neurodegenerative disease. The brain undergoes structural atrophy. The brain matter shrinks and the number of synapses and neurons declines. Pathological structural features, neuritic plaques and neurofibrillary tangles, appear. Both structures are ordered aggregates of protein fragments. Both are easily visualized in sections of postmortem brain material. The demonstration of plaques and tangles in brain sections provides the conclusive diagnosis of Alzheimer's disease. However, the specific nature of the memory and cognitive loss, together with imaging studies and measurements of disease-related markers in the CSF, allow physicians to diagnose Alzheimer's disease in living patients with over 95% accuracy.

The biochemical analysis of neuritic plaques together with the identification of specific genes that cause Alzheimer's disease has led to a widely accepted concept of the disease mechanism, referred to as the amyloid hypothesis. This hypothesis puts the amyloid precursor protein (APP) and its fragment (Aβ) into the center of the pathological process. Detailed studies of the function and processing of this protein have identified a small number of highly attractive putative drug targets. The discussion of these targets takes up a large fraction of this chapter, since they are expected to lead to disease-modifying drugs that slow down or even stop the degenerative processes and the resulting memory loss. The currently available drugs, to be discussed first, modify synaptic actions in the brain and provide only palliative remedy without affecting the underlying disease process.

9.2 CHOLINERGIC DEFICIT AND ACETYLCHOLINESTERASE INHIBITORS

In advanced Alzheimer's disease ventricles and the fluid-filled spaces of the cerebral sulci are enlarged at the expense of brain matter. The number of nerve cells is massively reduced, in the cerebral cortex in particular as well as in the associated areas such as the hippocampus. It is difficult to imagine how any therapeutic approach might be successful in such advanced stages of degeneration. However, at early stages of the disease the neuronal populations are not uniformly affected. The cholinergic neurons of the basal forebrain are a prominent neuronal population that undergoes atrophic changes at the beginning of the disease. The cell bodies of these neurons are located in the septum and the nucleus basalis, a loosely defined structure at the base of the forebrain. These neurons provide a divergent projection to the hippocampus and all cortical areas. The hippocampus plays a prominent role in memory processes. Lesions of the hippocampus strongly impair memory in animals and humans. Long-term potentiation (LTP), the enhancement of synaptic strength following multiple uses, is a common feature in the hippocampus and is believed to be linked to memory. Hippocampal LTP is regulated by cholinergic afferents. Selective lesions of the cholinergic input in animals impair memory performance while leaving other behavioral functions intact. Pharmacological studies provide a bridge from animals to humans. Antagonists of cholinergic receptors, atropine and scopolamine, impair memory in all species. Scopolamine has a notorious reputation because it has been used to disturb the memory of prisoners during interrogations in order to extract more confidential information from them. Together, these observations make a convincing case that cholinergic neurons of the basal forebrain are important for memory functions.

The realization that the cholinergic neurons are among the earliest neuronal populations affected in Alzheimer's disease and that they are involved in memory functions has led to the hypothesis that cholinergic neurotransmitter replacement therapy might be beneficial in Alzheimer's disease. Early efforts reflected the successful experience in Parkinson's disease and attempted to increase the synaptic concentration of acetylcholine by providing the metabolic precursor molecules. Choline, the immediate precursor of acetylcholine, and lecithin, a natural lipid and food component that contains choline were tried in animals and taken into exploratory clinical studies. While encouraging findings emerged in animal experiments, human studies did not substantiate the expectations. The second approach, increasing acetylcholine levels by blocking its enzymatic degradation, turned out to be more successful. Inhibitors of acetylcholinesterase, the enzyme uniquely responsible for terminating the synaptic action of acetylcholine, provide marginal, but statistically significant improvements of memory functions in Alzheimer's patients (Fig. 9.1). In absence of more effective drugs, they are widely prescribed.

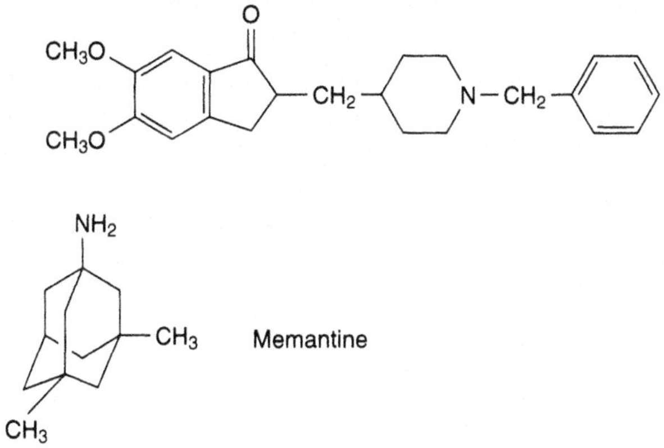

Figure 9.1 Drugs currently approved for the treatment of Alzheimer's disease. Donepezil is one of several approved inhibitors of acetylcholinesterase.

Acetylcholinesterase inhibitors potentiate cholinergic synaptic functions throughout the body. Complete blockage of the enzymatic activity in the synapses of the autonomic nervous system produces multiple, severe adverse effects that are ultimately fatal. Acetylcholinesterase inhibitors are among the most toxic compounds known, and they have been generated in large amounts for potential use as war poisons. The adverse effects drastically limit the doses that can be given to Alzheimer patients for therapeutic effects on their memory functions. It is possible that stronger cholinergic stimulation in the hippocampus might produce more robust effects on memory. Cholinergic receptors selectively expressed in the hippocampus thus represent attractive putative drug targets. The hippocampus is rich in muscarinic M1 receptors and $\alpha4\beta2$ or $\alpha7$ nicotinic receptors. Observations at M1 knockout mice suggest selective involvement of this receptor in memory functions. Several selective M1 agonists have been generated that enhance memory functions in animal assays. The M1 receptors thus represent an attractive putative drug target for palliative treatment of Alzheimer's disease (Anagnostaras et al., 2003). Subtype selective nicotinic receptor agonists are appealing as well, although the supportive evidence is not as strong as that for M1 muscarinic agonists. A compound with limited subtype selectivity for receptors containing the $\beta4$ subunit enhanced memory functions in rodents and primates (Schneider et al., 2003).

The cholinergic neurons of the basal forebrain express TrkA receptors for nerve growth factor (NGF), the initially discovered member of the neurotrophin protein family. The expression is highly selective in the brain. Besides the forebrain cholinergic neurons, and a few small populations of thalamic neurons, only the peripheral sympathetic and sensory neurons express TrkA and respond to NGF. The selectivity of the expression has prompted the speculation that administration of NGF into the brain may counteract the cholinergic neuron degeneration in Alzheimer's disease and so restore some of their memory functions (Lad et al., 2003). In animals, NGF stimulates the synthesis of proteins that support synaptic functions of cholinergic neurons and increases their ability to recover from injury and age-related atrophy. Improved memory functions reflect these molecular effects. Very limited clinical trials in which NGF was infused into the cerebral ventricles of Alzheimer patients, however, revealed pain as an adverse effect. The bulk of the NGF given into the ventricles appears to be rapidly transported to the central canal of the spinal cord, where it may induce hypertrophy of TrkA-expressing sensory neurons that mediate pain. To be useful therapeutically, NGF will thus have to be given locally to the forebrain cholinergic neurons. Attempts to deliver NGF by cell therapy or gene therapy into the basal forebrain are currently being pursued (Tuszynski and Blesch, 2004). The attempts to use NGF in Alzheimer's disease is an example of intracerebral neurotrophic factor therapy, a strategy to be discussed further in Chapter 10 on Parkinson's disease.

The clinical experience with acetylcholinesterase inhibitors supports further efforts toward treatments that enhance cholinergic neuron survival and function. Since the degeneration of the cholinergic neurons is an early event in Alzheimer's disease pathology, the resulting drugs will be useful for initial stages of the disease. Cholinergic replacement strategies are not expected to modify the progression of the disease or to be effective at advanced stages, when many other neuron populations have degenerated. Observations on transgenic animal models of Alzheimer's disease that reflect the disease process suggest that the cholinergic neuron deficit is a secondary event (German et al., 2003). Much more significant benefits than those obtained through cholinergic strategies are thus expected from drugs that modify the disease mechanism as discussed below.

9.3 AMYLOID HYPOTHESIS AND DISEASE-MODIFYING DRUGS

Alzheimer's disease presents the most convincing example in support of the view that the study of disease mechanisms map out the direct way to the identification of drug targets. The analysis of pathological brain structures in the brain of patients together with genetic studies of familial forms of Alzheimer's disease have led to a convincing concept of the disease mechanism and to novel drug targets. In 1984, Glenner and collaborators, working at the University of California, San Diego, published the amino acid sequence of a peptide they isolated from the brain of Alzheimer disease patients. The peptide, now called Aβ, was recognized to be a major component of neuritic plaques and identified as a fragment of an abundant brain protein, called amyloid precursor protein (APP). Just a few years later, in 1992, several research groups published that rare familial forms of Alzheimer's disease were caused by mutations of the *APP* gene. In 1996, additional mutations were identified in an enzyme that processes APP and generates the Aβ peptide. The mutations occurred in proteins called presenilin-1 and -2 (PS1 and PS2) that are part of a multimeric complex with proteolytic activity. The initially independent genetic and pathological investigations merged into common concepts and molecular biological approaches to further elucidate the disease mechanism.

Many additional studies around the essential initial findings have generated a detailed picture of the disease pathways in Alzheimer's disease. This concept, typically referred to as the amyloid hypothesis, ascribes the central role to the Aβ peptide. APP, from which Aβ is derived, is a neuronal protein that is expressed at high levels throughout the nervous system. It is a transmembranal protein located on intracellular membranes and the plasma membrane. APP is necessary for normal nervous system function, since gene knockout mice show a gradual loss of synaptic structures with increasing age. Three proteases are able to cleave APP (Fig. 9.2). α-Secretase cleaves APP just outside of the single transmembranal sequence and within the Aβ peptide. This enzymatic step thus precludes the formation of the Aβ peptide. β-Secretase, also called β-site APP cleaving enzyme-1 (BACE1), performs the *N*-terminal cleavage of Aβ on the extracellular or lumen side of the membrane. γ-Secretase, the third enzyme, is an intramembranal protease that cleaves the *C*-terminal end of Aβ. The γ-secretase enzyme is not entirely specific since it produces two forms of Aβ that differ by two amino acids, Aβ1-40 and Aβ1-42.

Once formed, the Aβ peptide quickly aggregates and forms oligomers that further assemble to larger polymeric complexes and finally to the highly ordered aggregates of

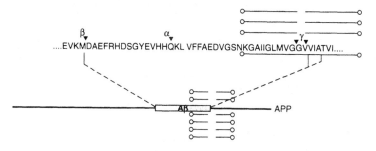

Figure 9.2 Cleavage of APP and formation of the Aβ peptide. Cleavage by the β-secretase generates the *N*-terminus of the peptide. The intramembrane cleavage by the γ-secretase generates the *C*-terminus of the two forms of Aβ, Aβ$_{1-40}$, and Aβ$_{1-42}$. Cleavage by the α-secretase generates a soluble fragment of APP and precludes the formation of Aβ.

the plaques. Aβ monomers and oligomers, also called Alzheimer's disease diffusible ligands (ADDLs), are believed to exert toxic effects on synaptic and cellular functions that ultimately lead to cell death (Gong et al., 2003). The exact mechanism of this toxicity remains to be established. No selective receptor has been identified for Aβ monomers, which is linked to cell degeneration and death. Toxic effects in cell cultures require concentrations higher than those expected to occur in the brain. Aβ oligomers, the ADDLs, may thus be the actual culprit, since they are toxic at low concentrations. At the early stages of Alzheimer's disease, the toxic effects of Aβ monomers or oligomers are believed to lead to synaptic dysfunction and the degeneration of specific, highly vulnerable cells. The further progress of the disease brings degenerative changes, and ultimately death, to many more populations of neurons, in particular, those of the cerebral cortex and the associated areas. Dementia, the behavioral consequence of Alzheimer's disease, is caused by the progressive loss of synapses and neurons. According to the amyloid hypothesis, the formation of neuritic plaques has no direct consequence. They are believed to be inactive deposits of excessive Aβ. The plaques are not metabolically inert, but Aβ contained in them can rapidly exchange with free Aβ peptide. The second pathological structure seen in the Alzheimer brain, the neurofibrillary tangles, are believed to be by-products of neuronal atrophy and degeneration.

The cascade of events predicted by the amyloid hypothesis is illustrated in Figure 9.3. The strongest support for the this view of events is provided by transgenic mice that express the mutated human forms of APP, PS1, or PS2 that cause Alzheimer's disease. Various strains of such mice have been generated. They share the reproduction of the determining feature of Alzheimer's disease. They all have significant deposits of plaques, the density of which increases over time. In the most rapidly progressing strains, plaque

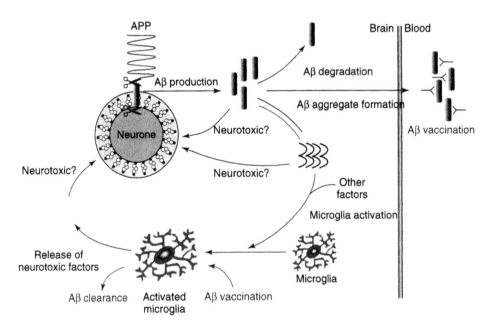

Figure 9.3   The amyloid hypothesis of the disease mechanism in Alzheimer's disease and drug targets identified by it. Inhibition of production, aggregation and toxic effects of Aβ is expected to slow down disease progression. The removal of Aβ with antibodies represents an attractive alternative strategy. (Reprinted with permission, Dominguez and Stooper, 2002, Elsevier)

accumulation is visible after a few months only. In all of them plaques become abundant after 12 months, in the second half of the animal's life span. Increased levels of Aβ can be measured in the brain even before plaque deposition occurs. Some, but not all, of the strains show behavioral deficits. These deficits tend to be small and require specific memory test settings to become evident. Some, but not all, of the strains show changes in synaptic density, whereas neuronal deficits have not been convincingly demonstrated in any of the strains so far. Some investigators reported that the behavioral and synaptic deficits precede the accumulation of plaques. These finding clearly supports the view that Aβ monomers or oligomers rather than the neuritic plaques are the main culprit of the disease.

9.3.1 β-Secretase Inhibitors

The amyloid cascade hypothesis identifies a small number of obvious drug targets (Fig. 9.3) (Dominiguez and de Stooper, 2002; Selkoe and Schenk, 2003). The most attractive among them is β-secretase, the protease that selectively cleaves APP to form the *N*-terminal of the Aβ peptide. Prevention of this catalytic event precludes the formation of Aβ and is thus expected to stop the Alzheimer's disease cascade. β-Secretase is a membrane bound aspartyl protease that is highly expressed in the brain. Its function seems to be specific for APP processing. Knockout mice are unable to generate the Aβ peptide, but they do not have any evident morphological or biochemical deficits. Possibly a highly homologous enzyme, BACE2, that does not cleave APP compensates for physiological functions of β-secretase in the knockout animals.

The selectivity of β-secretase for APP is an enormous advantage from a point of view of drug discovery, since it reduces the probability of mechanism-based adverse events. Many biopharmaceutical companies have embraced this unique target opportunity. Several peptidic inhibitors have been identified that are based on the amino acid sequence of APP sequence around the β cleavage site. The most potent ones incorporate the amino acid sequence of an Alzheimer's disease causing mutation, the so-called Swedish mutation, which changes two amino acids in the cleavage area and increases the catalytic efficacy of β-secretase. Modified peptides have been generated with high affinity for β-secretase and able to inhibit Aβ formation in cell culture assays. However, to be clinically useful β-secretase inhibitors will have to penetrate the blood-brain barrier, something the peptidic inhibitors are unable to do. The crystal structure of β-secretase suggests that the inhibitors assume an extended confirmation when bound to the enzyme. This creates a difficult situation for small molecule inhibitors that typically are more easily found for three-dimensional binding pockets. The search for a brain penetrant β-secretase inhibitor thus represents a most challenging and most rewarding goal for medicinal chemists (Wolfe, 2001).

9.3.2 γ-Secretase Inhibitors

γ-Secretase is the second obvious drug target suggested by the amyloid cascade hypothesis. It is necessary for the cleavage of the *C*-terminal of the Aβ peptide, and its inhibition alone will preclude the formation of the Aβ peptide. Although the catalytic domain of the γ-secretase contains two aspartates that also identify it as an aspartyl protease, its molecular nature and pharmacological specificity is very different from β-secretase. The catalytic domain is contained in the sequences of the presenilins, PS1 and PS2. However, to be catalytically active, the presenilins require the additional proteins nicastrin, Aph-1 and Pen-2, which together form a multimeric enzyme complex. In contrast to the β cleavage site of APP, which is just outside of the plasma membrane, the γ cleavage site is within the membrane. The γ-secretase enzyme is not specific for APP but cleaves several other proteins that are important for cell functions. Among them are notch, a signaling molecule that is important in immune functions, and ErbB4, a tyrosine kinase receptor mediating the actions of members of the epidermal growth factor family. The multiple roles of presenilins are reflected in a very severe phenotype of the knockout mice, with malformations of multiple organs.

Several peptidic and nonpeptidic inhibitors of γ-secretase have been characterized. They are effective in reducing Aβ levels in cultures of neuronal cells as well as in transgenic mouse models of Alzheimer's disease. Some of these compounds have excellent pharmacokinetic properties and effectively reduce Aβ levels in the brain of transgenic animal models with subcutaneous or oral administration (Lanz et al., 2003). γ-Secretase thus seems to be a more approachable, or more easily "drugable" target than β-secretase. Several compounds are in clinical development towards the ultimate test of the amyloid hypothesis in humans.

The relative lack of specificity is a significant problem for the clinical use of γ-secretase inhibitors. The inhibition of notch signaling in particular generates a serious concern since normal function of notch is required for the maintenance of hemopoetic stems cells and the further differentiation of immune cells in the adult organism (Lewis et al., 2003). Inhibiting the important functions of notch and of other γ-secretase substrates may generate severe adverse effects in the adult. Several strategies are feasible to overcome this limitation. First, partial inhibition of γ-secretase and partial reduction of Aβ formation may be sufficient for a beneficial clinical result in Alzheimer's disease. Such partial inhibition of notch processing may be without detrimental consequences to immune functions, making it possible to define a clinically effective dose of a γ-secretase inhibitor not associated with adverse effects. Second, it may be possible to identify drug receptors sites on the γ-secretase complex that regulate the substrate selectivity of the enzyme. The interactions of PS1 and PS2 with nicastrin, Aph-1, and Pen-2 are necessary for catalytic function and may also determine its substrate specificity. The molecular complexity of γ-secretase is likely to offer multiple drug receptor sites that influence the catalytic activity in distinct ways.

Intriguing clinical observations have suggested a direct approach to the identification of molecules that may affect γ-secretase activity to lower Aβ formation without adverse effects. Epidemiological analyses of large numbers of Alzheimer patients have revealed that the long-term consumption of some NSAIDs to reduce pain also reduces the risk for Alzheimer's disease. With a delay of several years, the NSAIDs prevent the development of the disease. Specific NSAIDs reduce γ-secretase activity in tissue culture studies and reduce Aβ levels in the brain of transgenic Alzheimer mice. This effect is independent of the NSAIDs' ability to inhibit the cyclooxygenase enzymes that mediate their pain-relieving properties. The receptor site and the mechanism of action that mediates the beneficial effects of NSAIDs for Alzheimer's disease remain to be elucidated. Once identified, this yet to be discovered receptor site is a highly intriguing putative target for novel drugs to treat Alzheimer's disease. Even in absence of understanding the receptor site, it has been possible to identify enantiomers of clinically used NSAIDs that do not inhibit cyclooxygenase but lower Aβ levels. These compounds do not exhibit the gastrointestinal toxicity associated with cyclooxygenase inhibition and are thus safe for long-term use. One of them, R-flurbiprofen, has been taken into clinical trials. If successful, these compounds and the receptor site mediating their beneficial actions may represent an astonishing shortcut to effective medication for Alzheimer's disease (Eriksen et al., 2003).

9.3.3 Aβ Antibodies

Active and passive immunization strategies attempt to remove Aβ from the brain by changing the dynamic equilibrium between the various compartments in which it is contained. The Aβ peptide occurs within and outside of the brain, and it can be measured in accessible fluids such as CSF and blood. The dynamics of exchange of Aβ between various organs and the various forms of aggregation appear rather complex and are not fully understood. Aβ is produced within neurons by cleavage from APP located in intracellular membranes. The mechanism of release remains to be defined. Aβ can also be generated directly in the extracellular space by cleavage from APP located at the plasma membrane. Aggregation to oligomers and polymers is believed to occur in the extracellular fluid but may also occur within the cell. Measurable levels of Aβ exist in the CSF. These levels are believed to reflect Aβ levels in the extracellular fluid of the brain, but the transport mechanisms remain to be characterized. The Aβ in the blood is believed to originate from the brain, since APP is predominantly expressed in the central nervous system, but contributions from the peripheral nervous system and other organs cannot be excluded. As illustrated in Figure 9.4, it is reasonable to assume that the various pools of Aβ are in a dynamic equilibrium with each other, and this, in consequence, offers a unique opportunity to lower Aβ levels in the brain. According to this concept the blood compartment represents a sink for brain Aβ. Removing Aβ from the blood will result in accelerated efflux of Aβ from the brain and reduce the Aβ contained in oligomeric and polymeric aggregates.

Active immunization studies in transgenic mouse have played an important role in establishing the rationale for the anti-Aβ approach to Alzheimer's disease (Schenk et al., 1999). Transgenic Alzheimer mice immunized against Aβ had much reduced levels of Aβ in the brain and did not develop the neuritic plaques. Immunization of mice that had already developed plaques resulted in removal of the plaques. Furthermore immunization reversed memory deficits of the mice before reducing Aβ levels and plaque density in the brain (Dodart et al., 2002).

The spectacular findings on Alzheimer mice models led to human trials with active immunization strategies. Unfortunately, several of the patients in these trials developed

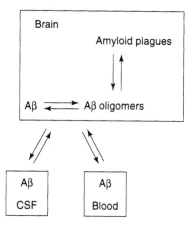

Figure 9.4 Dynamic equilibrium of Aβ in various aggregate forms and compartments.

severe adverse reactions, an inflammatory reaction of meningeal and brain tissues (Hock et al., 2003). These highly disturbing results mandated the immediate cessation of the trials. The cause for the adverse reactions remains unclear. It has been speculated that some of the anti-Aβ antibodies penetrated the brain where they bound to APP and disrupted its normal function. Antibodies normally do not penetrate through the blood-brain barrier; therefore this speculative explanation implies the opening of the barrier in Alzheimer patients. The inflammatory reaction may have been caused by a T-cell response to Aβ and T-cell invasion of brain tissue. Additional speculative explanations are linked to vascular Aβ deposits that occur in vessel walls of many Alzheimer patients, a condition described as cerebral amyloid angiopathy (Beckmann et al., 2003). Removal of these deposits by anti-Aβ antibodies might affect the integrity of the blood-brain barrier and thus facilitate antibody and brain penetration to the brain.

Despite this initial defeat, immunization strategies remain highly attractive for finding effective therapy against Alzheimer's disease. The tentative behavioral analysis of patients in the first trial with active immunization suggests a beneficial effect. Given the severe adverse effects observed in this study, passive immunization appears more attractive, where antibodies against Aβ are generated outside of the human body and given to patients by systemic injections. They are less likely to create adverse effects, since they do not activate the host's immune system and will not cause the generation of antibodies against other natural proteins. Antibody technologies have made enormous progress in recent years, and antibody therapy has become a standard feature for cancer and rheumatoid arthritis. It is possible now to routinely generate monoclonal humanized or human antibodies in sufficient quantities for therapeutic use in humans. It will be possible to design anti-Aβ antibodies that do not recognize APP and thus have a reduced potential to generate adverse effects. Like the inhibitors of β- and γ-secretases, active or passive immunization against Aβ will directly test the amyloid hypothesis in humans. Clinical success in any of the three approaches will increase the value of the other two.

9.3.4 Anti-Aggregation Molecules

The neuritic plaques in the brain of Alzheimer patients consisting of Aβ aggregates are one of several amyloid bodies that exist as pathological structures in human disease states (Merlini and Bellotti, 2003). Amyloid deposits in Parkinson's disease, the Lewy bodies, consist of α-synuclein; those in bovine spongiform encephalitis are composed of prion protein. In all these amyloid bodies, an ordered, repetitive aggregate is formed by antiparallel assemblies of peptide strands. The ordered structure allows specific molecules to intercalate in well-defined orientations that reflect the amyloid structure. If these molecules are dyes, such as Congo red, the resulting ordered stacking of the molecules confers birefringence, an optical property seen in polarized light. Birefringence of dyes such as Congo red or thioflavin-S serves as valuable diagnostic tools in the postmortem analysis of Alzheimer brain tissue.

The existence of highly specific intercalating agents leads to the hypothesis that chemical derivatives might selectively impair the amyloid assembly. In Alzheimer's disease, such anti-aggregation molecules are expected to change the equilibrium toward more soluble Aβ and, in consequence, to enhanced efflux of Aβ from the brain. It is conceivable, however, that liberation of Aβ from the functionally inert plaques can increase the pool of toxic, monomeric, or oligomeric Aβ and have detrimental consequences. The search for selective anti-aggregate inhibitors has generated several peptides that are highly effective in vitro. For therapeutic utility, brain-penetrant small molecules will have to be identified. As an alternative to this difficult approach, metal chelators have been proposed, based on data suggesting that aggregation of amyloid structures requires bivalent metal ions such as Cu^{2+}, Fe^{2+}, and Zn^{2+}. Clorquinol, a compound discovered as antibiotic but hampered with significant adverse effects, is an effective chelator of bivalent metal ions and inhibits amyloid aggregation in transgenic mouse models (Bush, 2002). Metal chelators with acceptable adverse effect profiles may thus be useful for the treatment of Alzheimer's disease.

9.3.5 Regulators of Cholesterol Metabolism

The discovery that a specific allele of ApoE is a risk factor for Alzheimer's disease has prompted speculations about a functional link to Aβ formation. ApoE is a blood plasma protein that is responsible for the transport of cholesterol between the liver and the other organs of the body. The ε4 allele is susceptibility or risk factor for Alzheimer's disease when compared with the other two existing ε2 and ε3 alleles. Complex transgenic mice have been generated, with knockout mutations for the mouse ApoE genes, carrying various combinations of human ApoE transgenes as well as human Alzheimer's disease genes. They have become highly useful tools for investigating the functions of the three alleles. The early findings suggest that all three forms of human ApoE facilitate the formation of plaques in the mice and that expression of different alleles change the synaptic loss seen in these mice (Buttini et al., 2002). The precise mechanisms of the different allele effects remain to be elucidated, and no drug target has emerged as yet that can provide a way to decelerate the progression of the disease pathways.

ApoE's function as a cholesterol transporter has triggered speculations that cholesterol levels may influence the Alzheimer's disease mechanisms. Indeed, retrospective studies with cholesterol-lowering drugs (inhibitors of β-hydroxy-β-methylglutaryl-coenzyme A, the statins) suggest that they might reduce the risk for Alzheimer's disease. Lowering cholesterol in cell culture media reduces the formation of Aβ from cells expressing APP. Administration of statin drugs to transgenic Alzheimer mice lowers brain Aβ levels. However, to be effective in these experimental systems, cholesterol had to be reduced to much lower levels than those achieved by statins in humans. The speculative link of cholesterol to Aβ remains very tantalizing, in particular, because cholesterol levels can be effectively manipulated in humans through the existing drugs (Puglielli et al., 2003).

The study of disease mechanisms and the amyloid hypothesis have identified a small number of highly attractive drug targets that are vigorously pursued by many biopharmaceutical companies. If the amyloid hypothesis for the disease mechanism is correct, they are likely to yield drugs that successfully modify the progression of the disease. Vice versa, positive effects of such drugs will provide the conclusive validation of the amyloid hypothesis. The focused progress in the Alzheimer field illustrates the power of drug discovery based on disease mechanisms.

9.4 NEUROFIBRILLARY TANGLES AND Tau

Neurofibrillary tangles are the second cardinal feature of Alzheimer's neuropathology. They consist of phosphorylated tau protein that is aggregated in unique structures called paired-helical filaments. Tau is one of several microtubule-associated proteins that regulates the assembly of microtubules and thus plays a crucial role in axonal growth and regeneration. The activity of tau is regulated by phosphorylation. Excessive phosphorylation, hyperphosphorylation, has been observed in postmortem brain material from several neurological diseases, including Alzheimer's disease. A specific form of inherited dementia, frontotemporal dementia, has been linked to mutations in the tau gene. The mutations change the interactions of tau with microtubules. When expressed in transgenic animals, the mutated tau appears hyperphosphorylated. The identification of tau disease genes prove that changes in tau function can directly cause neurodegenerative events in the brain, some of them associated with dementia (Hardy, 2003).

The relationship between the formation of plaques and tangles and between the formation of Aβ and the hyperphosphorylation of tau remains to be elucidated. Animal models with transgenes that cause plaques do not show neurofibrillary tangles, nor do the transgenic mice with tau mutations generate plaques in the brain. Thus changes in Aβ processing and tau phosphorylation appear to be alternative pathways to neurodegeneration and to dementia. The association of tau mutations to frontotemporal dementia, a disease clearly distinct from Alzheimer's disease, supports this view. The findings strengthen the belief that the amyloid cascade is the causative pathway leading to the typical Alzheimer cases and that neurofibrillary tangles are formed as a secondary process because of the neuronal degeneration.

Hyperphosphorylated tau has been observed in several neurodegenerative diseases including Alzheimer's disease, frontotemporal dementia, and Parkinson's disease. The familial forms of frontotemporal dementia demonstrate that hyperphosphorylation can be the primary event in neurodegenerative processes. Strategies to prevent this step may thus be able to prevent the loss of neurons in other disease conditions and provide at least partial or temporary benefits. Several protein kinases are able to phosphorylate tau, including extracellular regulated kinases-1 and -2 (ERK1 and ERK2), cycline-dependent kinase-5, and glycogen synthase kinase-3α and -3β (GSK-3α and GSK-3β). Inhibition of the most relevant kinases may prevent hyperphosphorylation of tau and the formation of neurofibrillary tangles in humans suffering from related diseases. The GSK-3 kinases are particularly interesting because they have been linked to the activity of γ-secretase. They may thus provide the so far elusive link between the two major pathological structures of Alzheimer's disease. GSK-3 kinases are inhibited by Li^+, the ion that is therapeutically effective in the treatment of bipolar disease. This unique situation makes it possible to directly test the hypothesis that inhibiting GSK-3 will delay neuronal loss in Alzheimer's and other neurodegenerative disease (Phiel et al., 2003). Successful verification will direct drug discovery programs to kinase inhibitors with higher selectivity and less toxicity than Li^+.

9.5   MEMORY-ENHANCING DRUGS

The degeneration of cholinergic neurons in Alzheimer's disease, which has led to the first therapeutically useful drugs, is now considered an event secondary to the overproduction and aggregation of Aβ. Although these drugs only marginally improve the medical condition, they show that enhancing the function of specific synapses can have beneficial effects on memory. Is it possible to enhance memory in Alzheimer's patients by influencing synaptic mechanisms other than the cholinergic ones? If such drugs can be found, they might improve memory performance in normal humans, not suffering from any dementia. It is conceivable that they might enhance aspects of intellectual abilities beyond dementia. Improving intellectual functions ranks among the impossible dreams of humans.

But many other activities we now consider normal, flying and genetic engineering, for example, were among the impossible dreams not too long ago. The concept of cognition enhancers has been explored pharmacologically before. A specific drug, piracetam, has been advertised as "memory booster" and approved for the treatment of dementia in several countries. Piracetam has been heralded as the first drug in a new class called "nootropics" from the Greek meaning "acting on the mind" (Giurgea, 1972). The mechanism of action of piracetam is not clear and its beneficial actions in humans are marginal at best. Despite these early and exaggerated claims, the search for memory-enhancing drugs is a worthwhile and not necessarily unreachable goal.

9.5.1 Hippocampal Circuits

The early attempts to find memory-enhancing drugs relied on random testing of compounds in behavioral animal assays. Since then, research on memory mechanisms has made very significant advances, through the combined application of genetic, molecular, electrophysiological, and behavioral techniques to this problem. Many investigations have focused on the hippocampus, given very strong evidence for a crucial role of this brain structure in memory. Experimental lesions of the hippocampal selectively interfere with memory processes in animals. Bilateral destruction of the hippocampus in humans precludes the formation of new memories. The hippocampal circuitry is understood in detail (Fig. 9.5). Synapses participating in several of its pathways exhibit long-term potentiation (LTP) or long-term depression (LTD), changes in synaptic transmission that reflect previous activity. This synaptic plasticity is believed to be a necessary element of the processes that make it possible to deposit and retrieve memories. Hippocampal LTP is influenced by cholinergic afferents from the basal forebrain, providing a physiological basis for the positive effects of cholinergic therapeutics. Both muscarinic and nicotinic receptors are abundant in the hippocampus and represent attractive putative targets for memory-enhancing drugs. The most intriguing finding that the $A\beta$ peptide binds to and inhibits the normal function of $\alpha7$ nicotinic receptors makes them a particularly appealing target (Wang et al., 2003).

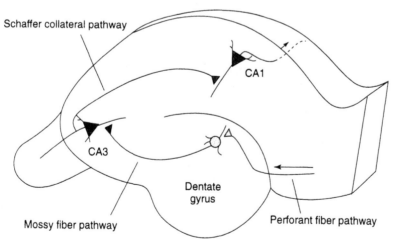

Figure 9.5 Hippocampal circuitry. The major excitatory pathways are shown. In addition the hippocampus receives various inputs from modulatory systems, including serotonergic, noradrenergic, and cholinergic afferents, and it contains GABAergic interneurons.

Besides the cholinergic neurons there are several other hippocampal modulatory systems that might lead to drug targets for memory-enhancing drugs. Galanin is one among these additional synaptic modulators. Galanin is a neuropeptide that activates three G-protein-coupled receptors, GALR1, GALR2, and GALR3. Mutant mice unable to form galanin have deficits in memory processes, and they also exhibit atrophic changes of the cholinergic neurons that innervate the hippocampus. Galanin exerts an inhibitory influence on the cholinergic hippocampal afferents. Thus galanin receptor antagonists might stimulate the cholinergic input to the hippocampus and provide an approach to finding memory enhancers (Counts et al., 2003).

The hippocampus is abundant in GABAergic inhibitory interneurons. While most subtypes of GABA-A receptors are represented in the hippocampus, those containing the $\alpha5$ subunit are particularly abundant and their large number provide an opportunity to selectively influence hippocampal function. Compounds that reduce the activity of GABA-A$\alpha5$ containing receptors selectively reduce the activity of the inhibitory circuits of the hippocampus. The diminished inhibition facilitates the formation of LTP hippocampal synapses and increases memory performance in animal assays. Strong support for this concept is provided by studies on knockout mice with deletions of the $\alpha5$ receptor gene, which perform better than wild-type mice in assays testing memory functions. As discussed in more detail in Chapter 4, the benzodiazepine receptor site offers an opportunity to modify the $\alpha5$ containing GABA-A receptors in the desired way. Inverse agonists for GABA-A$\alpha5$ receptors decrease the opening frequency of these receptors, and diminish the inhibitory action of the GABAergic interneurons in the hippocampus. Inverse agonists for the benzodiazepine receptor site on GABA-A$\alpha5$ receptors thus represent a captivating approach to finding compounds that enhance memory performance in humans (Collinson et al., 2002).

Glutamate is the dominant neurotransmitter within the hippocampus, and most of the efferent projections from the hippocampus use glutamatergic synapses to influence the target neurons. Ionotropic and metabotropic glutamate receptors are abundant in the hippocampus and its target areas, offering many target opportunities but little guidance for a further selection process. The NMDA type of ionotropic glutamate receptor plays a central role in hippocampal memory formation. NMDA antagonists disrupt hippocampal LTP and memory in animal behavioral assays. Several studies with transgenic animals including elegant investigations on mice with deletions of the NMDA receptors restricted to a subfield of hippocampal neurons confirm the essential contribution of NMDA receptors (Nakazawa et al., 2003). It is not surprising that complete blockade or removal of the most influential type of glutamate receptor is functionally disruptive. Agonistic or antagonistic drugs for the crucial receptor type will influence hippocampal processes in excessive ways that are not expected to be therapeutically useful. The complexity of the glutamatergic synapse, however, will offer many opportunities for more subtle influences that may enhance synaptic plasticity and memory functions.

Subtle influences on NMDA receptors are likely to underlie the therapeutic efficacy of memantine, a compound recently approved for the treatment of Alzheimer's disease. Memantine binds with relatively low affinity to NMDA receptors at the same site as the much more potent antagonist MK-801. The blockade of NMDA receptors by memantine is voltage dependent, thus increasing the magnitude of its effects during periods of high synaptic activity (Danysz and Parsons, 2003). The compound has been taken into clinical development based on the vague speculation that the activity of glutamatergic synapses is increased in diseases such as Alzheimer's disease and that partial inhibition of NMDA receptors might have positive effect. In carefully designed clinical studies, memantine showed mild improvements in rating scales that reflect the general function of Alzheimer patients. There was no effect on memory as measured by the Mini Mental State Exam rating scale, which is typically considered standard for Alzheimer trials (Reisberg et al., 2003). Memantine has been prescribed for Alzheimer's disease for more than a decade in several European countries and has recently been approved in the United States. The vast clinical experience makes it clear that is efficacy is as marginal as that of the cholinesterase inhibitors. The need for truly effective disease-modifying therapy in Alzheimer's disease remains as strong as ever.

The NMDA receptors in the hippocampal glutamatergic synapses are surrounded by other ionotropic glutamate receptors that mediate synaptic functions in concordance with NMDA receptors. The AMPA family of ionotropic receptors is affected by a group of compounds called ampakines (Lynch, 2002). Ampakines are selective modulators of AMPA receptors. They potentiate the actions of glutamate on active receptors in a way comparable to the actions of benzodiazepines on GABA-A receptors. The ampakines delay the deactivation and desensitization of AMPA receptors following the pulse of stimulatory glutamate. In some hippocampal synapses, activation of AMPA receptors is necessary for NMDA receptors to become activated. Prolongation of AMPA receptor action through the ampakines will thus enhance NMDA receptor functions as well. Various ampakines have been generated that differ in specific kinetic properties. It may be possible to further improve selectivity by making them selective for specific subtypes of the AMPA receptor group. One of the nonselective ampakines, CX516, increases LTP of hippocampal synapses and improves memory functions in animal tests, and thus is being explored in human studies. Activation of glutamate receptors, if encompassing NMDA receptors and other central players, carries the danger of excessive stimulation and seizure induction. Subtype-selective ampakines appear safer and such compounds are appealing for further drug discovery and development efforts.

The hippocampal glutamatergic synapses are complex functional units that encompass many additional regulatory elements, each of which represents a potential drug target in the search of memory-enhancing drugs. Metabotropic glutamate receptors, located pre- or postsynaptically, influence the functions of NMDA and AMPA receptors. Each of these receptors or regulatory proteins represents a potential drug target in the search for memory-enhancing drugs. As in many other situations the abundance of attractive putative targets signifies enormous opportunity as well as the very difficult challenge to select the best ones.

9.5.2 Molecular Biology of Memory Functions

Many synapses besides those of the hippocampus are capable of long-term plasticity in the form of LTP or LTD. They include synapses in the amygdala, discussed in Chapter 8 in the context of fear potentiation, and cerebellar synapses that mediate reflex habituation, the gradual adaptation to repetitive sensory stimulus. Evolutionary efficiency makes it likely that the same molecular mechanisms are used by all these synapses and that there is a general molecular biology of memory formation in the nervous system. Rapid progress in research during the recent years indeed supports the view that fundamental mechanisms underlie memory functions in vertebrate and invertebrate species and that they might include elements suitable as drug targets.

Early animal studies and clinical observations led to the distinction of short-term and long-term memory. Any event experienced by an animal or human is first kept in short-term memory, whereas only some of the events are stored more permanently. Short-term memory can be disrupted in humans through trauma or electric shock and is thus believed to rely on specific activity patterns in synaptic circuits. This information storage decays within a few minutes unless transferred into long-term memory. Active gene expression is necessary for long-term memory formation. It is blocked by inhibitors of protein synthesis. In a similar way LTP is sometimes separated into early-LTP and late-LTP that is dependent on protein synthesis. Memory mutations in *Drosophila* have been instrumental in depicting the molecular biology of these processes. They identified a small number of regulatory molecules necessary for memory formation. The fundamental principles of these memory pathways were verified in studies with transgenic mice at the electrophysiological and behavioral level.

The sequence of events depicted in Figure 9.6 has emerged from the molecular investigations of memory mechanisms. The sensory experiences to be remembered are initially reflected by patterns of synaptic activity, with glutamatergic synapses playing the major role. Activation of the postsynaptic neurons through NMDA and other glutamate receptors changes the ionic composition on the postsynaptic side and results in the influx of Ca^{2+}. The ionic changes generate an excitatory postsynaptic potential and participate in the regulation of the postsynaptic neuronal activity. The influx of Ca^{2+} has additional metabolic consequences. It stimulates several intracellular signaling pathways, including the activation of calmodulin, calcineurin, and protein kinase A. Protein kinase A is trans-

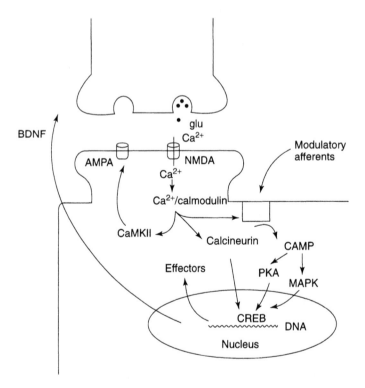

Figure 9.6 Molecular mechanisms of memory formation. NMDA receptor activation stimulates Ca^{2+} influx and various secondary events including the activation of calmodulin kinase II (CaMKII), protein kinase A (PKA), and Map-kinase (MAPK). Modulatory afferents influence these processes. The pathways converge in the activation of CREB (cAMP-responsive element-binding protein), which regulates the synthesis of many effector proteins. Secreted effectors, including BDNF (brain-derived neurotrophic factor) are able to regulate the function and morphology of the synapse. (Adapted from Kandel, 2001)

ported to the nucleus where it phosphorylates and activates the cAMP-responsive element-binding (CREB) protein. CREB is a transcriptional regulator that induces the synthesis of many proteins, including mediators of synaptic function. The altered synaptic composition changes the functional properties of the synapse that make possible late-LTP and long-term memory. The activation of CREB through synaptic activity and the subsequent changes in protein expressions are now believed to represent the crucial molecular steps for memory (Kandel, 2001; Tully et al., 2003).

It is tempting to think that activators of CREB might represent memory-enhancing drugs. Unfortunately, CREB participates in many regulatory pathways, including growth-amplifying pathways of some forms of cancer. CREB activators might be effective as memory enhancers but at the price of a severe adverse effect profile. Alternative indirectly acting regulators thus seem more attractive. CREB activation through protein kinase A is counteracted by phosphodiesterase 4. An inhibitor for this enzyme with poor selectivity, rolipram, was discovered many years ago and evaluated in several human disease conditions. Rolipram and, more recently discovered, selective inhibitors of phosphodiesterase 4 improve memory performance in animal models. The existing clinical experience with rolipram has not revealed any substantial effect on memory in humans, but the clinical trials were not designed to detect benefits related to memory. Positive effects may have been masked by actions of rolipram on other receptor sites. Phosphodiesterase 4 inhibitors have the potential to be mildly efficacious but safe enhancers of memory performance.

CREB activation stimulates the synthesis of brain-derived neurotrophic factor (BDNF) among many other proteins. While discovered as a neurotrophic factor, BDNF also plays a role as synaptic modulator. It is released upon synaptic activation from the postsynaptic dendrite and appears to act as retrograde messenger that enhances the function of the presynaptic side. An important role of BDNF in memory processing is supported by various studies on transgenic animals as well as human mutations (Egan et al.,

Table 9.1 Current and future drugs and targets for Alzheimer's disease

---

Current Drugs

AChE inhibitors
Memantine (NMDA inhibitor)

Future Drugs and Targets

Disease-Modifying Drugs
β-secretase inhibitors
γ-secretase inhibitors
Aβ antibodies
Anti-aggregation molecules
Tau protein kinase inhibitors (GSK-3)

Memory Enhancers
Regulators of AMPA receptors (ampakines)
Regulators of NMDA receptors
GABA-Aα5 inverse agonists
ORL1 antagonists
BDNF mimetics
Cholinergic muscarinic agonists
Cholinergic nicotinic agonists

2003). Potentiation of BDNF actions thus provides an intriguing potential approach toward memory-enhancing drugs. However, as discussed in more detail in Chapter 10, protein growth factors represent a difficult challenge for central nervous system drug discovery. They do not pass the blood-brain barrier, and small-molecule activators or potentiators have so far been elusive. In addition the neurotrophic actions of BDNF may mediate unacceptable adverse effects in addition to the desired benefits on synaptic function.

The study of the molecular biology of memory, together with the investigations on hippocampal synaptic circuitry has identified several highly attractive putative drug targets that are vigorously pursued in the biopharmaceutical industry. The potential rewards in this field are enormous since memory enhancers would benefit Alzheimer's disease patients and many of the elderly. However, the level of difficulty and challenge in this field seems particularly high.

9.6   ANIMAL MODELS

Two kinds of transgenic animal models are used in drug discovery for Alzheimer's disease, animals expressing human mutant genes that cause the disease and transgenic animals reflecting specific features of memory mechanisms. The disease-causing mutants include mutants of APP, and mutants of PS1 and PS2 of the γ-secretase complex. Various strains have been produced and characterized. Most widely used are those combining an APP and PS1 or PS2 mutations in the same mouse. Table 9.2 lists the best characterized strains. They differ in the speed of plaque deposition, synaptic loss, and magnitude of memory deficits. While these transgenic animals support the amyloid hypothesis for the disease mechanism, it should not be forgotten that they represent artificial organisms. Most humans suffering from Alzheimer's disease are caused by factors other than these mutations. The relatively rare cases of familial Alzheimer's disease are caused by a single mutation rather than a combination of mutated disease genes. Despite these limitations the transgenic Alzheimer mice have been extremely important for drug discovery related to the amyloid hypothesis (Wong et al., 2002).

Further refinement of the transgenic mice models is likely. The existing transgenic strains are being crossbred in mice that express the various isoforms of human ApoE. The

Table 9.2   Animal models for Alzheimer's disease

Transgenic Mice with Human Disease Genes
APP Alzheimer's disease mutations
PS1/PS2 Alzheimer's disease mutations
APP and PS1/PS2 combinations
Humanized ApoE mice
APP and PS1/PS2 mutations combined with ApoE mice
Tau frontotemporal dementia disease mutations

Animals Used for Study of Memory Mechanisms
Lesion-Generating Selective Replicating Memory Deficits
Hippocampal lesions
Neurotoxin lesions of hippocampal cholinergic afferents

Transgenic Mice with Enhanced Memory Functions
Hippocampus-specific overexpression of active CREB
GABA-Aα5 knockouts
ORL1 knockout

---

stepwise replacement of mouse genes with human genes that are part of the Alzheimer disease cascade gradually approach the exact steps occurring in the human brain. The human tauopathies have been recreated in transgenic mice through the expression of mutated human genes that cause these conditions. Combining them with APP/PS1 mutant mice generates animals that exhibit neuritic plaques and neurofibrillary tangles, comparable to the pathological appearance of the human Alzheimer brain. However, the combination of several disease genes in a single organism represents a highly artificial situation that might generate molecular interactions different from those in the human disease.

Several animal models exist that reflect the cholinergic deficit of Alzheimer's disease. Lesions of the septum, selective destruction of cholinergic neurons by targeted toxins, or the administration of cholinergic receptor inhibitors produce animals with impairment in memory. They are useful in drug discovery programs that aim at improving the cholinergic therapy and at identifying synaptic mechanisms regulated by the cholinergic input. Cholinergic lesion models replicate a defined, partial feature of Alzheimer's disease only and have thus limited utility.

The elucidation of molecular mechanisms of memory has produced several animals with memory deficits. Similar to animals with cholinergic lesions, these mutant mice cannot be considered models of Alzheimer's disease, but they do have utility for specific drug discovery programs toward memory enhancers. Since memory is complex process involving many proteins, it is not surprising that many gene knockouts have memory deficits. It is easier to destroy than to build, and removal of a single element is often able to disrupt a complex process. Nevertheless, knockout mice with memory deficits are very useful when it is necessary to distinguish between the specific effects of a drug candidate and those mediated by off-target activities. From a point of view of defining molecular mechanism of memory, the most interesting knockout or transgenic mice are those with improved memory function. Besides the GABA-Aα5 receptor knockouts, knockout mice of the opioid receptor-like 1 (ORL1) receptor for the neuropeptide nociceptin show enhanced memory performance (Mamiya et al., 2003). Such unexpected observations may provide a shortcut to target identification for memory-enhancing drugs.

9.7 CLINICAL TRIALS AND TRANSLATIONAL MEDICINE

Alzheimer's disease has an insidious onset and progresses gradually over several years. As in other age-related neurodegenerative diseases, the changes are superimposed on more subtle modifications that occur in the normal population. The performance of humans in tests of memory performance peaks between 20 and 30 years, then declines very subtly over the decades. The rate of decline seems to accelerate after 50 years, with significant drop between 50 and 60 years, and a further acceleration of decline after 80 years. These are average figures, and the individual rates vary significantly. Subtypes of memory differ in the rate of decline. Nevertheless, the decline of memory and cognitive functions is a well-documented phenomenon.

Drugs useful for the treatment of Alzheimer's disease may affect memory functions in multiple ways as illustrated in Figure 9.7. Memory-enhancing compounds, if they can be found, might elevate the performance of normal humans, elderly humans with mild cognitive impairment (MCI), and Alzheimer patients. Disease-modifying drugs are expected to slow the rate of progression of the disease and perhaps even reverse it to normal levels. Preventative drugs will postpone the average onset of the disease. The various ways drugs may modify Alzheimer's disease make the design of clinical trials a challenging enterprise. The

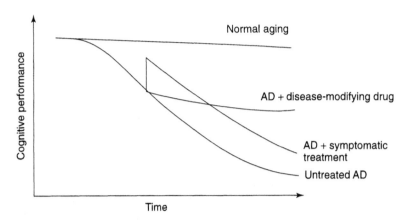

Figure 9.7 Possible drug effects on Alzheimer's disease.

expected type of effect has to be given careful consideration when selecting the patient population and the number of patients necessary for meaningful results.

The effects of memory-enhancing effects are evaluated with short-term drug treatment and the help of well-established behavioral tests. Several simple tests have been characterized to monitor the relatively severe cognitive dysfunction of Alzheimer's disease. The Mini Mental State Exam test, which relies on a very simple questionnaire, is most widely used. The currently available drugs for Alzheimer's disease, acetylcholinesterase inhibitors and memantine, produce very subtle effects in these tests only. More elaborate memory tests, such as the Cantab test system, tests humans in highly standardized situations to reveal verbal and visual memory (Blackwell et al., 2004). In absence of truly effective memory-enhancing drugs, a group of young normal humans is included in the test to serve as positive control group. Disease-modifying drugs require trials of several months, even years duration, because of the large variability among patients and the very gradually progression rate. Several hundred patients and a treatment period of more than six months is considered minimally necessary to establish a positive outcome. Prevention trials require yet larger number of patients and longer observation times to have a chance to produce a significant result.

The massive efforts and costs of clinical trials for disease-modifying or preventative drugs have triggered the search for alternative approaches and surrogate endpoints. Dementia is the medically relevant condition that needs to be corrected, and drugs have to ameliorate this behavioral condition to be useful for the patients. However, any other functional parameter that more directly reflects the drug's mechanism of action will be enormously useful during the early phases of drug development. Readouts that reflect the pharmacological effects of the drug will allow investigators to ascertain that it produces the desired effect at the molecular level. The amyloid hypothesis ascribes the central role to elevated Aβ levels. While brain Aβ levels cannot be measured directly in humans, it is possible to monitor CSF concentrations of the peptide. The average CSF concentration of Aβ is elevated in Alzheimer's disease patients, and these levels are sometimes used for confirmatory diagnostics in Alzheimer's disease. The interindividual differences are very high, however, providing considerable uncertainty for the individual diagnosis. Individual CSF levels may nevertheless be useful to establish efficacy of drugs that inhibit Aβ formation. A small number of elderly people suffer from elevated intracerebral pressure and are implanted with chronic ventriculoperitoneal shunts. These patients might be suitable for monitoring the gradual reduction of Aβ CSF levels that are expected to occur following the administration of secretase inhibitors (Silverberg et al., 2002). Similarly dynamic changes of Aβ concentrations in plasma might be useful to monitor the actions of specific drugs.

Imaging studies have played an important role in Alzheimer research for many years as additional diagnostic tool. MRI shows ventricular enlargement and cortical shrinkage in living patients, but significant values are typically obtained at advanced stages of the disease only. More recently functional changes that parallel the decline in memory functions have been demonstrated with fMRI techniques. Most exciting progress has come from the combination of imaging techniques with specific dyes that bind to pathological structures typical for Alzheimer's disease. Molecules that selectively intercalate in the structures of neuritic plaques and carry an appropriate label group might be visualized with PET techniques (Bacskai et al., 2003).

Clinical trial Alzheimer's disease rely on established and well-tested designs that take into considerations the many possible outcomes. Behavioral tests that reflect the medically relevant parameters have been largely standardized but are further refined. Methods to measure drug efficacy at the molecular level in vivo that have started to emerge will provide most useful surrogate markers for short and decisive proof-of-principle clinical trials.

9.8 CONCLUSIONS

Alzheimer's disease is an age-related, chronic, and progressing illness that represents a major medical and societal problem. Loss of synapses and neurons and the formation of pathological structures, neuritic plaques, and neurofibrillary tangles are its cardinal features. The currently available drugs, acetylcholinesterase inhibitors and the NMDA receptor antagonist memantine, offer only marginal behavioral improvement. Very significant progress in the treatment is expected to occur in the foreseeable future because of rapid advances in the understanding of the disease mechanisms.

The combination of biochemical studies on postmortem brain with the discovery of disease genes has led to the formulation of the amyloid hypothesis, a unifying conceptual view of the disease cascade. It ascribes the central function to the Aβ peptide, which is cleaved by the β- and γ-secretase from the precursor protein. The amyloid hypothesis identifies several putative approaches for drug discovery that are very actively pursued by the biopharmaceutical companies and show high promise. Inhibitors of the secretases are efficacious in animal models of the disease. Capturing Aβ in the blood by anti-Aβ antibodies reduces brain levels of the peptide. Tentative evidence in support of this approach has been obtained in clinical studies. It may be possible to reduce brain Aβ levels by drugs that prevent the formation of the neuritic plaques that consist of Aβ aggregates. In addition to these approaches that are expected to be successful, there are alternative attempts to prevent the formation of the neurofibrillary tangles consisting of hyperphosphorylated tau protein. Specific inhibitors for kinases that phosphorylate tau may interfere with some of the pathological steps of Alzheimer's disease.

Loss of memory is the dominant behavioral feature of Alzheimer's disease, and mild memory loss occurs frequently with normal aging. Drugs that improve memory functions would be useful for both conditions. Genetic and molecular biological research of the recent years has identified fundamental mechanisms of memory. The crucial roles have been ascribed to glutamatergic synapses that exhibit long-term plasticity and to intracellular changes of protein expression regulated by the transcriptional factor CREB. The complexity of glutamatergic synapses offers multiple drug target opportunities. Specific regulatory steps upstream or downstream of CREB activation provide putative drug targets. Many of the molecules involved participate in processes other than memory, making selectivity a central problem in the discovery of memory-enhancing drugs.

Several highly useful transgenic animal models have been generated for Alzheimer's disease in order to replicate the disease mechanism, as outlined by the amyloid hypothesis. Transgenic animals with modifications of specific molecular elements of memory formation have been produced that serve as test systems for drug candidates acting on these targets. Clinical trials for disease-modifying drugs and memory enhancers use memory tests as primary endpoint. Trials needed to establish a change in progression of the disease require large patient populations and long observation times. Methods to measure $A\beta$ levels during drug treatment or to visualize the $A\beta$ aggregates in the brain are very actively pursued to obtain pharmacological readouts of drug efficacy. These methods will hopefully also provide surrogate markers for short and decisive proof-of-principle clinical trials.

Alzheimer's disease represents one of the most rapidly progressing, exciting, and promising fields of modern drug discovery. Drug trials over the near future years will hopefully validate the targets chosen and provide the many patients with effective medication.

REFERENCES

Further Reading

BUSH, A.I. Metal complexing agents as therapies for Alzheimer's disease. *Neurobiol. Aging* 23: 1031–1038, 2002.

COUNTS, S.E., PEREZ, S.E., GINSBERG, S.D., DE LACALLE, S., and MUFSON, E.J. Galanin in Alzheimer's disease. *Mol. Intervent.* 3: 137–156, 2003.

DOMINGUEZ, D.I., and DE STOOPER, B. Novel therapeutic strategies provide the real test for the amyloid hypothesis of Alzheimer's disease. *Trends Pharmacol. Sci.* 23: 323–330, 2002.

HARDY, J. The relationship between amyloid and tau. *J. Mol. Neurosci.* 20: 203–206, 2003.

KANDEL, E.R. The molecular biology of memory storage: A dialogue between genes and synapses. *Science* 294: 1030–1038, 2001.

LAD, S.P., NEET, K.E., and MUFSON, E.J. Nerve growth factor: structure, function and therapeutic implications for Alzheimer's disease. *Curr. Drug Targ. CNS Neurol. Disc.* 2: 315–334, 2003.

LYNCH, G. Memory enhancement: the search for mechanism-based drugs. *Nature Neurosci.* 5 (suppl.): 1035–1038, 2002.

MERLINI, G., and BELLOTTI, V. Molecular mechanisms of amyloidosis. *N. Eng. J. Med.* 349: 583–596, 2003.

PUGLIELLI, L., TANZI, R.E., and KOVACS, D.M. Alzheimer's disease: The cholesterol connection. *Nature Neurosci.* 6: 345–351, 2003.

SELKOE, D.J., and SCHENK, D. Alzheimer's disease: molecular understanding predicts amyloid-based therapeutics. *An. Rev. Pharmacol. Toxicol.* 43: 545–584, 2003.

TULLY, T., BOURTCHOULADZE, R., SCOTT, R., and TALLMAN, J. Targeting the CREB pathway for memory enhancers. *Nature Rev. Drug Disc.* 2: 267–277, 2003.

WOLFE, M.S. Secretase targets for Alzheimer's disease: Identification and therapeutic potential. *J. Med. Chem.* 44: 2039–2060, 2001.

WONG, P.C., CAI, H., BORCHELT, D.R., and PRICE, D.L. Genetically engineered mouse models of neurodegenerative diseases. *Nature Neurosci.* 5: 633–639, 2002.

Citations

ANAGOSTARAS, S.G., MURPHY, G.G., HAMILTON, S.E., MITCHELL, S.L., RAHNAMA, N.J., NATHANSON, N.M., and SILVA, A.J. Selective cognitive dysfunction in acetylcholine M1 muscarinic receptor mutant mice. *Nature Neurosci.* 6: 51–58, 2003.

BACSKAI, B.J., HICKEY, G.A., SKOCH, J., KAJDASZ, S.T., WANG, Y., HUANG, G.F., MATHIS, C.A., KLUNK, W.E., and HYMAN, B.T. Four-dimensional multiphoton imaging of brain entry, amyloid-binding and clearance of an amyloid-B ligand in transgenic mice by using multiphoton microscopy. *Proc. Natl. Acad. Sci. USA* 100: 12462–12467, 2003.

BECKMANN, N., SCHULER, A., MUEGGLER, T., MEYER, E.P., WIEDERHOLD, K.H., STAUFENBIEL, M., and KRUCKER, T.

Age-dependent cerebrovascular abnormalities and blood flow disturbances in APP23 mice modeling Alzheimer's disease. *J. Neurosci.* 23: 8453–8459, 2003.

BLACKWELL, A.D., SAHAKIAN, B.J., VESEY, R., SEMPLE, J.M., ROBBINS, T.W., and HODGES, J.R. Detecting dementia: novel neuropsychological markers of preclinical Alzheimer's disease. *Dement. Geriatr. Cogn. Disord.* 17: 42–48, 2004.

BUTTINI, M., YU, G.Q., SHOCKLEY, K., HUANG, Y., JONES, B., MASLIAH, E., MALLORY, M., YEO, T., LONGO, F.M., and MUCKE, L. Modulation of Alzheimer-like synaptic and cholinergic deficits in transgenic mice by human apolipoprotein E depends on isoform, aging, and overexpression of amyloid β peptides but not on plaque formation. *J. Neurosci.* 22: 10539–10548, 2002.

COLLINSON, N., KUENZI, F.M., JAROLIMEK, W., MAUBACH, K.A., COTHLIFF, R., SUR, C., SMITH, A., OUT, F.M., HOWELL, O., ATACK, J.R., McKERNAN, R.M., SEABROOK, G.R., DAWSON, G.R., WHITING, P.J., and ROSAHL, T.W. Enhanced learning and memory and altered GABAergic synaptic transmission in mice lacking the alpha 5 subunit of the GABA-A receptor. *J. Neurosci.* 22: 5572–5580, 2002.

DANYSZ, W., and PARSONS, C.G. The NMDA receptor antagonist memantine as a symptomatological and neuroprotective treatment for Alzheimer's disease: Preclinical evidence. *Int. J. Geriatr. Psychiat.* 18: S23–32, 2003.

DODART, J.D., BALES, K.R., GANNON, K.S., GREENE, S.J., DeMATTOS, R.B., MATHIS, C., DeLONG, C.A., WU, S., WU, X., HOLTZMAN, D.M., and PAUL, S.M. Immunization reverses memory deficits without reducing brain Abeta burden in Alzheimer's disease model. *Nature Neurosci.* 5: 452–457, 2002.

EGAN, M.F., KIJIMA, M., CALLICOTT, J.H., GOLDBERG, T.E., KOACHANA, B.S., BERTOLINO, A., ZAITSEV, E., GOLD, B., GOLDMAN, D., DEAN, M., LU, B., and WEINBERGER, D.R. The BDNF val66met polymorphism affects activity-dependent secretion of BDNF and human memory and hippocampal function. *Cell* 112: 257–269, 2003.

ERIKSEN, J.L., SAGI, S.A., SMITH, T.E., WEGGEN, S., DAS, P., McLENDON, D.C., OZOLS, V.V., JESSING, K.W., ZAVITZ, K.H., KOO, E.H., and GOLDE, T.E. NSAIDs and enantiomers of flurbiprofen target gamma-secretase and lower Abeta 42 in vivo. *J. Clin. Invest.* 112: 440–449, 2003.

GERMAN, D.C., YAZDANI, U., SPECIALE, S.G., PASHBAKHSH, P., GAMES, D., and LIANG, C.L. Cholinergic neuropathology in a mouse model of Alzheimer's disease. *J. Comp. Neurol.* 462: 371–381, 2003.

GIURGEA, C. Pharmacology of integrative activity of the brain. Attempt at nootropic concept in psychopharmacology. *Actual Pharmacol. (Paris)* 25: 115–156, 1972.

GONG, Y., CHANG, L., VIOLA, K.L., LACOR, P.N., LAMPERT, M.P., FINCH, C.E., KRAFFT, G.A., and KLEIN, W.L. Alzheimer's disease-affected brain: Presence of oligomeric A beta ligands (ADDLs) suggest a molecular basis for reversible memory loss. *Proc. Natl. Acad. Sci. USA.* 100: 10417–10422, 2003.

HOCK, C., KONIETZKO, J.R., TRACY, J., SIGNORELLI, A., MULLER-TILLMANNS, B., LEMKE, U., HENKE, K., MORITZ, E., GARCIA, E., WOLLMER, M.A., UMBRICHT, D., DE QUERVAIN, D.J.F., HOFMANN, M., MADDALENA, A., PAPASSOTIROPOLOULOS, A., and NITSCH, R. Antibodies against β-amyloid slow cognitive decline in Alzheimer's disease. *Neuron*, 38: 547–554, 2003.

LANZ, T.A., HIMES, C.S., PALLANTE, G., ADAMS, L., YAMAZAKI, S., AMORE, B., and MERCHANT, K.M. The gamma-secretase inhibitor *N*-[*N*-(3,5-difluorophenyl)-lacetyl)-L-alanyl]-*S*-phenylglycine *t*-butyl ester reduces A beta levels in vivo in plasma and cerebrospinal fluid in young (plaque-free) and aged (plaque-bearing) Tg2576 mice. *J. Pharmacol. Exp. Ther.* 305: 864–871, 2003.

LEWIS, H.D., PEREZ REVUALTA, B.I., NADIN, A., NEDUVELIL, J.G., HARRISON, T., POLLACK, S.J., and SHEARMAN, M.S. Catalytic site-directed gamma-secretase complex inhibitors do not discriminate pharmacologically between Notch S3 and beta-APP cleavages. *Biochemistry* 42: 7580–7586, 2003.

MAMIYA, T., YAMADA, K., MIYAMOTO, Y., KONIG, N., WATANABE, Y., NODA, Y., and NABESHIMA, T. Neuronal mechanism of nociceptin-induced modulation of learning and memory: involvement of *N*-methyl-D-aspartate receptors. *Mol. Psych.* 8: 752–765, 2003.

NAKAZAWA, K., SUN, L.D., QUIRK, M.C., RONDI-REIG, L., WILSON, M.A., and TONEGAWA, S. Hippocampal CA3 NMDA receptors are crucial for memory acquisition of one-time experience. *Neuron* 38: 305–315, 2003.

PHIEL, C.J., WILSON, C.A., LEE, V.M.Y., and KLEIN, P.S. GSK-3α regulates production of Alzheimer's disease amyloid-β-peptides. *Nature* 423: 435–439, 2003.

REISBERG, B., DOODY, R., STOFFLER, A., SCHMITT, F., FERRIS, S., and MOBIUS, H.J. The Memantine Study Group. *N. Eng. J. Med.* 348: 1333–1341, 2003.

SCHENK, D., BARBOUR, R., DUNN, W., GORDON, G., GRAJEDA, H., GUIDO, T., HU, K., HUANG, J., JOHNSON-WOOD, K., KHAN, K., KHOLODENKO, D., LEE, M., LIAO, Z., LIEBERBURG, I., MOTTER, R., MUTTER, L., SORIANO, F., SHOPP, G., VASQUEZ, N., VANERVERT, C., WALKER, S., WOGULIS, M., YEDNOCK, T., GAMES, D., and SEUBERT, P. Immunization with amyloid-beta attenuates Alzheimer-disease-like pathology in the PDAPP mouse. *Nature* 400: 173–177, 1999.

SCHNEIDER, J.S., TINKER, J.P., MENZAGHI, F., and LLOYD, G.K. The subtype-selective nicotinic acetylcholine receptor agonist SIB-1553A improves both attention and memory components of a spatial working memory task in chronic low dose 1-methyl-4-phenyl-1,2,3,6-tetrahydropyridine-treated monkeys. *J. Pharm. Exp. Ther.* 306: 401–406, 2003.

SILVERBERG, G.D., LEVINTHAL, E., SULLIVAN, E.V., BLOCK, D.A., CHANG, S.D., LEVEREN, J.l, FLITMAN, S., WINN, R., MARCIANO, F., SAUL, F., HUHN, S., MAYO, M., and McGUIRE, I. Assessment of low-flow CSF drainage as a treatment for AD: results of a randomized pilot study. *Neurology* 59: 1126–1127, 2002.

TUSZYNSKI, M.H., and BLESCH, A. Nerve growth factor: from animal models of cholinergic neuron degeneration to gene therapy in Alzheimer's disease. *Prog. Brain Res.* 146: 441–449, 2004.

WANG, H.Y., LI, W., BENEDETTI, N.J., and LEE, D.H. Alpha 7 nicotinic acetylcholine receptors mediate beta-amyloid peptide-induced tau protein phosphorylation. *J. Biol. Chem.* 278: 31547–31553, 2003.

Chapter 10

Parkinson's Disease

In 1817 Dr. James Parkinson, a physician working in England, published an article to describe a clinical condition he called shaking palsy. Other neurologists began to accept the condition as a defined clinical entity and referred to it as Parkinson's disease, the name that now stands for a well-recognized neurological condition. To this day the initial behavioral description by James Parkinson provides the basis for the clinical diagnosis:

> *Involuntary tremulous motion, with lessened muscular power, in part not in action and even when supported; with a propensity to bend the trunk forwards, and to pass from a walking to a running pace; the senses and intellect being uninjured.*

The inability to move, the dominance of the symptoms related to motor functions, justifies the inclusion of Parkinson's disease in the group of movement disorders, although it has become clear that there are significant cognitive and emotional alterations. Parkinson's disease is not a fatal illness and, because of the existing drugs, manageable for many years. Nevertheless, it is a difficult and emotionally painful disease, in particular, when it progresses beyond the initial years. Celebrity cases, for example, Pope John Paul II, have brought the disease to common awareness and broad public understanding.

From the perspective of drug discovery, Parkinson's disease is uniquely attractive and uniquely difficult. The current drug treatment represents the first successful example of rationale drug discovery in the neuroscience, heralded in textbooks, lectures, prices, novels, and movies. Indeed, these drugs allow physicians to effectively treat the symptoms of Parkinson's disease for many years. They are a proud example of what drug discovery can do and promises to achieve for many other nervous system diseases. However, the current drugs do not prevent the progression of the disease and gradually become ineffective. Curative medication has remained elusive despite years of intense research and substantial discoveries. Strong supportive evidence exists for both, environmental and genetic causes. It seems possible to merge the two sets of data into a unifying hypothesis for the disease mechanism and to define obvious drug target opportunities. The search for disease-modifying drugs for Parkinson's disease thus remains one of the most challenging and rewarding goals for neuroscience drug discovery.

10.1 SYMPTOMS AND PATHOLOGY

Parkinson's disease affects approximately 1% of the population above 65 years of age. While there are rare cases of young Parkinson's disease patients, the typical age of onset is after the age of 45. Three cardinal symptoms, bradykinesia, rigidity, and tremor, allow

Drug Discovery for Nervous System Diseases, by Franz F. Hefti
ISBN 0-471-46563-1   Copyright © 2005 by John Wiley & Sons, Inc.

the neurologist to make the initial clinical diagnosis. Slowness of movement (brady-kinesia from Greek) presents itself as slow, shuffling gait, low and slurred speech, tiny handwriting, and general immobility. The body appears rigid. Forced movement of joints is not smooth but reminiscent of cogwheels. Tremor of the limbs occurs at rest but is suppressed during purposeful movements, when walking or grasping an object. The disease gradually advances over many years. The rate of progression is variable from patient to patient, but most of them reach an end stage within 15 to 20 years after diagnosis. Before the discovery of the symptomatic treatment the advanced cases required hospitalization or care in nursing homes, since they were immobile and unable to perform the basic functions of human life. Death occurred from respiratory and gastrointestinal complications, not from the disease itself.

Postmortem analysis provides the conclusive diagnosis of Parkinson's disease. There are two determining features, the selective loss of dopaminergic neurons in the substantia nigra and the occurrence of Lewy bodies. Dopaminergic neurons provide a dense innervation to the motor nuclei of the basal ganglia, the caudate nucleus and putamen in particular. They also innervate in more diffuse manner structures associated with emotional and cognitive functions such as cerebral cortex, nucleus accumbens, amygdala, and hippocampus. The dopaminergic cell bodies are located in the zona campacta of the substantia nigra and in the ventral tegmentum. In primates and humans the dopaminergic neurons are heavily pigmented, appearing black in sections of unstained brain. The name substantia nigra (black substance) directly reflects this property. In Parkinson's disease pigmentation is substantially reduced or completely absent. Underlying this macroscopic difference, the number of dopaminergic cell bodies is typically reduced to less than 20% of the normal population.

The Lewy bodies are a unique histopathological feature, intracellular inclusions that are stained with eosin, the classical dye for cytoplasmic components. The Lewy bodies tend to be ball-shaped and, at further microscopic analysis, have an amorphous core with radiating fibrils. They occur in the remaining dopaminergic neurons of the substantia nigra but also in nondopaminergic neurons of other brain areas. The protein α-synuclein is the principal component of Lewy bodies. α-Synuclein is a soluble monomeric protein that is abundant in neuronal synapses and is believed to be important for the presynaptic function. The demonstration of substantial dopaminergic neuron loss in the midbrain and the existence of Lewy bodies provide the conclusive postmortem diagnosis of Parkinson's disease.

In addition to the motor symptoms, Parkinson's disease is often associated with emotional and cognitive symptoms such as fatigue, depression, and slowness in thinking (bradyphrenia). In addition there are problems in functions mediated by the autonomous nervous system. Sleep disturbance, numbness and tingling and other sensory disturbances, bladder dysfunction, and constipation are common complaints of Parkinson patients. Over the years these nonmotor symptoms can become the most significant problem of patient care. In elderly patients cognitive decline is frequent, leading often to a diagnosis of Parkinson's and Alzheimer's disease. However, the two diseases are clearly distinct and believed to reflect different diseases pathways. Parkinson's disease is now recognized as a complex neurological disease with behavioral components beyond the initially described motor symptoms (Fahn, 2003).

10.2 SYMPTOMATIC DOPAMINE REPLACEMENT THERAPY

The dopaminergic neurons that degenerate in Parkinson's disease constitute only a tiny fraction of all neurons in the human brain. The total number of mesencephalic dopaminergic neurons in the human brain has been estimated at 0.5 to 1.0 million. Assuming the rough estimate of 100 billion for the total number of neurons in the human brain, dopaminergic neurons represent the small fraction of only 0.001%. It seems surprising that the loss of such a minor proportion can cause a major neurological disease, in particular, when comparing it with the typically negligible consequences of cortical lesions of similar size. However, the unique and crucial role of dopaminergic neurons is very well documented. Neuropathological studies over an entire century have confirmed the correlation between dopaminergic neuron loss and disease symptoms (Jellinger, 2002). While other neuronal systems may show degenerative changes at advanced stages of the disease, they are not as severe or as consistent as those of the dopaminergic neurons.

Animal studies strongly support the view that the loss of mesencephalic dopaminergic neurons is responsible for the behavioral symptoms of Parkinson's disease. Selective toxins are available to destroy dopaminergic neurons in the living brain. 6-Hydroxydopamine is a close analogue of dopamine with a high oxidative potential. Following direct injection into the brain, it is transported by the dopamine and norepinephrine transporters into the catecholaminergic neurons, where its oxidative capacity leads to rapid degenerative changes and cell death. Local bilateral injections of 6-hydroxydopamine into the substantia nigra selectively destroy dopaminergic neurons and generate animal models that accurately reproduce the cell loss in Parkinson's disease. Animals with complete bilateral 6-hydroxydopamine lesions of the substantia nigra are immobile. A second toxin, 1-methyl-4-phenyl-1,2,3,6-tetrahydropyridine (MPTP), passes the blood-brain barrier and is oxidized to 1-methyl-4-phenyl-pyridinium (MPP$^+$) through the catalytic action of monoamine oxidase (MAO). MPP$^+$ is a selective substrate for the dopamine transporter and accumulates selectively in the dopaminergic neurons, where it interferes with mitochondrial mechanisms, leading to dopaminergic cell death. Rodents, primates, and even humans exposed to MPTP are hypokinetic and rigid in a similar way as parkinsonian patients.

Efficacy of dopamine replacement therapy most convincingly demonstrates the central role of the dopaminergic deficit in Parkinson's disease. The history of the discovery of dopamine as neurotransmitter and of the conceptualization of dopamine replacement therapy is well known (Carlsson, 2002). The selective loss of neurons in the substantia nigra, and the realization that these provide the major dopaminergic innervation to the forebrain, suggested that the symptoms are caused by the absence of dopamine and that replacing the missing transmitter might be therapeutically effective. Exploratory studies made clear that dopamine was ineffective because it did not cross the blood-brain barrier. Systemic administration of the brain penetrant precursor, L-DOPA, provided some improvement but also severe cardiovascular adverse effects because the bulk of it was decarboxylated to vasoactive dopamine before passing through the blood-brain barrier. Two, independently working pharmaceutical industry research groups at Roche, in Basel, Switzerland, and Merck & Co., in West Point, Pennsylvania, produced combination drugs in which L-DOPA is combined with a non–brain penetrant inhibitor of the enzyme that catalyzes the conversion to dopamine (Bartholini and Pletscher, 1968; Lotti and Porter, 1970). The combination of L-DOPA with peripheral inhibitors of aromatic amino acid decarboxylase (AADC) produces substantial elevations of dopamine levels in the brain without cardiovascular side effects (Fig. 10.1). These drugs provide very effective,

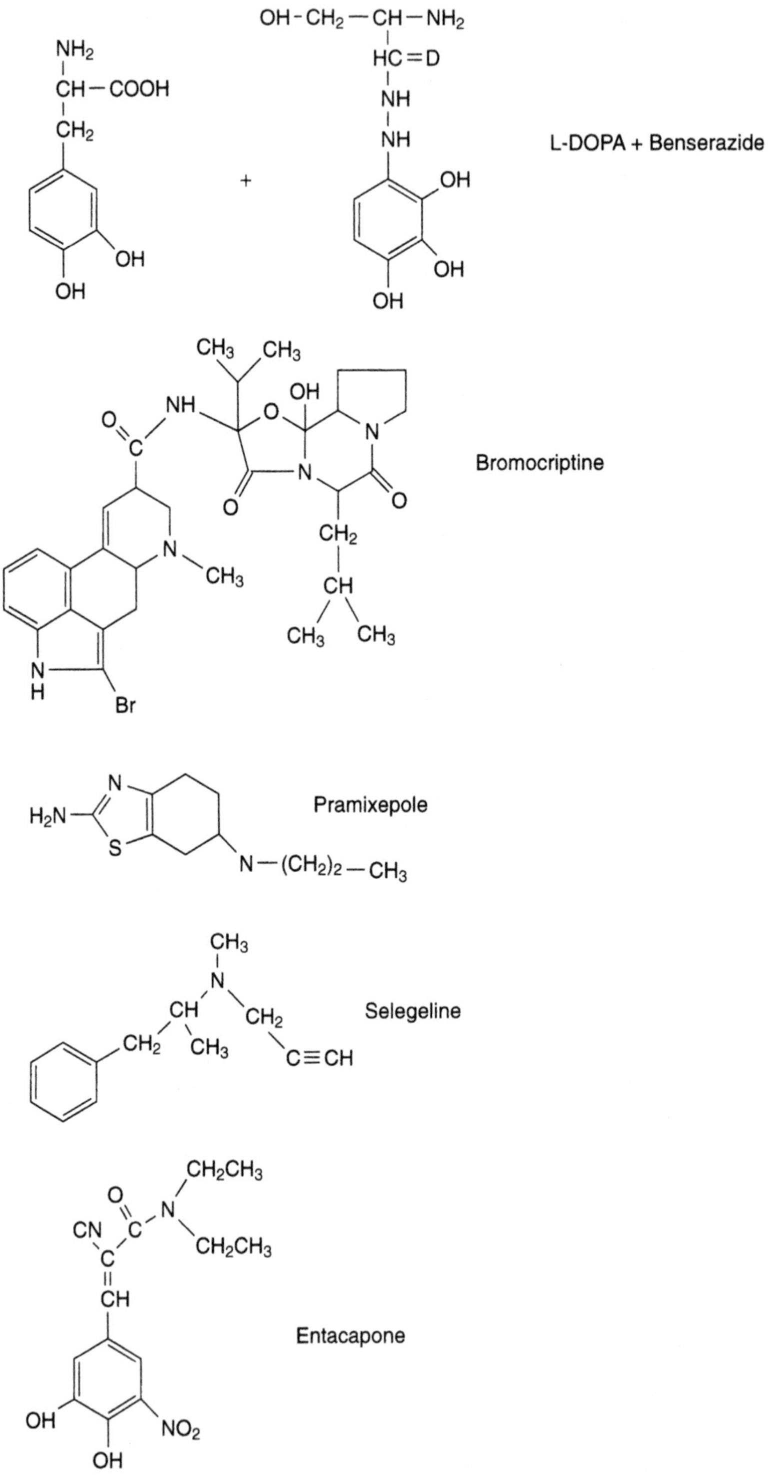

Figure 10.1 Current drugs for Parkinson's disease (L-DOPA and benserazide, an inhibitor of peripheral AAAD are given as combination drug). Bromocriptine and pramexipole are dopamine receptor agonists; selegeline is an inhibitor of MAO, entacapone an inhibitor of COMT.

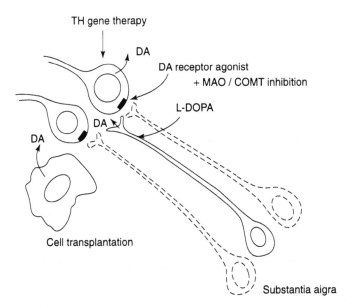

Figure 10.2 Dopamine substitution therapy. The degeneration of dopaminergic neurons decreases dopamine release in the target areas. Precursor therapy with L-DOPA generates dopamine in the surviving neurons. Inhibition of dopamine metabolism with MAO and COMT inhibitors increase the synaptic levels of dopamine. Direct dopamine receptor agonists replace the missing dopamine. Transplantation of cells able to release dopamine into the target areas provides a local source of dopamine. Gene therapy with the synthetic enzyme TH generates the synthetic machinery in the target area.

sometimes miraculous relief of the symptoms of Parkinson's disease, in particular, during the first few years after the initial diagnosis.

Following the introduction of L-DOPA, the molecular characterization of the dopaminergic synapse has identified alternative drug targets for dopamine substitution therapy (Fig. 10.2). Several directly acting dopamine receptor agonists have been discovered and introduced into clinical practice. The first one, bromocriptine, was followed by pergolide, ropinirole, and pramipexole. These compounds are all agonists on the D_2 receptor subtype but differ in their affinity to other dopamine receptor subtypes. Bromocriptine is a selective D_2 agonist. Pergolide also stimulates D_1 receptors, whereas ropinirole and pramipexole are agonists on D_2 and D_3 receptors. The contribution of D_1 and D_3 receptor activation to the clinical efficacy has remained controversial. The clinical efficacy of bromocriptine documents that D_2 activation is sufficient for the therapeutic effect. Tentative evidence has been obtained that D_3 receptor co-activation has a beneficial effect on the adverse effect profile. Selective D_1 agonists have been reported to be efficacious in animal models of Parkinson's disease, but none of these compounds have reached clinical practice. Thus D_1 and D_3 receptors remain potential drug targets for Parkinson's disease.

The synaptic concentration of dopamine is controlled by release, re-uptake, and degradation of the transmitter. Inhibitors of catabolic enzymes, MAO and catechol-*O*-methyltransferase (COMT), have found utility as drugs. Selegeline and entacapone, respectively, are approved drugs inhibiting these enzymes. They have marginal efficacy by themselves but are useful as adjunct drugs to L-DOPA and dopamine agonists. While theoretically useful, drugs that affect release and reuptake of dopamine are not prescribed because of their abuse potential. Amphetamine, a compound that releases dopamine and

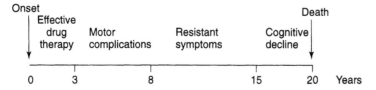

Figure 10.3   Gradual loss of efficacy of dopamine replacement therapy.

other catecholamines, and cocaine, which selectively blocks the dopamine transporter (DAT), induce excessive behavioral stimulation and have a very high abuse potential.

Dopamine replacement therapy effectively controls parkinsonian symptoms during the first years of the disease. Invariably, however, patients experience problems (Fig. 10.3). The drug treatment gradually becomes less efficacious, a situation clinical described as "wearing off phenomenon." Some patients experience disturbing fluctuations between periods of drug efficacy and absence of benefit. Some of the patients can shift within a few minutes from full motor activity to complete immobility. The molecular basis of this on–off phenomenon is unclear. The wearing-off and on–off phenomena prompt patients to increase the drug doses, very often at the price of dopaminergic overstimulation that manifests itself in involuntary movements, called dyskinesia.

The gradually occurring complications of dopamine replacement therapy is believed to reflect the underlying progression of the disease. Dopaminergic neurons continue to degenerate. Their terminals disappear over time, and the death of the cell body completes the process. The progressing loss of dopaminergic innervation increases the burden carried by the pharmacotherapy. Patients typically start therapy with L-DOPA or a dopamine receptor agonist alone and then gradually increase the dose. At later stages they combine the two, and finally add MAO and COMT inhibitors as adjunct therapy. The fine-tuning or titration of dopaminergic replacement therapy often requires an expert movement disorder specialist who supervises the patients during their exploration of various drug combinations and regimens.

The stimulation of dopaminergic receptors during several years with drugs may contribute to the wearing-off and on–off phenomena. It has been speculated that chronic L-DOPA therapy may have long-term toxic effects on the brain. If so, it would be best to start pharmacotherapy with dopamine agonists and to delay L-DOPA as long as possible. The question whether to start treatment with L-DOPA or with dopamine agonists has been a long-standing controversy in the Parkinson field. Up to this day it has remained unresolved and has retained its ability to generate heated discussions at scientific meetings. There is no conclusive data demonstrating that L-DOPA therapy, even over many years, reduces the function and viability of dopaminergic neurons in animals. Small-scale imaging studies in human patients suggest that dopaminergic marker proteins visualized with PET studies decline less rapidly in patients treated with agonists than in patients treated with L-DOPA (Marek et al., 2002). While the imaging studies are suggestive, they need to be replicated with larger patient populations and the behavioral significance of the observed changes has to be established before reliable conclusions can be drawn.

In some Parkinson patients long-term treatment with L-DOPA or dopamine agonists causes psychotic symptoms. This not surprising since dopamine D_2 antagonists are therapeutically useful in schizophrenia and since agents that enhance dopaminergic neurotransmission, amphetamine and cocaine, are known to induce psychosis. The dose as well as subtle differences in the mechanisms of dopaminergic stimulation determine the occurrence of psychotic symptoms in Parkinson patients. At sufficiently high doses every drug able to stimulate dopaminergic receptors induces psychotic symptoms. In Parkinson patients treated with L-DOPA, visual hallucinations and paranoia are common, rather than auditory hallucinations that are more widespread in schizophrenia. In elderly parkinsonian patients, it is often these psychiatric adverse effects that present the biggest problem in patient care.

Despite the long-term complications dopamine replacement therapy allows patients to live normally for many years (Guttman et al., 2003). Efforts continue to provide additional drugs with different degrees of selectivity and improved pharmacokinetic properties. It is possible that agonists with unique profiles of D_1, D_2, and D_3 receptor activation or agonists with different pharmacokinetic properties might have better therapeutic efficacy than the existing receptor agonists. The available experience, however, suggests that such improvements will only be marginal. Agonists with different receptor subtype profiles have been tested in patients, revealing only small differences in efficacy and adverse effect profiles. Several attempts with alternative formulations of L-DOPA to provide steady plasma concentrations failed to substantially improve the therapeutic benefits. Most patients optimize individually their intake of various medications for maximal therapeutic benefit. It is quite possibly that the currently available dopamine replacement drugs offer the maximal therapeutic benefits that can be achieved with this approach.

Dopaminergic cell transplantation is a variant of dopamine replacement therapy that generated very high hopes for many years. In animal models fetal dopaminergic neurons implanted into the target areas of dopaminergic neurons completely reverse the parkinsonian symptoms. Many years of clinical experimentation confirmed that beneficial effects can be obtained in humans. However, carefully controlled clinical studies showed relatively mild benefits only and long-term adverse effects in many patients (Olanow et al., 2003). The experience with fetal cell transplantation puts in question the efforts to produce engineered cells able to secrete dopamine or to generate dopaminergic cells from stem cells for transplantation studies. The results obtained with fetal transplantation make it likely that the maximal benefits to be obtained from such approaches will not supersede those obtained with drug-based dopamine replacement therapy. It tends to confirm the view that dopamine replacement therapy is close to the maximum possible with the existing drugs.

10.3 PALLIATIVE DRUGS ACTING ON OTHER TRANSMITTER SYSTEMS

The nigro-striatal dopaminergic projection is part of the extrapyramidal motor system, which makes an essential contribution to all motor behaviors (Fig. 10.4). The dopaminergic neurons modify the activity of the GABAergic and cholinergic neurons in the putamen and caudate nucleus (caudate-putamen in rodents), exerting a restraining influence on the GABAergic output pathways to the globus pallidus and the thalamus, which form the major inhibitory output pathways of the extrapyramidal system. Removal of the dopaminergic nigro-striatal pathway, by experimental lesions or through the influence of Parkinson's disease, reduces this inhibitory influence of dopamine and so generates hyperactivity in the GABAergic pathways. The resulting, more pronounced inhibition in the extrapyramidal systems is believed to underlie many of the behavioral features of Parkin-

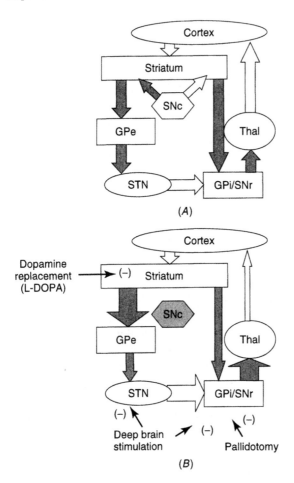

Figure 10.4 Extrapyramidal pathways and effect of dopaminergic neuron degeneration. (**A**) Under normal conditions the dopaminergic input to the striatum provides a balanced stimulation to the direct and indirect output pathways that regulate the motor nuclei. (**B**) Absence of dopaminergic neurons produces abnormal excitation in the indirect pathway and increased inhibition of the thalamic motor nuclei. Dopamine replacement therapy and neurosurgical interference in specific nuclei correct some of the misbalance. GPe: external globus pallidus; Gpi: internal globus pallidus; SNc: substantia nigra zona compacta; Snr: substantia nigra zona reticulata. STN: subthalamic nucleus; Thal: thalamus. (Reprinted with permission, Marino et al., 2003)

son's disease. It should thus be possible to find drugs that directly modify these systems and that compensate for the absence of the dopaminergic input. Such drugs might be able to complement the dopamine replacement therapy and reduce its adverse effects. In particular, they might be able to dampen any excessive stimulation caused by dopaminergic agents and so reduce the associated symptoms, hyperkinesias and psychosis.

Opposing the inhibitory effect of dopaminergic afferents, cholinergic interneurons in the putamen and caudate nucleus exert an excitatory influence on the GABAergic output neurons. By inhibiting the cholinergic influence, it is possible to compensate in part for the effects of dopaminergic denervation. Indeed, before the discovery of dopamine replacement therapy, antagonists for muscarinic cholinergic receptors, such as atropine, were frequently used in clinical practice of Parkinson's disease. They produce a mild beneficial effect only but are still added occasionally to the dopamine replacement therapy. Amantadine, a compound that entered clinical practice as an antiviral drug, has to be added to the list of clinical useful drugs. It has various affinities to cholinergic and glutamatergic receptors. Its modest therapeutic effects in Parkinson's disease are ascribed to its anticholinergic properties. It remains possible that selective cholinergic receptor antagonists have a more pronounced therapeutic effect in Parkinson's disease than the currently available nonselective ones. The very marginal efficacy of the nonselective drugs, however, dampens the enthusiasm for this approach.

Impressive neurosurgical contributions to Parkinson therapy provide strong support for the view that direct modulation of the activity of the extrapyramidal pathways is therapeutically effective. Precise stereotaxic lesions of specific thalamic nuclei provide effective relief of some parkinsonian symptoms, tremor in particular. Stereotaxic surgery has become an excellent treatment option for patients with poor response to dopamine replacement therapy and a predominance of tremor. In the recent years deep brain stimulation with surgically implanted electrodes has replaced the earlier lesion techniques. The precise mechanism of action of deep brain stimulation is not understood. High-frequency stimulation may activate glutamatergic pathways or, alternatively, desensitize inhibitory GABAergic pathways of the extrapyramidal motor system. The success of the neuro-surgical intervention provides indirect validation for drug targets that mediate pharmacological manipulation of the output pathways of the putamen and caudate nucleus.

Most GABAergic projection neurons from putamen and caudate nucleus innervate the globus pallidus. GABAergic transmission in the globus pallidus is modulated by glutamatergic neurons that influence GABA release at the presynaptic level. Anatomical and electrophysiological studies identified mGluR4 receptors as key mediators of this effect. mGluR4 agonists reduce the inhibitory actions of GABA. Allosteric mGluR4 agonists have been identified that reverse the sedative effects of reserpine, a drug that depletes catecholamines in the brain and provides a crude pharmacological model for parkinsonian immobility. Despite the need for further confirmation in appropriate animal models of Parkinson's disease, the available data identify the mGluR4 receptor as a highly attractive drug target for Parkinson's disease. The possibility to use allosteric modulators rather than direct activators is particularly attractive because modulators are less likely to produce excessive and detrimental stimulation of the receptors (Marino et al., 2003).

The identification of the mGluR4 receptor as drug target exemplifies target identification strategies that incorporates anatomical, physiological, and clinical knowledge of the function of the extrapyramidal motor system. The same approach is likely to identify additional targets that influence firing patterns in the extrapyramidal motor system. Involvement of other ionotropic and metabotropic glutamate receptors is expected. Those selectively involved in extrapyramidal motor functions will represent attractive drug targets. Selectively expressed receptors for modulatory neurotransmitters and neuropeptides may represent appealing alternatives. Adenosine A2A receptors have been pursued, since they are highly expressed in several parts of the basal ganglia. In the globus pallidus they potentiate the release of GABA, in support of the view that A2A antagonists might be therapeutically useful. Clinical studies with A2A antagonists showed mild improvements of therapeutic efficacy of L-DOPA, but the effect was not at a level making a convincing case for the underlying concept (Bara-Jimenez et al., 2003). It is possible that effects on A2A receptors outside of the extrapyramidal system limit the therapeutically useful effects. Receptors uniquely located in the extrapyramidal system represent more suitable drug targets. The search for such receptors remains an exciting and promising approach to improved antiparkinsonian therapeutics.

10.4 DISEASE-MODIFYING DRUGS

None of the currently available drugs prevent the progression of Parkinson's disease. Future detailed comparative studies may reveal minor differences in the rate individual adverse effects appear with the chronic use of specific palliative drugs. The problems remains, though, that the majority of Parkinson patients reach a state of "burnout" several years after the initial diagnosis of the disease. The loss of dopaminergic neurons progresses despite the treatment, gradually raising the hurdle the therapeutics have to overcome. Fortunately, because of recent significant scientific breakthroughs, the Parkinson field is now poised to identify drugs that might be able to stop the loss of dopaminergic neurons. The breakthroughs include the discovery that Parkinson's disease can be caused by environmental toxins as well as by genetic mutations, and that mitochondrial dysfunction plays a central role in the disease process. A unified hypothesis for the Parkinson's disease mechanism, similar to the amyloid hypothesis in Alzheimer's disease, is emerging. Optimal drug targets remain to be identified, but the aspects discussed below are likely to become integral components of the final picture (Dauer and Przedborski, 2003).

10.4.1 MPTP

The discovery of the dopaminergic neuron toxin MPTP makes an astounding story, both for its societal significance and its impact on Parkinson research. Details have been narrated extensively (Langston, 1996), so the essentials may suffice for this chapter. In 1982 MPTP was generated involuntarily during illegal synthesis of a heroin substitute sold as street drug in San Jose, California. A small number of drug users developed parkinsonian symptoms and found their ways to Parkinson's disease specialists. Scientific investigations in the style of the now widely popular Crime Scene Investigation television shows provided initial evidence that MPTP destroyed the dopaminergic cells and caused parkinsonian symptoms in the drug users. The subsequent broad effort of many research laboratories firmly established the mechanisms of action of this compound (Fig. 10.5). Following intravenous administration, MPTP passes the blood-brain barrier and is converted to 1-methyl-4-phenylpyridinium (MPP^+) through the catalytic action of MAO-A. MPP^+ is a selective substrate for the dopamine transporter DAT and accumulates selectively within dopaminergic neurons. Its chemical structure, which includes a delocalized positive charge, favors accumulation in the mitochondria, where it inhibits the function of complex I. The resulting mitochondrial deficiency causes cell death of the dopaminergic neurons. The symptoms the patients manifest are indistinguishable from those of Parkinson's disease.

The MPTP story remains the best illustration for dangers of street drugs and serves wonderfully well to scare susceptible teenagers. What is the significance for Parkinson drug discovery? The discovery that a single toxic event can cause Parkinson's disease prompted a flurry of speculations on environmental toxins potentially responsible for the majority of the cases. Suggestive observations pointed to higher incidence in geographical areas with intense agriculture. It was emphasized that Parkinson's disease was first

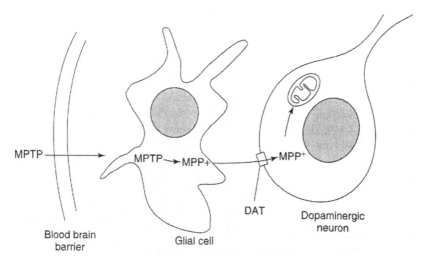

Figure 10.5 Mechanism of action of MPTP. The toxin is able to pass the blood-brain barrier. It penetrates into glial cells where it is converted to MPP⁻, which is selectively taken up into dopaminergic neurons by the dopamine transporter DAT. Within the dopaminergic neurons it inhibits mitochondrial function by blocking complex I.

described in early industrial England, during the first period in history when human-made chemicals (xenobiotics) were produced in large quantities. More detailed epidemiological studies, however, failed identify the expected geographical pockets of Parkinson's disease. The distribution is surprisingly uniform over the entire globe. Citations from old literature emerged that suggested the existence of Parkinson's disease well before the industrial revolution. For example, the Roman physician Galen described ". . . a kind of paralysis which prevents people from walking straight . . . , failing to lift the foot and pulling back instead, like walking up a steep decline," a picture immediately invoking a Parkinson patient. Despite intensive searches it proved impossible to identify specific compounds that might be responsible for the majority of Parkinson's disease cases. The structural requirements are very strict for a compound to have MPTP-like toxicity. Several criteria have to be fulfilled by a single molecule. It has to be bioavailable, following oral or cutaneous exposure, pass the blood-brain barrier, be a substrate for DAT, and it has to be a mitochondrial toxin. Only MPTP itself and a few very close analogues fulfill all these criteria (Michel, 1989). The mechanism of action of MPTP speaks against the possibility that the majority of Parkinson cases are caused by exposure to a specific dopaminergic neurotoxin. Nevertheless, it is possible that toxic exposures might make a significant contribution to the disease process. Two molecules, paraquat and rotenone, which have structural similarity to MPTP and are mitochondrial toxins are able to destroy dopaminergic neurons when infused chronically into animals (Betarbet et al., 2000). In cell cultures they do not selectively destroy dopaminergic neurons and evidence for nonselective toxicity has been observed also in vivo. It is, however, possible that the dopaminergic neurons are more vulnerable to mitochondrial inhibition than some of the nondopaminergic neurons and that the loss of dopaminergic neurons is clinically more significant than that of other neurons. The studies with rotenone and paraquat are compatible with the view that long-term exposure to environmental toxins is a contributing factor to the parkinsonian disease mechanism.

10.4.2 Mitochondrial Dysfunction

The inhibition of complex I by MPTP or other mitochondrial toxins reduces the formation of ATP and may thus result in energy failure and death by dopaminergic neurons in extreme situations. Even with partial inhibition, however, complex I inhibition results in overflow of electrons, and the increased production of free radicals and reactive oxygen species. This condition is often referred to as "oxidative stress" and is believed to be a contributing or even causative factor for neuronal death (Cohen, 2000). Experimental manipulations that reduce the levels of free radicals and reactive oxygen species in animals attenuate MPTP toxicity in animals. For example, transgenic overexpression of superoxide dismutase, a free radical scavenger enzyme, increases the tolerance to MPTP. Mice with null mutations of neuronal nitric oxide synthase, the enzyme responsible for the formation of the highly reactive peroxynitrite, are also less responsive to MPTP. Depletion of glutathione, a molecule deactivating reactive oxygen species, increases the toxicity. Oxidative damage can affect many cellular molecules and processes. Specific proteins malfunction and the patterns of gene expression change. For example, poly-ADP-ribose polymerase, a DNA repair enzyme that is highly ATP dependent, is induced. Knockout mice of this gene are less vulnerable to MPTP toxicity. The combination of ATP depletion and oxidative damage appears to lead to cell death following the inhibition of complex I by MPTP.

Tentative findings are available that mitochondrial dysfunction and free-radical damage participate in the disease process of human Parkinson's disease. Some of the familial forms of Parkinson's disease appear to be associated with mitochondrial deficiencies. A single-nucleotide polymorphism in NADH dehydrogenase of complex I affects the risk of Parkinson's disease in Caucasian populations (van der Walt et al., 2003). Additional, more speculative observations lend support. The substantia nigra is rich in Fe^{2+}, an ion that catalyzes oxidative reactions. Chelators of ion prevent MPTP toxicity (Kaur et al., 2003). Exposure to high doses of manganese can cause a condition similar to Parkinson's disease. Mn^{2+} ions may accelerate catalytic processes normally supported by Fe^{2+}. While very speculative, these considerations suggest the possibility that free-radical scavengers or ion chelators may be beneficial in the treatment of Parkinson's disease. In the mitochondria, coenzyme Q_{10} accepts the electrons released by complex I and serves as natural antioxidant. Inhibition of complex I could exceed the capacity of the available coenzyme Q_{10}, a condition that might be overcome by external administration of coenzyme Q_{10} or other suitable antioxidant molecules. An initial clinical study with high doses of coenzyme Q_{10} indeed provided evidence for decreased progression of the disease (Shults et al., 2002). Confirmation of these beneficial effects of coenzyme Q_{10} will hopefully validate the antioxidant approach to Parkinson's disease and strengthen an attractive field for drug discovery.

10.4.3 Disease Genes: α-Synuclein, Parkins

The discovery of several forms of familial Parkinson's disease has shifted the focus of attention from environmental causes to genetic causes. The first autosomal dominant mutation causing Parkinson's disease was identified in α-synuclein, a protein that constitutes the major component of Lewy bodies (Polymeropoulos et al., 1997). Similar to other aggregating proteins, α-synuclein is able to form fibrils composed of antiparallel β-sheet structures. This discovery had enormous impact on Parkinson research, since it proves that a single molecular event can cause the two major pathological features, dopaminergic cell degeneration and the formation of Lewy bodies. α-Synuclein is predominantly located in the presynaptic terminals of neurons where it is believed to play a role in docking and recycling of synaptic vesicles. Deletion of the gene in mouse has few if any functional consequences, making it unlikely that the human mutation cause Parkinson's disease because of a lack of function. Two disease-causing mutations have been detected, both of which increase the propensity of α-synuclein to aggregate into oligomers and to form protofibrils. Two kindreds with familial Parkinson's disease are caused by multiplication of the α-synuclein gene. The carriers succumb to an accelerated form of the disease, including loss of dopaminergic neurons, formation of Lewy bodies, and severe neuronal loss in brain areas other than the substantia nigra (Farrer et al., 2004). Overexpression of mutant α-synuclein in mice causes various pathological changes, including the formation of Lewy body-like cellular inclusions. In some models small reductions in dopaminergic neuron numbers have been detected. But these changes are far less significant than those in Parkinson's disease, and they are not selective for the dopaminergic cells. Selective dopaminergic neuron degeneration has been observed in *Drosophila* expressing the human mutant α-synuclein gene, providing further support for the view that α-synuclein mutations are able to cause selective dopaminergic cell loss (Eriksen et al., 2003).

A second mutation causing Parkinson's disease, discovered soon after α-synuclein, is an autosomal recessive mutation in a gene called parkin. The encoded protein is part of the proteasome protein degradation complex. It functions as an E3 ubiquitin ligase that links misfolded proteins to ubiquitin and leads them to degradation. Several parkin mutations have been discovered that inactivate the enzymatic function. These findings prompt the hypothesis that parkin mutations prevent the degradation of misfolded α-synuclein and accelerate the formation of Lewy bodies and subsequent dopaminergic cell death. Several other Parkinson's disease genes have been discovered following the description of α-synuclein and parkin. An attempt to generate a standardized nomenclature has assigned the code name "park 1" to α-synuclein, "park 2" to parkin, and "park 3–10" to the other genes identified as loci for disease-causing mutations. The park 5 locus encodes ubiquitin C-terminal hydrolyse-L1, another enzyme of the proteasome protein degradation complex. Park 7 encodes DJ-1, a protein tentatively associated with mitochondrial functions and the inactivation of free radicals. The proteins encoded by the other park loci remain to be characterized.

10.4.4 Tentative Integrated Hypothesis and Drug Targets

The link of disease genes to protein degradation and mitochondrial functions, while still very tentative, prompts tantalizing speculations about the disease mechanism of Parkinson's disease (Dawson and Dawson, 2003). Figure 10.6 and Table 10.1 represent an attempt to depict a scheme that incorporates information gained from the mechanism of toxicity of MPTP as well as from the disease mutations. It has to be emphasized, though, that this scheme is speculative and awaiting confirmation by experimental studies. It has not been possible as yet to fit all disease-causing mutations and environmental toxins into a unified hypothesis or to replicate the full disease profile in transgenic animals. Substantial uncertainty remains, and additional research will be necessary before a unified hypothesis can be considered as plausible as the amyloid hypothesis for Alzheimer's disease.

Further research has to explain the selective vulnerability of dopaminergic neurons in

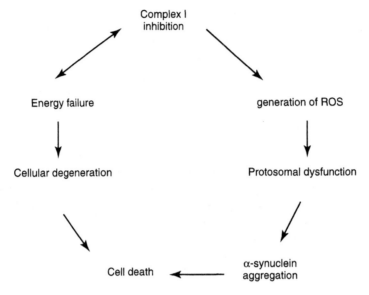

Figure 10.6 Unified hypothesis for disease mechanism. Mitochondrial failure initiates different cascades that lead to α-synuclein aggregation and cell death. Accelerated aggregation of α-synuclein in familial Parkinson's disease can directly cause cell death.

Table 10.1 Current and future drug targets for Parkinson's disease

---

Current Targets

Aromatic amino acid decarboxylase (conversion of L-DOPA to dopamine)

Dopamine receptors

D_2 receptors, contributions from D_1 and D_3 receptors

Catechol-*O*-methyltransferase (COMT)

Monoamine oxidase (MAO)

Future Drugs and Targets

D_1, D_3 dopamine receptors (selective agonists)

Glutamate receptors

mGluR4 receptors

AMPA receptors

Adenosine receptors

Reactive oxygen species

Fe^{2+} chelators

free-radical scavengers

α-Synuclein

anti-aggregation molecules

Proteasome complex

GDNF receptor (c-ret/GFRα1)

direct receptor activators

downstream regulators (e.g., Jnk inhibitors)

Parkinson's disease. It is tempting to speculate that the nature of the neurotransmitter, dopamine, may be a significant factor. Catecholamines, dopamine, and norepinephrine are reactive chemicals, and it is the dopaminergic and noradrenergic neurons that degenerate in Parkinson's disease. The very similar monoaminergic neuronal population, using the slightly less reactive transmitter substance serotonin, do not degenerate. Dopaminergic and noradrenergic neurons, but not serotonergic neurons, are pigmented in the human brain. Those neurons with high melanin content are particularly vulnerable. The absence of pigment in the rodent brain may explain the lack of success in replicating dopaminergic cell loss in transgenic animals. Melanin may play a significant but highly underestimated role in the disease process (Zecca, 2003).

The tentative hypothesis for a disease mechanism depicted in Figure 10.6 suggests a number of putative drug targets. Molecules that absorb the excessive reactive oxygen species, such as coenzyme Q_{10}, have received tentative clinical validation. Chelators of divalent ions such as Fe^{2+} may be useful. Effects of antioxidants or ion chelators will not be selective for dopaminergic neurons, generating significant concerns about general toxicity. Specific inhibitors of α-synuclein aggregation might prevent the formation of Lewy bodies. Hopefully, the recently discovered disease mutations will identify additional, and selective, putative drug targets. In absence of such discoveries, general strategies, such as those based on neurotrophic factors discussed below, may decrease the vulnerability of dopaminergic neurons to the disease process.

10.4.5 Neurotrophic Factor Therapy

Neurotrophic factors are crucial regulators of neuronal survival and maturation during development. In the adult nervous system these processes are no longer operational under normal conditions. However, the pharmacological administration of neurotrophic factors often increases the resistance of adult neuronal populations to toxic insults and disease processes and promotes their capacity for compensatory adaptations. Dopaminergic neurons of the mesencephalon respond to several neurotrophic factors. In the neurotrophin family, BDNF and neurotrophin-4/5, both of which activate the TrkB tyrosine kinase receptors, have mild beneficial effects in animals with experimentally induced degeneration of the dopaminergic cells. More robust effects are obtained with members of the glial cell-derived neurotrophic factor (GDNF) protein family. GDNF and neurturin, which activate receptor complexes composed of the protein kinase c-ret and, respectively, glycosylphosphatidylinositol-anchored GDNF family receptors $\alpha 1$ and $\alpha 2$ (GFRα1 and GFRα2), are beneficial in various lesion models of Parkinson's disease. As proteins, the neurotrophic factors do not pass the blood-brain barrier and require intracerebral administration to be effective. In an initial clinical trial, GDNF was infused into the ventricles of Parkinson patients through chronically implanted shunts and infusion pumps. This effort was abandoned because of various adverse effects and the absence of positive effects on parkinsonian symptoms. A second attempt, where GDNF was infused directly into the target areas of dopaminergic neurons, provided the first tentative evidence for clinical efficacy (Gill et al., 2003). Carefully controlled clinical studies will have to verify this approach.

Growth factor therapy, similar to stereotaxic surgery, may become useful for a subset of patients, but because of the invasive nature it is not suitable for general medical practice. The robust actions of neurotrophic factors have triggered the search for mimetics, small molecules that stimulate neurotrophic factor receptors or that modify their pathways

(Pollack and Harper, 2002). Selective, direct activators for Trk receptors so far have been elusive. While several research groups have reported initial progress toward such molecules, they have not been able to obtain sufficient potency or selectivity to make them suitable for clinical use. Transmembrane kinase receptors seem to represent a particular difficult challenge for drug discovery. While it is possible to make selective antagonists, a breakthrough is still awaited for direct activators or potentiators.

Events downstream of the neurotrophic factor receptors offer various putative drug targets that appear more drugable than the neurotrophic factors themselves (Fig. 10.7). Neurotrophic factors activate several pathways, some of which overlap with the so-called intracellular stress pathways that are activated by inflammatory cytokines and agents noxious to cells. The protein kinase c-Jun *N*-terminal kinase (Jnk) is believed to be a key mediator of these pathways. Inhibition of Jnk and kinases upstream of Jnk attenuates the toxic effects of MPP+ on dopaminergic neurons in cell culture. Most of the existing kinase

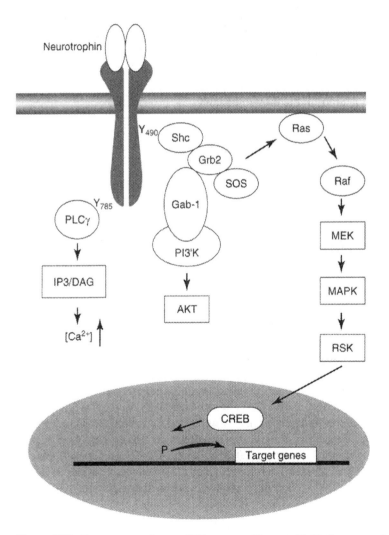

Figure 10.7   Downstream pathways of Trk receptors. Neurotrophin binding causes dimerization of Trk and phosphorylation of tyrosine residues at position 490 and 785. They bind the signaling molecules Shc and PLCγ and stimulate three distinct pathways, the Ras/Map kinase cascade, PI3 kinase and Akt, and IP3-mediated Ca^{2+} release. (Reproduced with permission, Segal, 2003)

inhibitors are not selective and interfere with the activity of several other kinases. One of them, CEP1347, identified by researchers at Cephalon Inc., West Chester, Pennsylvania, inhibits Jnk and attenuates MPTP toxicity in animal models of Parkinson's disease (Saporito et al., 2002). This compound is currently in clinical trials. A positive outcome will further validate the neurotrophic factor approach and will identify specific kinases as attractive drug targets.

During development the neurotrophic factors regulate the survival of responsive neurons by suppressing apoptotic mechanism. There is no conclusive evidence for an apoptotic component of the gradual loss of dopaminergic neurons in Parkinson's disease. However, it cannot be excluded that individual neurons go through degenerative events in very brief time intervals typical for apoptosis rather than, as is generally assumed, gradually loose functionality over many years. Apoptotic cell loss in slowly progressing neurodegenerative diseases might be comparable to radioactive decay where the gradual reduction of a population is caused by the rapid decay of individual atoms at different times. In cell culture systems the toxic effects of MPP+ on dopaminergic neurons are prevented by inhibitors of caspases, the proteases catalyzing protein degradation during apoptosis (Bilsland et al., 2002). It will be interesting to explore apoptotic mechanisms and the efficacy of apoptosis inhibitors in the emerging animal models of Parkinson's disease that reflect the gradually progressing cell loss.

Other drug discovery approaches related to neurotrophic factors include attempts to increase the synthesis of BDNF and to modify the function of immunophilins, proteins that have been linked to axonal regeneration in the nervous system. Ligands for immunophilins have been taken into clinical trials for Parkinson's disease, based on tantalizing but not entirely consistent effects in animal models of Parkinson's disease. In a search for compounds able to stimulate the synthesis of neurotrophic factors endogenous to the brain, specific ampakines, potentiators of the AMPA glutamate receptors, have been identified that are able to enhance the synthesis of BDNF. These compounds promote the survival of dopaminergic neurons in animal exposed to MPTP. The complex actions of ampakines on systems other than the dopaminergic neurons may limit their utility in Parkinson's disease. The animal studies do point out that it is possible to discover small, brain-penetrant molecules able to cross the blood-brain barrier and to stimulate neurotrophic factor mechanisms in the brain. Molecular pathways upstream and downstream of neurotrophic factors are likely to offer several attractive putative targets for disease-modifying drugs.

10.5 ANIMAL MODELS AND EXPERIMENTAL MEDICINE

Several well-characterized animal models are available that reproduce the dopaminergic deficit in Parkinson's disease (Beal, 2001; Table 10.2). They are useful for the discovery of symptomatic treatments, including both, compounds that replace dopamine and compounds that modify the activity of other pathways of the extrapyramidal system. The models are acute injury models and do not reproduce the pathological process that leads to gradually degeneration of dopaminergic neurons in Parkinson's disease. The first of these models, reserpine-treated rodents, provides a simple pharmacological test for drugs that counteract dopamine depletion. Reserpine interferes with the function of the vesicular catecholamine transporter VMT2 and prevents normal synaptic functions of dopaminergic, noradrenergic and serotonergic neurons. Reserpine-treated animals are immobile, hypothermic, and have diarrhea. The behavioral immobility largely reflects the absence of dopaminergic neurotransmission, since it can be counteracted with L-DOPA and dopamine

Table 10.2 Animal models for Parkinson's disease

Animal Models Reflecting Advanced Parkinson's Disease and Useful for Evaluating Symptomatic Drugs

Reserpine-treated rodents

Rats with unilateral or bilateral 6-hydroxydopamine injections into the substantia nigra or caudate-putamen

Mice treated systemically with MPTP

Monkeys treated i.v. with MPTP

Animal Models Reflecting the Disease Process and Useful for Evaluating Disease-Modifying Drugs

Transgenic mice expressing human disease genes (α-synuclein, parkins)

Transgenic *Drosophila* flies expressing human disease genes

Monkeys with chronic rotenone exposure

---

receptor agonists. Data obtained in the reserpine model have only tentative significance for Parkinson's disease and should be confirmed in one of the following lesion models, which more accurately reflect the dopaminergic neuron degeneration of Parkinson's disease.

Animals with 6-hydroxydopamine lesions of the substantia nigra specifically replicate the dopaminergic cell loss of the substantia nigra of Parkinson's disease. Bilateral lesions cause hypokinesia in rodents. Complete lesions produce total immobility. Direct and indirect dopamine agonists restore the normal behavior. Rats with unilateral 6-hydroxydopamine lesions of the substantia nigra represent the most widely used animal model for testing drugs that compensate for a dopaminergic deficit. The unilateral lesions cause functional hypersensitivity of the denervated striatum, resulting in asymmetrical posture of the animals, and rotational behavior in response to dopamine agonists. The frequency of rotations provides an easily quantifiable readout of dopamine agonist activity. In honor of the inventor, the model is often called the Ungerstedt model. It is a standard feature of every laboratory where dopaminergic mechanisms are studied.

MPTP treatment of mice results in a partial destruction of dopaminergic terminals and cell bodies. The extent of the destruction is dependent on the animal strain and the dosage. MPTP-treated animals are hypokinetic, and dopamine agonists restore normal function. The most accurate reproduction of Parkinson's disease is obtained by treating monkeys intravenously with MPTP, a procedure that accurately reproduces the initial human experiences. MPTP-treated monkeys have selective lesions of dopaminergic neurons, and all the cardinal behavioral features of Parkinson's disease. They respond to dopamine replacement therapy in a very similar way as human patients. These monkeys are most useful in the search for novel agents that provide dopamine replacement therapy and for the evaluation of drugs that regulate the actions of other extrapyramidal pathways. Brains of MTPT-treated monkeys, however, do not contain Lewy bodies and thus are not a reliable model to study the disease mechanism of Parkinson's disease.

There are no reliable animal models as yet that replicate the parkinsonian disease process. Chronic infusions of rotenone or paraquat into monkeys cause degenerative changes in dopaminergic system but also affect other neuronal populations. None of the transgenic mice expressing human disease genes so far replicates the human pathology. Aggregations similar to Lewy bodies have been observed in some transgenic strains, but, degeneration of dopaminergic neurons in the mice has been minor or completely absent.

The ongoing worldwide efforts to characterize the function of the various Parkinson's disease genes will likely bring rapid progress and gradually improved replication of the disease pathology. Understanding of disease mechanisms will march forward hand in hand with the development of more accurate transgenic mouse models.

Transgenic *Drosophila* flies have become a most intriguing and useful test system to study Parkinson's disease mechanisms (Auluck et al., 2002). Expression of human disease genes in the flies causes degeneration of dopaminergic neurons and a fly-specific behavioral phenotype that can be reversed with L-DOPA. The dopaminergic cell loss is accompanied by the appearance of α-synuclein aggregates. *Drosophila* genetics provides an elegant and rapid tool to study the influence of various genes of the proteasome pathway on the dopaminergic neuron and α-synuclein pathology. Combinations of various disease genes can be studied within short time periods. Using *Drosophila* transgenic studies to guide the more time-consuming evaluations in transgenic mice represents a most attractive strategy toward understanding the disease mechanism and development of a reliable mammalian model.

Clinical trials are relatively simple for drug candidates expected to have symptomatic effects only. The effects of dopamine replacement therapy become manifest within a few hours, making it easy to establish clinical efficacy. Given the existence of many efficacious drugs, new candidates have to be given initially as addition to existing drugs. Long observation periods are necessary to establish long-term adverse effects. Clinical trials are complex for disease-modifying drugs, and they require observation times of one year or more. Nevertheless, clinical trial design is well established to detect such changes. The progression of the underlying disease can be established during brief periods of withdrawal of dopamine replacement medicine. Trials for disease-modifying drugs are often done with newly diagnosed patients, and the time interval between first diagnosis and the need for dopamine replacement therapy serves as an endpoint. Past experience with failed and successful trials has established confidence that efficacy of disease-modifying drugs can be established in decisive clinical trials (Shults et al., 2002).

Imaging technologies are very actively pursued as diagnostic tools and alternative readouts for disease-modifying drugs. Several PET ligands have been characterized, each of which monitors a unique aspect of dopaminergic neuron structure and function. Fluoro-DOPA is converted to fluoro-dopamine, which then accumulates predominantly in vesicles of catecholaminergic neurons. The resulting signal thus reflects the catalytic capacity of the aromatic amino acid decarboxylase as well as the storage capacity of catecholaminergic neurons. Labeled compounds that bind to the vesicular transporter VMAT2 and cell membrane transporter DAT, respectively, provide a more direct measurement of structural integrity of the dopaminergic synapses than fluoro-DOPA. PET studies with a labeled dopamine receptor antagonist such as raclopride provides a functional readout of synaptic activity, since the released endogenous dopamine displaces the labeled antagonists. Imaging techniques have the potential to provide an accurate measurement of dopaminergic neuron degeneration during the progression of Parkinson's disease. Their use is limited by high costs, and unless they provide a clear advantage over the standard behavioral assessment of Parkinson's disease, they are unlikely to find general use.

10.6 CONCLUSIONS

Parkinson's disease is an age-related, frequent movement disorder that receives only inadequate treatment from the existing drugs. Its symptoms, slowness of movement and rigidity, are caused by the degeneration of dopaminergic neurons in the mesencephalon, the dominant pathological feature of the disease. Intracellular aggregations, Lewy bodies, in dopaminergic neurons and other neuron populations, represent the second characteristic pathological feature of the disease. The disease progresses gradually and leads to severe disability in one to two decades after the initial diagnosis.

Highly effective dopamine replacement therapy is available that provides excellent symptomatic relief of parkinsonian symptoms during the early years of the disease. The available drugs include the dopamine precursor L-DOPA in combination with a peripherally acting enzyme inhibitor that prevents the formation of dopamine outside of the brain, several directly acting dopamine receptor agonists, and inhibitors of the catabolic enzymes monoamine oxidase and catechol-O-methyltransferase. L-DOPA or a dopamine agonist is typically sufficient at the beginning of the illness. Combinations of drugs become necessary with the progression of the disease, but even optimal treatment gradually looses efficacy. After several years of treatment, adverse effects, dyskinesias and psychosis, overshadow beneficial effects. It may be possible to further improve the dopamine replacement therapy with variants of the existing drugs. However, it seems likely that the currently available palette of directly and indirectly acting dopamine agonists yield the maximal benefits to be achieved with dopamine replacement therapy.

The dopaminergic neurons affected in Parkinson's disease are an element of the extrapyramidal motor system in the brain. Degeneration of the dopaminergic pathway results in hyperactivity of inhibitory output pathways that regulate motor behaviors. Drugs that directly modulate the output pathways might be able to compensate for the absence of the dopaminergic projection. The success of neurosurgical stimulation and lesion techniques in treating Parkinson patients provides strong support for the view that direct modulation of the activity of the extrapyramidal pathways is therapeutically effective. Neurotransmitter receptors or ion channels that are selectively expressed on neurons of the extrapyramidal motor systems thus represent highly attractive putative targets for symptomatic drugs with a mechanism of action different from the currently used dopaminergic agents.

There is evidence for environmental and genetic causes of Parkinson's disease. MPTP, an ingredient of a street drug, causes selective destruction of dopaminergic neurons and produces the cardinal behavioral features of Parkinson's disease. The structural requirements are very strict for a compound to have MPTP-like neurotoxicity and the search for generally present dopaminergic neurotoxins has failed to identify chemicals that could be responsible for general Parkinson's disease. However, toxins less selective than MPTP might contribute to the vulnerability of dopaminergic neurons. MPTP destroys these cells by interfering with mitochondrial function that causes energy failure and overproduction of reactive oxygen species. Tentative clinical evidence supports the view that compounds able to inactivate the reactive oxygen species might decelerate the progression of Parkinson's disease.

Several disease genes have been discovered that cause familial forms of Parkinson's disease. One of them, α-synuclein, provides the major component of Lewy bodies. Mutations causing familial Parkinson's disease increase the propensity of α-synuclein aggregation into fibrillary structures. Two other disease genes code for enzymes that belong to the proteasome protein degradation complex, suggesting the possibility that they might impair the removal of misfolded α-synuclein. The rapid progress in the characterization of disease genes makes it likely that an integrated hypothesis of Parkinson disease mechanism will emerge soon and will include aspects of mitochondrial and proteasome functions. It is expected that drug targets with high probability of success will emerge from these studies.

The search for disease-modifying drugs includes the evaluation of neurotrophic factor mechanism. GDNF promotes survival of dopaminergic neurons in various experimental conditions and has been found effective in exploratory clinical trials. Proteins that regulate the synthesis of neurotrophic factors or form part of the receptor-mediated signaling cascade thus represent attractive putative drug targets. Exploratory clinical studies with such agents are under way and will help to assess the validity of the neurotrophic factor approach.

Animal models that replicate the dopaminergic cell loss of Parkinson's disease are well characterized and routinely used in the discovery of drugs to counteract the symptoms of the disease. There are no animal models as yet that replicate the progressive nature of the disease and provide utility in the search for disease-modifying drugs. Rapid progress in studies of transgenic mice is likely to provide such models in the foreseeable future. Well-established clinical trial designs are available to test symptomatic and disease-modifying drugs in Parkinson patients.

Parkinson's disease represents a significant medical need as well as one of the most attractive areas for drug discovery. The search for symptomatic drugs relies on the success of the existing dopamine replacement therapies. Very active research on genes and toxins that are known to cause the disease are likely to identify targets for novel disease-modifying drugs.

REFERENCES

Further Reading

BEAL, M.F. Experimental models of Parkinson's disease. *Nature Rev. Neurosci.* 2: 325–332, 2001.

CARLSSON, A. Treatment of Parkinson's with L-DOPA: The early discovery phase, and a comment on current problems. *J. Neural. Transm.* 109: 777–787, 2002.

COHEN, G. Oxidative stress, mitochondrial respiration, and Parkinson's disease. *An. N.Y. Acad. Sci.* 899: 112–120, 2000.

DAUER, W., and PRZEDBORSKI, S. Parkinson's disease: mechanisms and models. *Neuron* 39: 889–909, 2003.

DAWSON, T.M., and DAWSON, V.L. Molecular pathways of neurodegeneration in Parkinson's disease. *Science* 302: 819–822, 2003.

ERIKSEN, J.L., DAWSON, T.M., DICKSON, D.W., and PETRUCELLI, L. Caught in the act: α-Synuclein is the culprit in Parkinson's disease. *Neuron* 40: 453–456, 2003.

FAHN, S. Description of Parkinson's disease as a clinical syndrome. *An. N.Y. Acad. Sci.* 991: 1–14, 2003.

GUTTMAN, M., KISH, S.J., and FURUKAWA, Y. Current concepts in the diagnosis and management of Parkinson's disease. *Can. Med. Assoc. J.* 168: 293–301, 2003.

JELLINGER, K.A. Recent developments in the pathology of Parkinson's disease. *J. Neural. Transm.* (suppl.) 62: 347–376, 2002.

LANGSTON, J.W. The etiology of Parkinson's disease with emphasis on the MPTP story. *Neurology* 47: S153–160, 1996.

POLLACK, S.J., and HARPER, S.J. Small molecule Trk receptor agonists and other neurotrophic factor mimetics. *Curr. Drug Target CNS Neurol. Disord.* 1: 59–80, 2002.

Citations

AULUCK, P.K., CHAN, H.Y., TROJANOWSKI, J.Q., LEE, V.M., and BONINI, N.M. Chaperone suppression of alpha-synuclein toxicity in a *Drosophila* model for Parkinson's disease. *Science* 295: 865–868, 2002.

BARA-JIMENEZ, W., SHERZAI, A., DIMITROVA, T., FAVIT, A., BIBBIANI, F., GILLESPIE, M., MORRIS, M.J., MOURADIAN, M.M., and CHASE, T.N. Adenosine A(2A) receptor antag-

onist treatment of Parkinson's disease. *Neurology* 61: 293–296, 2003.

BARTHOLINI, G., and PLETSCHER, A. Cerebral accumulation and metabolism of C14-dopa after selective inhibition of peripheral decarboxylase. *J. Pharmacol. Exp. Ther.* 61: 14–20, 1968.

BETARBET, R., SHERER, T.B., MACKENZIE, G., GARCIA-

OSUNA, M., PANOV, A.V., and GREENAMYRE, J.T. Chronic systemic pesticide exposure reproduces features of Parkinson's disease. *Nature Neurosci.* 22: 2637–2649, 2000.

BILSLAND, J., ROY, S., XANTHOUDAKIS, S., NICHOLSON, D.W., HAN, Y., GRIMM, E., HEFTI F., and HARPER, S.J. Caspase inhibitors attenuate 1-methyl-4-phenylpyridinium toxicity in primary cultures of mesencephalic dopaminergic neurons. *J. Neurosci.* 22: 2637–2649, 2002.

FARRER, M., KACHERGUS, J., FORNO, L., LINCOLN, S., WANG, D.S., HULIHAN, M., MARAGANORE, D., GWINN-HARDY, K., WSZOLEK, Z., DICKSON, D., and LANGSTON, J.W. Comparison of kindreds with parkinsonism and asynuclein genomic multiplications. *An. Neurol.* 55: 174–179, 2004.

GILL, S.S., PATEL, N.K., HOTTON, G.R., O'SULLIVON, K., McCARTER, R., BUNNAGE, M., BROOKS, D.J., SVENDSEN, C.N., and HEYWOOD, P. Direct brain infusion of glial cell line-derived neurotrophic factor in Parkinson's disease. *Nature Med.* 9: 589–595, 2003.

KAUR, D., YANTIRI, F., RAJAGOPALAN, S., KUMAR, J., MO, J.Q., BOONPLUEANG, R., VSWANATH, V., JACOBS, R., YANG, L., BEAL, M.F., DIMONTE, D., VOKITASKIS, I., ELLERBY, L., CHERNY, R.A., BUSH, A.I., and ANDERSEN, J.K. Genetic or pharmacological iron chelation prevents MPTP-induced neurotoxicity in vivo: a novel therapy for Parkinson's disease. *Neuron* 37: 899–909, 2003.

LOTTI, V.J., and PORTER, C.C. Potentiation and inhibition of some central actions of L(−)-DOPA by decarboxy-lase inhibitors. *J. Pharmacol. Exp. Ther.* 172: 406–415, 1970.

MAREK, K., JENNINGS, D., and SEIBYL, J. Do dopamine agonists or levodopa modify Parkinson's disease progression? *Eur. J. Neurol.* (suppl.) 3: 15–22, 2002.

MARINO, M.J., WILLIAMS, D.L. JR., O'BRIEN, J.A., VALENTI, O., McDONALD, T.P., CLEMENTS, M.K., WANG, R., DiLELLA, A.G., HESS, J.F., KINNEY, G.G., and CONN, P.J. Allosteric modulation of group III metabotropic glutamate receptor 4: A potential approach to Parkinson's disease treatment. *Proc. Natl. Acad. Sci. USA* 100: 13668–13673, 2003.

MICHEL, P., DANDAPANI, B.K., SANCHEZ-RAMOS, J., EFANGE, S., PRESSMAN, B.C., and HEFTI, F. Toxic effects of potential environmental neurotoxins related to 1-methyl-4-phenylpyridinium (MPP$^+$) on cultured rat dopaminergic neurons. *J. Pharmacol. Exp. Ther.* 248: 842–850, 1989.

MURRAY, T.K., WHALLEY, K., ROBINSON, C.S., WARD, M.A., HICKS, C.A., LODGE, D., VANDERGRIFF, J.L., BAUMBARGER, P., SIUDA, E., GATES, M., OGDEN, A.M., SKOLNICK, P., ZIMMERMAN, D.M., NISENBAUM, E.S., BLEAKMAN, D., and O'NEILL, M.J. LY503430, a novel alpha-amino-3-hydroxy-5-methylisoxazole-4-propionic acid receptor potentiator with function, neuroprotective and neurotrophic effects in rodent models of Parkinson's disease. *J. Pharmacol. Exp. Ther.* 306: 752–762, 2003.

OLANOW, C.W., GOETZ, C.G., KORDOWER, J.H., STOESSLY, A.J., SOSSI, V., BRIN, M.F., SHANNON, K.M., NAUERT, G.M., PERL, D.M., GODBOLD, J., and FREEMAN, T.B. A double-blind controlled trial of bilateral fetal nigral transplantation in Parkinson's disease. *An. Neurol.* 54: 403–414, 2003.

PARKINSON, J. *An Essay on the Shaking Palsy.* Sherwood, Neely, and Jones, London, 1817.

POLYMEROPOULOS, M.H., LAVEDAN, C., LEROY, E., IDE, S.E., DEHEJIA, A., DUTRA, A., PIKE, B., ROOT, H., RUBINSTEIN, J., BOYER, R., STENROOS, E.S., CHANDRASEKHARAPPA, S., ATHANASSIADOU, A., PAPAPETROPOULOS, T., JOHNSON, W.G., LAZZARINI, A.M., DUVOISIN, R.C., DI IORIO, G., GOLBE, L.I., and NUSSBAUM, R.L. Mutation in the alpha-synuclein gene identified in families with Parkinson's disease. *Science* 276: 2045–2047, 1997.

SAPORITO, M.S., HUDKINS, R.L., and MARONEY, A.C. Discovery of CEP-1347/KT-7515, an inhibitor of the JNK/SAPK pathway for the treatment of neurodegenerative diseases. *Prog. Med. Chem.* 40: 23–62, 2002.

SEGAL, R.A. Selectivity in neurotrophin signaling: theme and variations. *An. Rev. Neurosci.* 26: 299–330, 2003.

SHULTS, C.W., OAKES, D., KIEBURTZ, K., BEAL, M.F., HAAS, R., PLUMP, S., JUNCOS, J.L., NUTT, J., SHOULSON, I., CARTER, J., KOMPOLITI, K., PERLMUTTER, J.S., REICH, S., STERN, M., WATTS, R.L., KURLAN, R., MOLHO, E., HARRISON, M., LEW, M., and the Parkinson Study Group. Effects of coenzyme Q$_{10}$ in early Parkinson disease: Evidence for slowing of the functional decline. *Arch. Neurol.* 59: 1541–1550, 2002.

VAN DER WALT, J.M., NICODEMUS, K.K., MARTIN, E.R., SCOTT, W.K., NANCE, M.A., WATTS, R.L., HUBBLE, J.P., HAINES, J.L., KOLLER, W.C., LYONS, K., PAHWA, R., STERN, M.B., COLCHER, A., HINER, B.C., JANKOVIC, J., ONDO, W.G., ALLEN, F.H. JR., GOETZ, C.G., SMALL, G.W., MASTAGLIA, F., STAJICH, J.M., McLAURIN, A.C., MIDDLETON, L.T., SCOTT, B.L., SCHMECHEL, D.E., PERICAK-VANCE, M.A., and VANCE, J.M. Mitochondrial polymorphisms significantly reduce the risk of Parkinson's disease. *Am. J. Hum. Genet.* 72: 804–811, 2003.

ZECCA, L., ZUCCA, F.A., COSTI, P., TAMPELLINI, D., GATTI, A., GERLACH, M., RIEDERER, P., FARIELLO, R.G., ITO, S., GALLORINI, M., and SULZER, D. The neuromelanin of human substantia nigra: Structure, synthesis and molecular behaviour. *J. Neural. Transm.* (suppl.) 65: 145–155, 2003.

Chapter 11

Ischemic Stroke, Brain and Spinal Cord Injury

Failure of the cardiovascular system is the leading cause of death in medically advanced societies, where the impact of fatal infectious diseases and accidents has been minimized. The major culprits are myocardial infarction, heart attack, and ischemic stroke of the brain, sometimes called brain attack. Ischemic stroke is caused by the occlusion or rupture of blood vessels supplying the nervous system. The location of the infarct determines the magnitude and the nature of the resulting behavioral deficits. Occlusion or rupture of major arteries or of vessels supplying centers of critical autonomic functions tends to be fatal. Strokes in capillaries or in less significant brain areas result in disabilities of various kind and magnitude. Very small strokes often go unnoticed but, when occurring in sequence, may produce behavioral deficits reminiscent of slowly progressing neurodegenerative diseases.

The events following an ischemic stroke follow a typical sequence. Symptoms become apparent abruptly, or they develop over several minutes to a few hours, in parallel with underlying degenerative changes of the brain tissue. Maximal deficits are evident within one to five days. A recovery phase of several days to weeks follows, which may restitute some of the lost functions. The behavioral consequences of minor strokes may resolve completely. In contrast, massive strokes, when not fatal, leave patients with chronic deficits such as motor paralysis, speech impairment, cognitive impairment, and other severe disabilities.

The rapid progress over the recent decades in the understanding of cardiovascular diseases has identified effective strategies for the prevention of myocardial infarction and ischemic stroke of the brain. Drugs that lower blood pressure prevent platelet aggregation, and lower blood cholesterol levels decrease the risk of heart and brain attacks. A single drug has been approved for intervention treatment during the acute phase of the stroke, plasminogen activator (tPA), an enzyme able to dissolve blood clots responsible for vessel occlusion. No drugs are available to stop the neuronal degeneration within infarcted brain tissue, and none are on hand that reliably promote neuronal regeneration and functional recovery.

Traumatic injuries to the brain and spinal cord have consequences similar to those of ischemic stroke. Injuries of the nervous system caused by traffic accidents or weapons occur frequently and result in degenerative changes of brain tissue by mechanisms similar to those operating after an ischemic stroke. Both produce long-lasting impairments and

Drug Discovery for Nervous System Diseases, by Franz F. Hefti
ISBN 0-471-46563-1   Copyright © 2005 by John Wiley & Sons, Inc.

human suffering and have remained without effective drug treatments. Drugs able to minimize the destructive consequences or to stimulate the regenerative processes in ischemic stroke are likely to benefit patients with traumatic injuries as well. Together, these conditions represent a most significant unmet medical need and opportunity for novel and innovative drug discovery.

11.1 MECHANISMS OF ISCHEMIC STROKE

Estimates of stroke incidence in industrialized countries suggest that each year approximately 0.5% of the population suffer an ischemic attack. The risk increases gradually with age. Approximately 1% of the population suffers from chronic disabilities because of a previous stroke. The causes for ischemic strokes of the brain, occlusion or rupture of a blood vessel, are the same as the causes for cardiac strokes. Both are the consequence of a multifactorial process with genetic and environmental components. While no specific genes have been conclusively identified, twin studies and family studies point to higher risk for stroke in some families. Elevated blood pressure, caused by genetic or environmental factors, and atherosclerosis, the blockade of arteries by lipid deposits, are the most significant risk factors. Medications that lower blood pressure and blood cholesterol levels substantially diminish the risk of cardiac and cerebral stroke.

The brain is highly dependent on the continuous provision of oxygen and nutrients, glucose in particular. Obstruction or rupture of a blood vessel deprives a specific brain area of nutrient and oxygen supply and causes rapid energy failure in the affected cells (Fig. 11.1). Mitochondrial malfunction and failure follows and results in the depletion of the cellular levels of ATP. Highly ATP-dependent processes, the various transporters in particular, are the first to be affected. The failure of Ca^{2+} transporters causes massive increases in intracellular Ca^{2+}, creating disturbances in a large number of regulatory systems. Since many cellular functions related to signaling, growth, differentiation, and motility are Ca^{2+}-dependent, an uncoordinated activation of energy-consuming processes is the consequence. Influx of Ca^{2+} into presynaptic terminals and the failure of ATP-dependent neurotransmitter uptake systems causes massive neurotransmitter overflow in the synapses. The unregulated release of the excitatory transmitter glutamate opens ionotropic receptors that contribute to the ionic imbalance within the cells. At least during the early phases of ischemic injury glutamate-stimulated NMDA receptors appear to play a major role. Exposure of neurons to glutamate in cell culture causes cell death comparable to events in the brain following a stroke. The concept that excitatory neurotransmitters are a gating event in the pathophysiology of stroke has dominated the field during the previous decade and is typically referred to as **excitotoxicity** (Lipton, 1999). It has become clear, though, that many other processes contribute to cell death in the infarcted area in addition to the damage that can be ascribed to glutamate toxicity.

Mitochondrial failure, in addition to causing ATP depletion, results in the formation of reactive oxygen species (ROS) that damage various proteins and nucleic acids (Lo et al., 2003). Damage of DNA activates repair enzymes that consume ATP at high rates. Oxidative stress produced by the ROS, together with the ionic imbalances and the mitochondrial release of cytochrome c, activates caspase enzymes that mediate the breakdown of DNA and apoptotic cell death. Evidence for both apoptotic and necrotic cell death has been obtained for stroke, pointing to several parallel and interacting pathways toward cell death. Additional components identified include Zn^{2+} that is stored in many synaptic vesicles, but tends to be toxic when released in excessive amounts, and reactive nitrogen

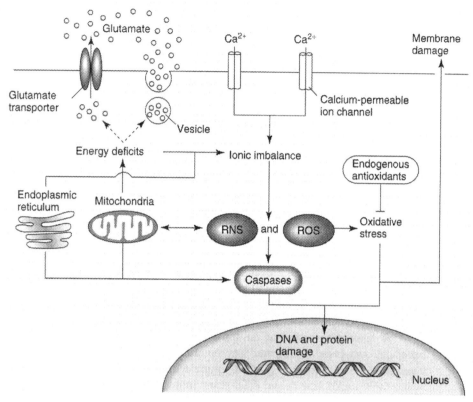

Figure 11.1 Mechanisms of ischemic cell death in the brain. Neural and glial cell death is caused by multiple. overlapping pathways, including excitotoxicity, ionic imbalance, oxidative stress, and mechanisms related to apoptotic pathways. RNS: reactive nitrogen species; ROS: reactive oxygen species. (Reprinted with permission. Lo et al., 2003)

species that are formed from the interaction of ROS with nitric oxide. Apoptotic pathways independent of the caspases are believed to play a role, involving molecules such as poly-(ADP ribose) polymerase, a DNA repair enzyme, and apoptosis-inducing factor (AIF) from the mitochondria. AIF translocates to the nucleus and promotes destructive processes. Ischemic energy failure also affects the endothelial cells forming the blood-brain barrier, opening the brain to various molecular and cellular players from which it is normally protected. Proteases including plasminogen activator and various metalloproteases may contribute to destructive processes. Mediators of immune functions, including various cytokines, penetrate into the infarcted area and are able to trigger secondary responses. The multitude of these possible events explains why it seems impossible to define a single pathway of cell death in ischemic stroke. The death of neurons and glial cells is thus reminiscent of the picture of "death by a thousand cuts" where a single dominant cause cannot be identified.

The pathways of cell death are likely to be different for various populations of cells in the infarcted area. Neurons are most vulnerable to loss of oxygen and nutrients; oligodendrocytes are very susceptible too, and astrocytes and endothelial cells are affected during more severe conditions. Among the neurons, hippocampal and cortical pyramidal cells, and Purkinje cells of the cerebellum are particularly sensitive. The differential sensitivity of neuronal populations may reflect size as well as diverse vulnerability to specific components of the destructive processes triggered by the ischemic stroke. The differential vulnerabilities of neuronal and nonneuronal cell populations further complicate the picture of stroke for drug discovery and development. Protective agents may be beneficial for some of the populations only.

For the cells in close proximity to the infarct, the cascade of events following energy failure evolves rapidly and leads to irreversible degeneration and death. Cells located more distant to the infarct, however, will not be affected to the same degree. Individual blood vessels, the small ones in particular, supply overlapping brain areas with nutrients and oxygen. In consequence there is a gradient in energy loss from the area with rapid and irreversible cell death, the **core** of the infarct, to the distant areas that are completely unaffected. Even rapid reperfusion, the restoration of blood flow, to the core fails to prevent cell death in this area. The term **penumbra** is used to describe the transition area, where only some loss of oxygen and nutrient supply occurs following the stroke. Dependent on the specific location of the vessel occlusion, the volume of the penumbra may be a small fraction of the core volume or may be much larger than the core. The penumbra evolves and disappears in the hours and days following the infarct. In some zones of it cells die and become part of the core, cells in other zones recover completely and become part of the surviving tissue. The penumbra is an important concept in drug discovery research because it seems possible to increase the likelihood of cellular survival in this area whereas less hope exists for cells dying rapidly in the core (Fig. 11.2).

Cell death in the brain and the spinal cord triggers various long-term responses, some beneficial and some detrimental for the restoration of lost behavioral abilities. Space vacated by dying neurons is gradually populated by glial cells, predominantly astrocytes, which form a glial scar tissue. Glial scars limit the ability of neurons to regenerate lost axonal connections and are believed to be a significant negative factor in traumatic brain and spinal cord injury. Neurogenesis may be able to gradually repopulate infarcted tissue with neurons. The recent exciting discoveries related to neurogenesis generate substantial hope, but these processes remain to be more thoroughly explored before their significance in stroke can be assessed. Axonal regeneration is rare in the central nervous system and will be discussed in more detail in the section on spinal cord injury. Of highest significance for stroke recovery are the processes of functional and morphologic rearrangements of neuronal connections in the surviving brain tissue. It is well established that training over several months is able to restore some of the lost functions. Size, location of the

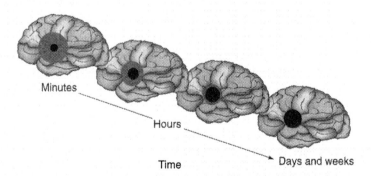

Figure 11.2 Evolution of the penumbra. The core of the infarct contains irreversibly dead neurons. In the penumbra, neuronal function is impaired. The neurons may revert to full functionality or become part of the core. (Reprinted with permission, Dirnagl et al., 1999, Elsevier)

infarct, as well as the age of the victim are the major determinants of the recovery. The ability to recover from stroke-induced damage gradually declines with age. The molecular and cellular basis of the recovery mechanism is very poorly understood, and they represent a most challenging area for drug discovery.

11.2 CURRENT TREATMENT

Stroke prevention is accomplished by drugs that reduce the risk of cardiac attacks. Available drugs able to lower blood pressure, including antagonists of β-adrenergic receptors, inhibitors of angiotensin-converting enzyme, and antagonists of the angiotensin II receptors, have been demonstrated in convincing studies to reduce the incidence of ischemic strokes to the brain. Inhibitors of cholesterol synthesis, the statins, make an effective contribution to stroke risk reduction by a different mechanism. By inhibiting the formation of lipid deposits in blood vessels they reduce the risk of vessel occlusions caused by detached fragments that initiate thrombus formation and vessel occlusion. Thrombus formation is directly suppressed by inhibitors of platelet aggregation, such as aspirin, which also reduce the risk of stroke. These drugs, alone and in combination, have major impact on medical care of the general population and are one of the reasons for the gradual increase in average life span in modern times. Further improvements, beyond the already impressive progress of cardiovascular pharmacotherapy, are possible and likely. The cardiovascular approaches are beyond the scope of this book and will not be further discussed here.

Intervention therapy attempts to restore blood supply to an infarcted area as soon as possible and to stop the cascade of events leading to cell death in nervous system tissue. If the infarct is caused by a thrombus obstructing a vessel, it is possible to treat patients with an intravenous injection of tPA, a protease that rapidly cleaves proteins in the clot and restores normal blood flow. To be clinically useful and effective, tPA has to be given within three hours after the onset of the stroke. Rapid diagnosis and well-trained rapid response medical teams are a prerequisite for success. Very often strokes are not recognized quickly enough or occur during sleep, and the time window closes before tPA therapy is available. The use of tPA is further restricted by the risk of bleeding caused by the potent proteolytic activity of the enzyme that enables it to attack weakened vessel walls. It may be possible to design more selective thrombolytic enzymes to decrease the bleeding risk, but the procedural issues, the short time window, and the need for rapid medical treatment create substantial barriers for this approach.

No drugs are currently available to stop the cascade of events that cause the death of neurons and glial cells after a stroke or to enhance the regenerative or adaptive processes that underlie restoration of function in the subsequent days and months. Given the enormous medical need, the search for such compounds is a major effort in many biopharmaceutical companies. Programmatic terms, such as **neuroprotection** and **neuroregeneration**, have been coined to support the endeavor. While intuitively attractive, these terms are vague from a scientific perspective and blur the fact that most molecular processes that increase survival of cells also enhance their regenerative capacity. The following sections therefore discuss specific molecular mechanisms and approaches that have been explored recently for stroke therapy, and more speculative ones that are suggested by studies of disease mechanism. Some of the attempts have generated intriguing signs for clinical efficacy, but none of the drug candidates tested so far has been approved for general use as marketed drug.

11.3 EXCITOTOXICITY AND GLUTAMATE ANTAGONISTS

The concept of excitotoxicity goes back to seminal observations made in the 1960s that monosodium glutamate, a frequently used flavor enhancer in food, causes brain lesions when used at very high concentrations (Olney, 1969). Many further studies confirmed that exposure of neurons to high concentrations of glutamate is toxic. Neurons kept in cell cultures die within minutes following rapid elevations of the glutamate concentration to high mM levels. Infusions of glutamate or glutamate receptor agonists into the brain cause structural lesions. The observation that glutamate levels are increased in the extracellular fluid in infarcted brain tissue closed the circle in support of the view that excessive excitatory stimulation is a key mediator of neuronal death in ischemic stroke.

The excitotoxicity hypothesis of stroke predicts that antagonists of glutamate receptors will prevent neuronal death in ischemia (Schwarcz and Meldrum, 1985). The initial attention was directed at the NMDA receptor subgroup because of the availability of a selective antagonist for this receptor family. Selective inhibitors of NMDA receptors reduce the infarct size in animal models of ischemic stroke in an effective way. Despite the difficult nature of the animal models for stroke, many research groups confirmed the robust beneficial effects of the NMDA antagonists. Active compounds include competitive inhibitors at the glutamate binding site, blockers of the ion channels, and antagonists binding to allosteric sites. A narrow time window limits the efficacy of the NMDA antagonists. In animal models, the compounds have to be given before, during, or immediately after the experimental ischemia to be efficacious. Treatment after a delay of more than approximately three hours is ineffective and neuronal death progresses as in untreated stroke. The time window established in the animal studies points out that excitotoxic processes are an important but transient feature in the disease mechanism of stroke.

More than 10 different NMDA antagonists were taken into clinical trials for the treatment of stroke, but none of them have been approved for general use. Several compounds were abandoned because of adverse effects; the others failed to show convincing efficacy. Three of the drug candidates were ineffective in large phase III clinical studies involving several thousand patients. At first impression, the totality of these studies seems to robustly refute the excitotoxicity hypothesis of stroke in humans. However, careful scrutiny of the clinical data undermines the validity of this conclusion. Some of the clinical trials were small studies only, with insufficient numbers of patients to reveal reliably an effect. Every human stroke is an individual event that occurs at a unique vascular site. The high degree of interindividual variability makes it necessary to include several hundreds of patients into each treatment group if statistically significant differences are to be detected. Some of the clinical studies allowed time intervals for treatment greater than three hours after stroke onset, the limit of efficacy established in most animal studies. Some of the compounds most likely had insufficient brain penetrance to effectively block NMDA receptors in the brain. Thus it is fair to argue that despite the large number of trials, the excitotoxicity hypothesis has not been adequately tested in the clinic. This is a very sobering and disturbing conclusion when considering the effort and expenses consumed. Rigorous standards have been formulated in response to the NMDA antagonist experience that will help increase the likelihood of success in future trials (Finkelstein et al., 1999).

The robust effects in animal models and the absence of conclusive clinical trials with NMDA antagonists keep alive the hope that glutamate receptor antagonists will find therapeutic utility in the treatment of stroke. Compounds that block specific NMDA receptor subtypes may have a lower risk for producing adverse effects than the ones clinically tested so far. In addition a variety of antagonists for AMPA and kainic acid receptor subtypes as well as for metabotropic glutamate receptor subtypes have beneficial effects in animal models of ischemic stroke. Transgenic variations of subunit expression are able to change the vulnerability of select populations of brain neurons. Detailed understanding of the expression patterns of specific subtypes in the human brain, combined with the studies of specific antagonists in animal models, will help clinical studies identify the drug targets with the highest likelihood of success.

11.4 BEYOND EXCITOTOXICITY

Unregulated release of neurotransmitter and excessive depolarization by excitatory amino acids is the key initial step in the cascade of events in stroke pathology but does not necessarily push the cells on an irrevocable path to death. Cell death may still be evitable if events downstream of glutamate receptor activation can be stopped. These downstream consequences evolve more slowly than the excitotoxicity and open a wider time window for therapeutic intervention. In many animal studies glutamate receptor antagonists reduce infarct volumes but do not fully prevent the loss of cells. In addition to the better time window, approaches directed to steps other than excitotoxicity may lead to drugs more effective than the glutamate receptor antagonists.

11.4.1 Ion Channel Modulators

Ionic imbalance is a direct consequence of energy loss and of glutamate receptor activation. The crucial role of Ca^{2+} in many cellular processes justifies the initial focus on this ion. Antagonists of Ca^{2+} channels that are used in the treatment of cardiac diseases have been reported to have beneficial effects in animal models of stroke. However, the clinical experience does not support the conclusion that these drugs improve the outcome in human ischemic stroke (Horn and Limburg, 2001). The general inhibition of Ca^{2+} channels may have detrimental effects since both excessively high and excessively low concentrations of Ca^{2+} appear to be detrimental for cell survival. The multitude and diversity of calcium channels in the brain and their differential expression patterns offer a wide and interesting area for further investigation. Selective inhibitors for subtypes may be able to clamp the intracellular Ca^{2+} concentrations at optimal levels. Similar arguments can be made for Na^+ and K^+ ion channels. Energy loss and glutamate receptor activation creates ionic imbalances also for these ions, and the various channel proteins all are attractive speculative drug targets for stroke therapy.

The number of ion channels is too large to sequentially sort through them with full-blown drug discovery programs. Several available experimental approaches and scientific speculations will help to identify the most promising channels. Channels specifically expressed by highly vulnerable populations of neurons may represent those with highest impact. Studies in transgenic animals with differential vulnerability to ischemic infarcts may identify specific channels contributing to ischemic cell death. It seems reasonable to speculate that channels playing modulatory roles may be more useful drug targets than those directly involved in neurotransmitter functions. For example, specific Ca^{2+}-dependent K^+ channels, called maxi-K channels, have been selected for further investigations because they prevent excessive neuronal depolarization when intracellular Ca^{2+} concentrations are high. Activators of these channels have beneficial effects in animal models of stroke (Gribkoff et al., 2001). The many ion channels offer a wide-open and attractive field for investigation in the stroke area.

11.4.2 Antioxidants and Ion Chelators

Parallel to the speculations outlined in the chapter on Parkinson's disease, it seems plausible that oxidative damage plays part in the degenerative events following an ischemic stroke. Energy loss and mitochondrial failure create an overflow of ROS and RNS able to damage proteins, nucleic acids, and other molecular components of the cells. Figure 11.3 shows the chemical pathways involved in the generation of ROS and RNS. Blood levels of vitamin C, an endogenous antioxidant, are reduced following a stroke. Damaged tissues with reduced levels of endogenous antioxidants or deactivating enzymes are particularly vulnerable to oxidative stress. In the heart and the kidney, oxidative damage appears to be one of the principal mediators of reperfusion injury following transient loss of blood supply. These findings and the associated speculations have supported a strong effort on antioxidant strategies for stroke in many companies during the past years (Gilgun-Sherki et al., 2002). Numerous publications reported beneficial effects of natural antioxidants in cell culture and animal stroke models. Compounds tested include vitamin C, vitamin E, coenzyme Q_{10}, α-lipoic acid, N-acetylcysteine, creatine, and glutathione. Many analogues of natural compounds and synthetic antioxidants were found efficacious, including vitamin E derivates, metallo-organic molecules that mimic the function of superoxide dismutase or glutathione peroxidase, spin-trap free-radical scavengers, and lazaroids, derivatives of natural steroids with antioxidant properties. Several of these molecules have been taken into clinical trials, but no convincing positive effects have been obtained as yet. Most of the trials were too small to provide a conclusive result. Most studies failed to include the demonstration that the drug candidate was sufficiently brain penetrant to effectively deactivate oxidative species at the site of the infarct. Thus, as for the NMDA antagonists, it is possible to argue that the antioxidant hypothesis for stroke therapy has not been adequately tested as yet. Indeed, several companies are continuing to pursue this

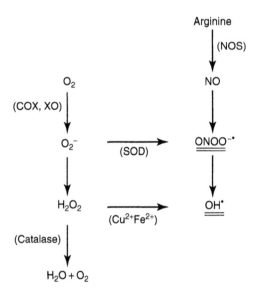

Figure 11.3   Synthetic pathways generating reactive oxygen species (ROS) and reactive nitrogen species (RNS). The principal reactive species, hydroxyl radical (OH·) and peroxynitrite anion (ONOO⁻), are underlined. COX: cyclooxygenase; NOS: nitric oxide synthase; SOD: superoxide dismutase; XO: xanthine oxidase.

approach and have taken new antioxidants into ongoing clinical trials. The extensive clinical trials with the lazaroids, which have not revealed meaningful benefits in extensive clinical trials in ischemic stroke or acute traumatic injury, tend to dampen the enthusiasm for this approach.

The research on Parkinson's disease illustrates the ability of Fe^{2+} and other metal ions to enhance oxidative damage following energy failure in the cells. For ischemic stroke, Zn^{2+} has become the focus of attention, prompted by intriguing observations on neuronal degeneration in the hippocampus. The granule cells contain high levels of Zn^{2+}, which is released synaptically and able to damage postsynaptic neurons at high concentrations (Sloviter, 1985). Subsequent studies confirmed the toxicity of Zn^{2+} in cell culture systems. Chelators of Zn^{2+} and related metal ions may thus be useful for stroke therapy, as has been speculated for antioxidants. Suitable compounds without toxicity will be necessary to adequately explore the metal chelator and antioxidant hypotheses. Extensive characterization of the pharmacological properties of the drug candidates before the clinical trials will increase the probability of success. The time window open for treatment has to be defined in animal models and be suitable large for practical clinical studies with newly diagnosed patients. A pharmacological marker for efficacy has to be identified, to determine a dose that indeed exerts the desired antioxidant effects in the human brain. Antioxidant strategies remain conceptually attractive if these practical hurdles can be overcome.

11.4.3 Apoptosis Inhibitors

Energy failure, excitotoxicity, ion imbalance, and oxidative stress initiate the sequence of molecular events that lead to structural disintegration and death of cells following ischemic stroke. At least some the neurons that die appear to follow the well-established pathways of apoptosis illustrated in Figure 11.4. The molecular components necessary for apoptotic degeneration are expressed in the adult brain. A primary role has been ascribed to caspase-3, because this enzyme regulates neuronal survival during development. Gene knockout mice lacking functional caspase-3 genes are born with larger brains and a higher number of neurons than normal mice. For these reasons several biopharmaceutical companies have actively pursued inhibitors of caspase-3 and other apoptotic mediators in the search of new stroke therapy.

Substantial support for apoptotic death in stroke has come from cell culture and in vivo studies. Mimicking the events of an ischemic stroke in cell culture by exposing neurons to reduced levels of glucose and oxygen or elevated concentrations of glutamate causes the activation of caspase-3. Inhibitors of caspases reduce neuronal degeneration in the cell culture models of ischemic stroke. Transgenic animals with null mutations of apoptosis mediators appear to be more resistant than control mice in experimental situations reflecting stroke. Such observations have been made with caspase-3 knockouts and with mice carrying null mutations of the upstream apoptosis inducing protein Bid. Caspase inhibitors infused intracerebrally into the brains of rodents have beneficial effects in animal stroke models.

Despite these captivating findings, the anti-apoptosis strategy for drug discovery provides no sure path to success. It has become clear that apoptosis plays a major role in ischemic injury in early development but not necessarily in the adult brain. Cell culture studies and at least some of the results obtained with transgenic animals reflect developmental functions. In the adult brain it has been difficult to robustly document key apoptotic events. Effects on regulators of the Bcl-2 family, release of cytochrome c from the

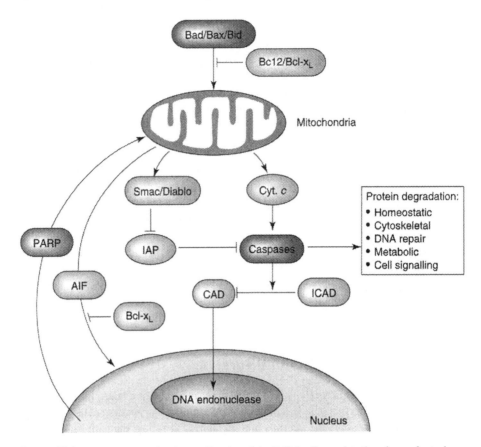

Figure 11.4   Apoptosis-related pathways. Proteins of the Bcl2 family regulate the release of cytochrome c from the mitochondria, which activates multiple pathways leading to cell degeneration. AIF: apoptosis-inducing factor; CAD: caspase-activated deoxyribonuclease; IAP: inhibitors of apoptosis; ICAD: inhibitor of caspase-activated deoxyribonuclease: PARP: poly-(ADP ribose) polymerase. (Reprinted with permission, from Lo et al., 2003)

mitochondria, caspase activation, and DNA fragmentation are not a ubiquitous feature of infarcted tissue. It has proved difficult to establish robust effects with inhibitors of caspases in animal models of stroke. These findings, together with the difficulty to generate brain penetrant inhibitors of caspases, have diminished the initial excitement about these strategies (Loetscher et al., 2001). Nevertheless, tentative evidence that apoptotic cell death is more abundant in the critical area of the penumbra and the possibility that apoptosis may proceed with molecular players other than the caspases is keeping alive a strong interest in this field.

11.4.4   Hypothermia and Vascular Approaches

The rate of biological reactions and the associated energy expenditure are highly dependent on temperature. A reduction in body temperature by 1°C reduces the oxygen and energy consumption by approximately 10%. Many animals take advantage of this situation during hibernation. Multiple reports of humans making a miraculous recovery after having been submersed in icy water make a strong case that hypothermia reduces the vulnerability of the brain to oxygen loss. In human patients suffering neurological damage after cardiac arrest, reduction of the body temperature by just a few degrees improves the behavioral recovery. Hypothermia reduces infarct size in animal models of stroke (Olsen et al., 2003). A few ice packs around the head and the chest might turn out to be as beneficial as drugs acting on specific molecular targets. While this thought is sobering for scientists engaged in drug discovery, the success of hypothermia therapy is by no means guaranteed, nor will it necessarily provide optimal therapy. Hypothermia tends to enhance dysfunctional aspects of the cardiovascular system in aged patients and, even if generally used in stroke therapy, will leave ample room open for further improvements by drugs preventing cellular degeneration.

Oxygen and glucose supply by the capillaries remaining functional in partially infarcted tissue determines cell survival in the penumbra. Several clinical trials and drug discovery programs explore the possibility to improve stroke outcome by increasing blood flow in these vessels. Inhibitors of platelet aggregation and thrombosis are expected to prevent secondary thrombus formation. Vasodilator drugs will ease the capillary resistance. Somewhat surprisingly, infusions of albumin increase blood flow during reperfusion and reduce infarct size in animal models of stroke (Belayev et al., 2001). Attempts to reduce energy demand of brain tissue or to increase blood flow following the infarct are sensible alternatives to those directed at neurons and glial cells.

11.5 ISCHEMIC PRECONDITIONING

Very brief periods of ischemia are without detrimental consequences for brain tissue. A gap of many minutes in oxygen and glucose supply is necessary for cell injury and loss to occur. The duration of ischemia, in addition to the size and location of the vessel occlusion, is a main determinant of the severity of the injury and the resulting behavioral deficits. Studies exploring the relationship between duration of ischemia and the functional consequences have revealed that short ischemic episodes diminish the effects of later episodes. The term ischemic preconditioning has been coined for this phenomenon. The resulting beneficial effects are referred to as **ischemic tolerance**. Other organs besides the brain show ischemic tolerance, including the heart, skeletal muscle, kidney, and the liver. Ischemic tolerance provides a tool to minimize the detrimental consequences of ischemia in surgical procedures. In cardiac surgery ischemic preconditioning is sometimes used to prepare the heart for later ischemic events during surgery on arteries that supply it with oxygen and nutrients. No comparable utility has been identified for brain surgery, but clinical experience in humans confirms the concept of ischemic tolerance. Multiple small strokes are less detrimental for behavioral functions than a single significant event. Time intervals of several hours to several months are effective depending on the severity of the initial transient ischemia (Abe and Nowak, 2003). Ischemic preconditioning must activate powerful pathways that allow the brain tissue to better resist later ischemic attacks.

Ischemic preconditioning offers a unique opportunity to identify molecular mechanisms that increase the resistance of brain tissue to episodes without oxygen and glucose (Kirino, 2002). It is perhaps one of the most rewarding parade grounds for technologies that survey the entire genome. Differential hybridization approaches, gene array technologies, and proteomic examinations are being actively pursued. Molecular players identified with the limited approaches so far include several neurotransmitter receptor proteins, glutamate and adenosine receptors in particular. Ischemic preconditioning upregulates the expression of heat shock proteins, and genes belonging to several intracellular kinase signaling pathways. Kinases, including Erk (extracellular signal-regulated kinase) and Akt, and the transcriptional regulators Elk and CREB, are activated. Proteins belonging to neurotrophic factors and their receptor families are differentially regulated. Among the activated transcription factors is NF-κB (nuclear factor-κB), which controls the expression of tumor necrosis factor-α and other mediators of inflammatory responses in tissues other than the nervous system. Ischemic preconditioning elevates the expression of uncoupling protein-2, a component of the mitochondria involved in the generation of ROS and resulting apoptotic events. Transgenic animals overexpressing uncoupling protein-2 show increased resistance in experimental ischemia (Matthiasson et al., 2003). The ongoing intense investigations on ischemic preconditioning are likely to embed these isolated observations into an encompassing picture of the events. The full analysis will point to the most appropriate future drug targets for stroke therapy.

11.6 TRAUMATIC BRAIN AND SPINAL CORD INJURY

Car accidents, sport accidents, and gunshot injuries are the dominant sources of traumatic brain and spinal cord injury in today's society. They cause fractures of the skull or vertebrae, direct mechanical damage to nervous system tissues, and further ischemic damage through injuries to the blood vessels. Mechanical compression damage and the secondary ischemia are believed to cause cell death by mechanisms similar to those operating in ischemic stroke. Evidence for efficacy of glutamate antagonists, antioxidants, and hypothermia in animal models of traumatic brain injury parallels that obtained in stroke models. Some of the NMDA antagonists developed for the stroke indication have also been tested in clinical trials with traumatic brain injury, with inconclusive results for the same reasons as those outlined for the stroke studies. It is likely that future drugs with efficacy in stroke will also be useful for the treatment of traumatic injury, and vice versa.

Spinal cord injury is one of the most devastating human accidents, especially because it most often strikes young people at the prime of their life. The finality of the deficits has remained immutable up to this day. No fully paraplegic patient bound to a wheelchair has regained the ability to walk as yet. The nature of the injury gives rise to special compassion that, together with the influence of celebrity victims, tends to create exaggerated expectations and substantial pressure on the researcher community. Spinal cord injury remains one of the highest hurdles for drug discovery research. The location and extent of the injury determine the deficits encountered in a precise and predictable way. Sensory perception and the voluntary neuromuscular control are lost below the injury. The voluntary override of autonomic reflexes such as bladder emptying has become impossible. Typically spinal cord damage is a contained injury where compression and shearing forces destroy the axons. Swelling of the tissue at the site of injury may cause additional compression damage, but clinical studies with steroid drugs to reduce edema, methylprednisolone in particular, have produced inconclusive results. Over several weeks after the injury, a scar tissue forms at the lesion site, which is comprised mainly of glial cells. The injured axons may extend local sprouts on the two sides of the scar, but no substantial regeneration takes place. Drug discovery approaches thus focus on removing glial inhibition to growth and enhancing the regenerative capacity of the descending projection neurons.

11.6.1 Removing Glial Inhibition

The glial scar at the site of injury forms a physical barrier that prevents axonal regeneration in the spinal cord. Surgical removal of the scar may be a necessary prerequisite for allowing regeneration in patients who sustained the injury several months or years ago. When glial scars are removed in animal models of spinal cord injury, axonal regeneration does not proceed beyond a few millimeters from the injury, because of additional barriers of molecular rather than physical nature. There is a principal difference between axonal regeneration in the central nervous system and the peripheral nervous system that was recognized by the early neuroscientists more than a century ago. Severed axons regenerate effectively within the glial and connective tissue of peripheral nerves, whereas regeneration in the brain and spinal cord occurs only rarely and to a very limited extent. The fact that motor neurons are able to regenerate axons in the periphery but not the spinal cord points to extrinsic factors as key determinants. Transplantation experiments confirm this concept in most elegant ways. When a bridge of peripheral nerve is grafted over the site of a spinal cord injury in experimental animals, the axons grow through the bridge tissue and innervate spinal cord areas proximal to the bridgehead on the other side (Davis and Aguyo, 1981). The peripheral nerve tissue thus provides a permissive environment for axonal degeneration, in contrast to the prohibitive environment of the spinal cord tissue. Many of the molecular factors that determine this difference are part of the myelin sheets. Peripheral myelin, generated by Schwann cells, but not the myelin provided by the central oligodendrocytes is permissive for axonal regeneration.

Research prompted by the transplantation experiments has identified molecular components responsible for the inhibition of regeneration by oligodendrocytes myelin sheets (Fig. 11.5). The Nogo receptor (NogoR) expressed by neurons mediates the action of several glial inhibitors. NogoR binds Nogo-A, the dominant splicing variant of Nogo expressed by oligodendrocytes. Antibodies against Nogo-A facilitate axonal growth in culture and in vivo and allow axons to overcome the inhibitory environment of oligodendrocytes (Caroni and Schwab, 1988). Myelin-associated glycoprotein and oligodendrocyte -myelin glycoprotein are additional proteins found in myelin that inhibit axonal growth. As Nogo-A, they bind to NogoR, most likely at overlapping binding sites. NogoR is expressed by neurons and found on the outer surface of axons. It is a glycosylphosphatidylinositol (GPI)-linked molecule without transmembranal domain and unable to provide an intracellular signal by itself. It associates with the low-affinity (p75) neurotrophin receptor that mediates at least part of the inhibitory actions of NogoR ligands. The precise sequence of downstream events remains to be elucidated, but initial evidence points to an important role for Rho kinase. Inhibitors of this enzyme stimulate axonal growth in vitro and in the spinal cord tissue in vivo. Many other aspects of the NogoR-mediated inhibition of axonal growth await clarification. It is not clear which of the three ligands is functionally the most important one. It is likely that the NogoR ligands are not the only players. Chondroitin sulfate proteoglycans that do not bind to this receptor are potent inhibitors of axonal growth (Morgenstern et al., 2002). Despite these gaps in knowledge it seems evident that NogoR is a highly attractive potential drug target. Molecules able to inhibit the binding of its ligands or to block the downstream signaling are expected to facilitate axonal regeneration in a significant way. While Rho kinase inhibitors are effective in animal models, multiple roles outside of the nervous system will limit its utility as drug target. The breakthroughs in molecular understanding of the inhibitory factors make this area one of the most attractive ones for nervous system drug discovery research (McGee and Strittmatter, 2003).

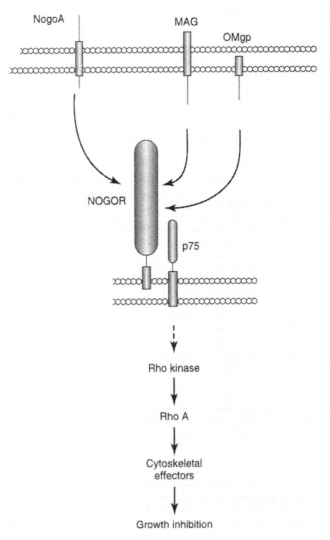

Figure 11.5 Nogo receptor and its ligands. The Nogo receptor (NogoR) is activated by Nogo-A, myelin-associated glycoprotein (MAG), and oligodendrocyte myelin glycoprotein (OMgp). NogoR interacts with the p75 neurotrophin receptor and activates Rho kinase and RhoA, leading to the inhibition of axonal growth.

11.6.2 Stimulating Axonal Growth

It seems possible to find drugs to directly enhance the regenerative capacity of neurons, in addition to removing the inhibitory action of glial proteins. Various growth factors, those of the neurotrophin family in particular, stimulate axonal elongation in culture, and some of them apparently also in the spinal cord of experimental animals. The association of the low-affinity (p75) neurotrophin receptor with NogoR is highly intriguing and prompts many speculations that are being experimentally explored. Axonal growth is stimulated by elevated intracellular levels of cAMP, encouraging speculations that phosphodiesterase inhibitors might have therapeutic utility in spinal cord injury (Neumann et al., 2002). In early development the spinal cord circuitry is established through complex, sequential

Table 11.1   Current and future drug targets

Current Targets

Prevention of Ischemic Stroke
Blood pressure-lowering drugs
Cholesterol synthesis inhibitors (statins)
Inhibitors of platelet aggregation

Intervention in Ischemic Stroke
tPA (a proteolytic enzyme to remove blood clots)

Future Targets

Intervention in Acute Ischemic Stroke and Traumatic Injury
Glutamate receptors
    NMDA, AMPA, and mGluR antagonists
Ion channels
    Ca^{2+}, Na^+ channel blockers
    maxi-K K^+ channel agonists
Reactive oxygen and nitrogen species
    antioxidants
Metal ions
    ion chelators
Apoptosis mechanisms
    caspase inhibitors
Targets identified from ischemic preconditioning studies

Stimulation of Axonal Regeneration in Spinal Cord Injury
Glial inhibitors
    Nogo receptor antagonists
    Rho kinase inhibitors
    chondroitin sulfate proteoglycans antagonists
Neurotrophic mechanisms
    neurotrophin mimetics
    phosphodiesterase inhibitors

molecular and cellular events that involve many growth factors and recognition proteins (Tanabe and Jessell, 1997). Prominent examples are the members of the ephrin and eph receptor families (Himanen and Nikolov, 2003). It may be possible to recreate the molecular conditions of early development to allow rebuilding of the severed spinal connections following injury in the adult. While this seems to be a daunting or even impossible task, the conjecture is sustained by the fact that spinal cord regeneration proceeds with ease in lower vertebrate species. Recent progress in research favors the optimistic view that it will be possible to find drugs that promote regeneration of the injured spinal cord (Table 11.1).

11.7   ANIMAL MODELS AND EXPERIMENTAL MEDICINE

Translation of experimental findings into clinical practice is very demanding in stroke and traumatic central nervous system injury. Animal model work requires a high degree of technical skill and is very labor intensive. Except for the cardiovascular approaches, the models are not validated because no efficacious drugs have been identified as yet. Clinical trials are very costly and require large numbers of patients. Experimental medicine approaches are only gradually emerging and await validation. Stroke, traumatic brain injury, and spinal cord injury each pose unique problems despite overlapping disease mechanisms.

11.7.1 Ischemic Stroke

Several well-characterized rodent models of stroke are generally used in drug discovery research. In the middle cerebral artery occlusion (MCAO) model, one of the major arteries supplying the forebrain is clamped or obstructed permanently, or transiently for various periods of time. MCAO causes a large ischemic infarct that encompasses cortical, striatal, and other subcortical areas. Histological techniques serve to establish the infarct size. Neuronal and glial cell survival is assessed using specific staining techniques. A frequently used enzymatic staining method uses 2,3,5-triphenyltetrazolium, a compound converted by mitochondrial enzymes to a red dye, and allowing the investigator to distinguish between metabolically active and inactive tissue. Behavioral measurements are sometimes added to assess the functional significance of drugs that minimize infarct size. Motor activity, quantitative measurements of walking or performance in simple tests of motor coordination, and various tests used for Alzheimer's disease research serve to measure cognitive activity. NMDA antagonists reliably reduce the infarct size and improve behavioral outcome measures in the MCAO model and serve as positive controls (Finklestein et al., 1999).

In earlier years investigators favored the gerbil as experimental animal species because it has an incomplete circle of Willis, the circular vessel at the base of the brain that bridges the blood supply of the left and right sides, thus making it possible to create a unilateral infarct by clamping one carotid artery. However, the desire to work with transgenic mice has made rats and mice into the favorite species, where reproducible unilateral infarcts can be produced with microsurgical techniques. Several additional methods are available to produce small and well-defined infarcts in cortical tissue. An elegant technique combines photosensitive dyes with laser illumination of surface blood vessels to generate reversible, localized vessel occlusion (Watson et al., 2002). Drug studies in primate models are sometimes advocated as necessary step before clinical trials, with the argument that cortical folding may be a major determinant of stroke mechanisms and that the lissencephalic rodents are inadequate to predict efficacy in the gyrencephalic human brain. While no differences in the early degenerative events have emerged as yet, monkeys may be more suitable to study the recovery processes following stroke, which occur much faster in rodents than in humans.

Experimental stroke models depend on sophisticated surgery and skilled investigators. The capacity of the models is very low. Even an experienced research group succeeds in running only a small number of animals per day. The variability in infarct size of individual animals is high, making it necessary to have at least 10 animals per experimental group to obtain a meaningful result. The capacity limitation explains why very few compounds have been adequately studied, with a full characterization of dose–response and time–response relationships, adequate positive controls, and sufficient power for convincing statistical analysis. An additional issue is the absence of clinical validation of the models. Except for the thrombolytic drug tPA, no drug efficacious in animal models has reached clinical approval. Many clinical trials will be necessary to settle this critical question.

Human strokes are individual events, every one of them is unique in location and the created behavioral deficits. The high variability makes in necessary to include large numbers of patients into clinical trials to obtain meaningful results. Short time windows open for treatment require rapid response units with well-trained medical personnel. These constraints make clinical stroke studies into long and expensive endeavors and tend to dampen the enthusiasm of decision makers in the pharmaceutical companies. Fortunately experimental medicine approaches with imaging techniques may be able to radically change this situation. Computed tomography (CT) and magnetic resonance imaging (MRI) are routinely used to localize infarcted tissue. Variations of these techniques may make it possible to visualize the penumbra (Fig. 11.2). Between the core of the infarct and the normal tissue visible with MRI, there typically is an area that appears normal in diffusion-weighted MRI, which reflects integrity of the tissue, but abnormal in perfusion-weighted MRI, which reflects blood flow. This area of **MRI diffusion–perfusion mismatch** has been operationally equated with the penumbra, because the tissue is alive despite impaired blood flow (Schlaug et al., 1999). Over time, zones ascribed to this area either become normal or become part of the core. Perfusion CT, which uses intravascular markers to image blood flow, has been proposed as an alternative technique for visualizing the penumbra (Wintermark et al., 2002). These methods are still experimental and cannot be considered definitive. Careful comparison between imaging readouts and histological definitions of the penumbra are necessary to test the hypothesis that zones defined by imaging techniques correspond to the histological definition of the penumbra, and that the evolution of these markers over time is predictive of the behavioral deficits. Initial studies suggest complex relationships (Fujioka et al., 2003). These efforts are well justified to proceed with high priority, since they may dramatically improve our ability to discover and develop stroke drugs. Imaging techniques visualizing the penumbra will make it possible to follow the evolution of a stroke and to define drug effects in individual patients. It will be possible to get conclusive data in trials with a small number of patients only, and to select the most promising drug candidates for the large clinical studies. Once these experimental clinical techniques are established, drug discovery research for stroke will become a most fruitful endeavor, whereas so far it has been a graveyard for many research projects.

11.7.2 Traumatic Brain Injury

In many aspects the situation of traumatic brain injury parallels that in stroke. Reliable and reproducible animal models have been established. Controlled weight drop onto brain tissue or fluid percussion pulses create local damage (Chen et al., 2003). Histological and behavioral markers serve as endpoints. As for stroke, these animal models are not validated, since no clinical trial has succeeded as yet. The interindividual variability of injuries in patients tends to be higher than in stroke, since skull fracture and bleeding provide additional confounding aspects. Definition of a penumbra is much more difficult than in stroke. For these reasons drug discovery for traumatic brain injury has remained an unattractive enterprise so far. Focus on ischemic stroke, with subsequent testing of successful drug candidates in traumatic brain injury, seems to be the most promising way forward.

11.7.3 Spinal Cord Injury

Spinal cord injury as it occurs in humans can be reliably reproduced in animals (Table 11.2). Weight drop and other contusion devices produce local damage and, with sufficient severity, cause complete injury to transversing axons (Khan et al., 1999). Full transections are useful when bridging tissue is implanted to overcome the gap (Bregman et al., 2002).

Table 11.2 Animal models

Ischemic Stroke
Middle cerebral artery occlusion (MCAO)
  transient or permanent (mice, rats)
Gerbil carotid artery ligation

Traumatic Brain Injury
Weight drop models
Fluid-percussion models

Spinal Cord Injury
Contusion models
Partial transection
Complete transection with bridging material

Partial spinal cord transactions leave a natural bridge through which regeneration may occur. Many variations of these methods are in use, often making it difficult to compare results among various research groups. Monitoring axonal regeneration with morphological techniques tends to be difficult because of the small number of axons responding. It is possible though to enhance the resolution with retrograde labeling techniques that identify the cell bodies projecting caudal to the spinal cord injury. Rodents show remarkable ability to recover spontaneously from partial spinal cord injury, suggesting an advantage of monkey models in this regard.

Clinical trial design and execution in spinal cord injury presents complex ethical and practical issues. Would it be ethical to test in a double-blinded fashion a drug that reduces neuronal loss in ischemic stroke, thereby denying newly injured patients a potentially beneficial drug? Once the injury is established and a glial scar has been formed, removal of the scar in addition to drug treatment might be necessary. Drug studies in patients with established partial spinal cord injury appears to provide the best way forward. Regeneration of axons into areas below the lesion is expected to restitute lost segmental functions that are easily monitored. Each patient would serve as his own control. Double-blinded crossover studies would provide all participating patients with potential drug benefits. These approaches will allow for the clinical testing of drug candidates and so sustain the current enthusiasm for drug discovery research on spinal cord injury.

11.8 CONCLUSIONS

Ischemic stroke, and traumatic brain and spinal cord injury, represent significant medical needs, but they are very difficult areas for drug discovery research. Impressive progress has been made in disease prevention with drugs that reduce the risk of thrombus formation and vessel occlusion. Drugs that reduce the risk of heart attacks also reduce the risk of ischemic stroke in the brain.

Drug discovery efforts focus on intervention therapy to limit the consequences of an ischemic attack. In special cases it is possible to restore circulation by administering tPA, a thrombolytic enzyme, but there is no approved therapy to directly prevent the loss of neurons and glial cells in infarcted brain tissue. During the hours after an infarct, brain tissue goes through a rapid sequence of events that includes overstimulation by excitatory neurotransmitters, intracellular ionic imbalances, generation of reactive oxygen species, followed by structural disintegration and death of cells. Despite many clinical trials there has been no conclusive demonstration that glutamate antagonists, which reliably reduce the infarct size in animal models of stroke, have beneficial effects in human patients. In their totality the trials have generated an inconclusive result. Glutamate antagonists and other molecules interfering with other events of the degenerative cascade, thus remain attractive approaches to stroke therapy. Ion channel blockers, antioxidants, and inhibitors of apoptosis are under active investigation.

Stroke drug discovery is highly dependent on a breakthrough in clinical trial design and execution. At present, many hundreds of patients are necessary for a conclusive trial. Emerging imaging techniques are expected to radically ease this burden and to make possible rapid testing of drug candidates. By providing an operational definition for the penumbra, the area partially infarcted only, these methods make it possible to directly monitor whether drugs improve cell survival during the hours after a stroke. The imaging methods are a critical requirement for success in drug discovery for stroke. They have the potential to transform this field from a painfully difficult to a most promising endeavor.

Many patients gradually recover from some of the deficits of stroke. The underlying mechanisms are poorly understood but believed to include neurogenesis, axonal regeneration, and functional rearrangements in surviving circuits. No drugs are currently available to enhance these processes. It is a difficult area for drug discovery, with only highly speculative approaches at the present time. Improving recovery from stroke represents a very high hurdle but important long-term goal for drug therapy.

Traumatic injury to the brain shares many common features with ischemic stroke but is further complicated by contusion, bleeding, and skull fractures. Mechanism of neuronal degeneration and recovery are believed to be very similar. Clinical trials in traumatic injury are as difficult as in stroke, and approaches of translational medicine appear yet more difficult. Using ischemic stroke to define drugs for use in traumatic injury thus appears to be the most fruitful strategy for this indication.

Spinal cord injury is dominated by axonal damage, pushing in the background the strategies to increase cell survival immediately after the injury. Central nervous system tissue normally provides insurmountable barriers to axonal regeneration. The recent discovery of the molecular basis for this inhibition provides substantial expectations for drug discovery research. NogoR, a receptor for several inhibitory molecules, represents an obvious putative drug target. Downstream mediators, including Rho kinase, present alternative target opportunities. In addition neurotrophic factor mimetics may be able to directly promote the neurons' capacity for regeneration. The recent breakthroughs in spinal cord research have made this area into one of the most promising and attractive ones for drug discovery research.

REFERENCES

Further Reading

BREGMAN, B.S., COUMANS, J.V., DAI, H.N., KUHN, P.L., LYNSKEY, J., MCATEE, M., and SANDHU, F. Transplants and neurotrophic factors increase regeneration and recovery of function after spinal cord injury. *Prog. Brain Res.* 137: 257–273, 2002.

DIRNAGL, U., IADECOLA, C., and MOSKOWITZ, M.A. Pathobiology of ischemic stroke: An integrated view. *Trends Neurosci.* 22: 391–397, 1999.

FINKELSTEIN, S.P., FISHER, M., FURLAN, A.J., GOLDSTEIN, L.B., GORELICK, P.B., KASTE, M., LEES, K.R., and TRAYSTMAN, R.J. Recommendations for standards regarding preclinical neuroprotective and restorative drug treatment. *Stroke* 30: 2752–2758, 1999.

GILGUN-SHERKI, Y., ROSENBAUM, Z., MELAMED, E., and OFFEN, D. Antioxidant therapy in acute central nervous system injury: current state. *Pharmacol. Rev.* 54: 271–284, 2002.

HIMANEN, J.P., and NIKOLOV, D.B. Eph signaling:

A structural view. *Trends Neurosci.* 26: 46–51, 2003.

KIRINO, T. Ischemic tolerance. *J. Cereb. Blood Flow Metab.* 22: 1283–1296, 2002.

LIPTON, P. Ischemic cell death in neurons. *Physiol. Rev.* 79: 1431–1568, 1999.

LO, E.H., DALKARA, T., and MOSKOWITZ, M.A. Mechanisms, challenges and opportunities in stroke. *Nature Rev. Neurosci.* 4: 399–415, 2003.

LOETSCHER, H., NIEDERHAUSER, O., KEMP, J., and GILL, R. Is caspase-3 inhibition a valid therapeutic strategy in cerebral ischemia? *Drug Dis. Today* 6: 671–680, 2001.

MCGEE, A.W., and STRITTMATTER, S.M. The nogo-66 receptor: focusing myelin inhibition of axon regeneration. *Trends Neurosci.* 26: 193–198, 2003.

TANABE, Y., and JESSELL, T.M. Diversity and pattern in the developing spinal cord. *Science* 274: 1115–1123, 1996.

Citations

ABE, H., and NOWAK, T.S., JR. Induced hippocampal neuron protection in an optimized gerbil ischemia model: Insult thresholds for tolerance induction and altered gene expression defined by ischemic depolarization. *J. Cereb. Blood Flow Metab.* 24: 84–97, 2003.

BELAYEV, L., LIU, Y., ZHAO, W., BUSTO, R., and GINSBERG, M.D. Human albumin therapy of acute ischemic stroke: Marked neuroprotective efficacy at moderate doses and with a broad therapeutic window. *Stroke* 32: 553–560, 2001.

CARONI, P., and SCHWAB, M.E. Antibody against myelin-associated inhibitor of neurite growth neutralizes nonpermissive substrate properties of CNS white matter. *Neuron* 1: 85–96, 1988.

CHEN, S., PICKARD, J.D., and HARRIS, N.G. Time course of cellular pathology after controlled cortical impact injury. *Exp. Neurol.* 182: 87–102, 2003.

DAVID, S., and AGUAYO, A.J. Axonal elongation into peripheral nervous system "bridges" after central nervous system injury in adult rats. *Science* 214: 931–933, 1981.

FUJIOKA, M., TAOKA, T., MATSUO, Y., MISHIMA, K., OGOSHI, K., KONDO, Y., TSUDA, M., FUJIWARA, M., ASANO, T., SAKAKI, T., MIYASAKI, A., PARK D., and SIESJÖ, B.K. Magnetic resonance imaging shows delayed ischemic striatal neurodegeneration. *An. Neurol.* 54: 732–747, 2003.

GRIBKOFF, V.K., STARRETT, J.E., JR., DWORETZKY, S.I., HEWAWASAM, P., BOISSARD, C.G., COOK, D.A., FRANTZ, S.W., HEMAN, K., HIBBARD, J.R., HUSTON, K., JOHNSON, G., KRISHNAN, B.S., KINNEY, G.G., LOMBARDO, L.A., MEANWELL, N.A., MOLINOFF, P.B., MYERS, R.A., MOON, S.L., ORTIZ, A., PAJOR, L., PIESCHL, R.L., POST-MUNSON, D.J., SIGNOR, L.J., SRINIVAS, N., TABER, M.T., THALODY, G., TROJNACKI, J.T., WIENER, H., YELESWARAM, K., and YEOLA, S.W. Targeting acute ischemic stroke with calcium-sensitive opener of maxi-K potassium channels. *Nature Med.* 7: 471–477, 2001.

HORN, J., and LIMBURG, M. Calcium antagonists for ischemic stroke: A systematic review. *Stroke* 32: 570–576, 2001.

KHAN, T., HAVEY, R.M., SAYERS, S.T., PATWARDHAN, A., and KING, W.W. Animal models of spinal cord contusion injuries. *Lab. Anim. Sci.* 49: 161–172, 1999.

MATTHIASSON, G., SHAMLOO, M., GIDO, G., MATHI, K., TOMASEVIC, G., YI, S., WARDEN, C.H., CASTILHO, R.F., MELCHER, T., GONZALEZ-ZULUETA, M., NIKOLICS, K., and WIELOCH, T. Uncoupling protein-2 prevents neuronal death and diminishes brain dysfunction after stroke and brain trauma. *Nature Med.* 9: 1062–1068.

MORGENSTERN, D.A., ASHER, R.A., and FAWCETT, J.W. Chondroitin sulphate proteoglycans in the CNS injury response. *Prog. Brain Res.* 137: 313–332, 2002.

NEUMANN, S., BRADKE, F., TESSIER-LAVIGNE, M., and BASBAUM, A. Regeneration of sensory axons within the injured spinal cord induced by intraganglionic cAMP elevation. *Neuron* 34: 885–893, 2002.

OLNEY, J.W. Brain lesions, obesity, and other disturbances in mice treated with monosodium glutamate. *Science* 164: 719–721, 1969.

OLSEN, T.S., WEBER, U.J., and KAMMERSGAARD, L.P. Therapeutic hypothermia for acute stroke. *Lancet Neurol.* 2: 410–416, 2003.

SCHLAUG, G., BENFIELD, A., BAIRD, A.E., SIEWERT, B., LOVBLAD, K.O., PARKER, R.A., EDELMAN, R.R., and WARACH, S. The ischemic penumbra: Operationally defined by diffusion and perfusion MRI. *Neurology* 53: 1528–1537, 1999.

SCHWARCZ, R., and MELDRUM, B. Excitatory aminoacid antagonists provide a therapeutic approach to neurological disorders. *Lancet* 20: 140–143, 1985.

SLOVITER, R.S. A selective loss of hippocampal mossy fiber Timm stain accompanies granule cell seizure activity induced by perforant path stimulation. *Brain Res.* 330: 150–153, 1985.

WATSON, B.D., PRADO, R., VELOSO, A., BRUNSCHIG, J.P., and DIETRICH, W.D. Cerebral blood flow restoration and reperfusion injury after ultraviolet laser-facilitated middle cerebral artery recanalization in rat thrombotic stroke. *Stroke* 33: 428–434, 2002.

WINTERMARK, M., REICHHART, M., THIRAN, J.P., MAEDER, P., CHALARON, M., SCHNYDER, P., BOGOUSSLAVSKY, J., and MEULI, R. Prognostic accuracy of cerebral blood flow measurement by perfusion computed tomography, at the time of emergency room admission, in acute stroke patients. *An. Neurol.* 51: 417–432, 2002.

Chapter 12

Other Neurodegenerative Disorders

Alzheimer's disease, ischemic stroke, and Parkinson's disease are the most prominent neurodegenerative diseases and are found on the activity list of most pharmaceutical companies. From a point of view of the patient population as well as scientific interest and attraction, several other neurodegenerative diseases deserve equal attention. They include multiple sclerosis, Huntington's and related glutamine-repeat diseases, amyotrophic lateral sclerosis (ALS), Creutzfeldt-Jakob and related prion diseases, and the neuropathies of the peripheral nervous system. For individually distinct reasons these ailments typically receive second priority by neuroscience drug discovery research groups. Multiple sclerosis has a dominant immune component and is habitually discussed and managed as part of the immunological and inflammatory diseases. Huntington's disease, ALS, and prion diseases affect fewer people than the dominant neurological diseases, thus facing higher obstacles in the allocation of limited resources. Peripheral neuropathies are typically discussed in the context of pain or diabetic disorders. Reflecting these circumstances, they are discussed in fewer words in this volume and combined into a single chapter.

12.1 MULTIPLE SCLEROSIS

Multiple sclerosis is a demyelinating disorder of the central nervous system that affects up to 0.1% of the population in some geographic areas. In the majority of the patients, typically the younger ones, the disease starts with individual attacks of demyelination and neurological deficits followed by partial to full recovery. This relapsing–remitting form of multiple sclerosis gradually evolves into the secondary, gradually progressive form of the disease in some of the affected. A minority of patients, typically the older ones, suffer from primary progressive multiple sclerosis, which advances steadily in absence of distinct episodes. The location and size of the demyelination plaques determine the clinical symptoms of the disease. Visual, sensory, or motor disturbances may prevail. Despite full recovery of the primary symptoms after the early episodes in the relapsing–remitting disease, the patients tend to remain more prone to physiological and psychological stress. At advanced stages of progressive multiple sclerosis, partial paralysis, impairments of digestive functions, and cognitive problems interfere with daily living (Compston and Coles, 2002).

The primary cause of multiple sclerosis has remained an enigma. There is a strong genetic component, since siblings of patients have a higher disease risk than the average

Drug Discovery for Nervous System Diseases, by Franz F. Hefti
ISBN 0-471-46563-1   Copyright © 2005 by John Wiley & Sons, Inc.

Table 12.1 Drugs and drug targets in multiple sclerosis

Current Drugs

Corticosteroids

Interferon β-1a and interferon β-1b

Glatimer acetate (random synthetic polypeptides)

Mitoxantrone (topoisomerase inhibitor)

Azathioprine (purine synthesis inhibitor)

Natalizumab (anti-VLA-4 antibody)

Future Drugs

Inhibitors of T-cell activation

Inhibitors of T-cell migration

Antagonists to pro-inflammatory cytokines

Oligodendrocyte differentiation and survival factors

population, and monozygotic twins have a higher concordance rate than dizygotic twins. No pedigrees with Mendelian traits and no susceptibility genes have been identified with certainty as yet, making it likely that many genes contribute. Epidemiological studies make an equally strong case for environmental contributions. Prevalence is highest among people living in Northern parts of Europe and America, and higher than in genetically comparable populations that migrated to other geographical areas.

Autoimmune mechanisms are a dominant feature of multiple sclerosis pathology. It is thus widely believed that the disease is caused by microbial pathogens sharing chemical components of human myelin and causing an autoimmune response by molecular mimicry. According to this view, multiple sclerosis is very similar to experimental autoimmune encephalitis (EAE), a condition that is easily created in animals by immunizing them against myelin components. An alternative view, however, suggests that oligodendrocytes degeneration is the primary event in multiple sclerosis, and that the formation of antimyelin antibodies is a consequence of metabolically inert myelin fragments that linger for prolonged periods of time after oligodendrocyte cell death. In support of this view, postmortem analysis of brain tissue from fresh lesions in young patients shows oligodendritic cell degeneration in absence of immune cell infiltration (Barnett and Prineas, 2004). The current drug therapy and drug discovery efforts concentrate on the autoimmune encephalitis part of the disease mechanism. The more recent pathological discoveries suggest intriguing alternative approaches.

12.1.1 Autoimmune Encephalitis and Related Drugs

The putative mechanisms of autoimmune encephalitis in multiple sclerosis are illustrated in Figure 12.1. According to this concept, antigen-presenting cells are activated by myelin fragments or molecules mimicking their immunogenic epitopes, and they initiate the formation of myelin-reactive T-cells. In a process involving α4-integrin, the T-cells migrate into brain tissue and interact with microglia cells that functions as local antigen-presenting cells. The secretion of various cytokines is a consequence of this interaction. The resulting local inflammatory response causes damage to oligodendrocytes and epithelial cells. Breakdown of the blood-brain barrier accelerates infiltration of myelin-reactive T-cells. Demyelination causes abnormal signal conduction in denuded axons. The loss of defined nodes of Ranvier disables the saltatory axon potential propagation and slows

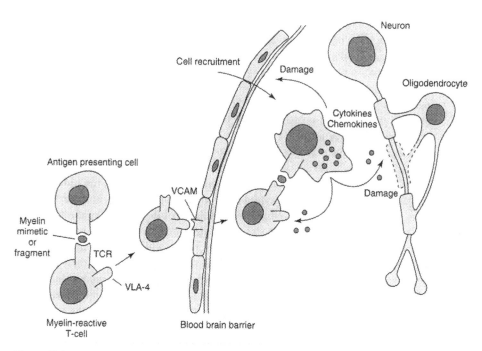

Figure 12.1 Mechanisms of autoimmune encephalitis. Presentation of myelin mimetics or fragments generates myelin-reactive T-cells, which pass into the brain through a process involving VLA-4 and vascular cell adhesion molecule (VCAM). They generate a local inflammatory response through the interaction with antigen-presenting microglia. Released cytokines and chemokines damage oligodendrocytes and causes the breakdown of myelin sheaths and axonal damage. Damage to the blood-brain barrier facilitates infiltration by further myelin-reactive T-cells.

down nerve conductance velocity. Spontaneous, aberrant axon potentials are generated in demyelinated axons and disrupt information encoding. Permanent damage and degeneration of axons is common with severe demyelination. In the remitting phase of the disease, the inflammatory response subsides and remyelination from residual oligodendrocytes or oligodendrocytes precursor cells gradually restores normal conduction in the surviving axons. Over several relapse-remission cycles the immune response broadens through epitope spreading and B-cell involvement.

The current therapeutic approaches to multiple sclerosis attempt to suppress the autoimmune response. Corticosteroids are given during the active relapse and reduce its duration, but they are unable to prevent long-term deficits and progression of the disease. Interferon β-1a and interferon β-1b, initially pursued as anti-viral strategies, slightly reduce the relapse rate despite the lack of evidence for a viral cause of the disease. The mechanism of action remains unclear and may involve suppression of the release of pro-inflammatory cytokines. A mild reduction of the relapse rate was demonstrated for glatimer acetate, a mixture of synthetic polypeptides believed to mimic sequences of myelin basic protein and able to prevent the binding of myelin basic protein to myelin-reactive T-cell receptors. Azathioprine, an immunosuppressant purine analogue, and mitoxantrone, a DNA repair inhibitor, are marginally effective drugs used in the treatment of aggressive forms of relapsing–remitting multiple sclerosis. The most significant effects on relapse rate and progression of the disease have been obtained with natalizumab, an antibody against the α4-integrin component of very late antigen-4 (VLA-4) that interacts with vascular cell adhesion molecule. Disruption of this interaction inhibits the migration of T-cells through the blood-brain barrier (Miller et al., 2003).

The autoimmune cascade suggests many additional approaches to drug discovery. Clinical trials with general suppressors of the immune response, such as cyclosporine, have revealed minor beneficial effects at the cost of significant adverse effects, thus directing future efforts toward more specific strategies. New attempts to block the interaction between myelin basic protein and reactive T-cells have not met with success as yet, but remain conceptually attractive. It seems feasible to identify the subtypes of polypeptides contained in glatimer acetate that bind to T-cell receptors and improve their affinity and specificity. The clinical success of natalizumab, the anti-VLA-4 antibody, validates blocking of T-cell migration as a successful strategy. Penetration of the blood-brain barrier is complex process that offers several conceptual opportunities for interference. Metalloproteases enzymes are involved in the breakdown of the extracellular matrix by the T-cells and present alternative putative targets for drug discovery. Several research groups have embarked on the genomic profiling of brain tissue with an active demyelinating autoimmune process. Several chemokines, cytokines, neuropeptides and their receptors, as well as enzymes involved in prostaglandin synthesis, are among molecules upregulated in demyelinating plaques (Steinman and Zamvil, 2003). Cytosolic phospholipase A$_2$ is expressed in EAE lesions, and inhibitors of this enzyme prevent the onset and the progression of EAE in mice (Kalvyvas and David, 2004). Many of the proteins overexpressed in plaque tissue represent attractive putative drug targets, but similar to the situation in depression and ischemic stroke, the number of speculative targets vastly exceeds the capacity of drug development programs and clinical studies (Zamvil and Steinman, 2003). Rigorous evaluation of drug candidates in the most appropriate animal models and confirmation of the mechanism in human tissue will help in the selection of the most promising approaches.

12.1.2 Remyelination and Prevention of Axon Degeneration

Remyelination occurs spontaneously during the remission from a multiple sclerosis relapse but seems to be incomplete. Residual oligodendrocytes as well as local oligodendrocytes progenitors contribute to this process. Stimulation of oligodendrocytes differentiation is expected to enhance remyelination and functional recovery of the patients. Encouraging results with cell therapy approaches in EAE animal models, such as transplantation of myelin-producing Schwann cells to the lesion site, lend support for related drug discovery efforts (Kohama et al., 2001). Receptors for oligodendrocyte-specific differentiation factors are attractive putative targets (Wilson et al., 2003). The breakdown of the blood-brain barrier at the sites of multiple sclerosis lesions may allow growth factors or biological mimetics to reach the brain following systemic administration. LPA1/edg2 G-protein-coupled receptors of the lysophospholipid receptor family are selectively expressed by oligodendrocytes and may offer an opportunity for a small molecule agonist approach, where brain penetration is more easily achieved (Weiner et al., 1998).

The myelin sheath provides trophic support for the embedded axons and contributes to their maintenance and survival. Persistent loss of axons in demyelinated plaques is a well-established feature of multiple sclerosis and may be the major determinant of irreversible functional disabilities. Possibly processes similar to those mediating neuron death in ischemic stroke and acute injury contribute to axonal degeneration in multiple sclerosis. Memantine, the NMDA glutamate receptor antagonist, is effective in the EAE model (Paul and Bolton, 2002). Glutamate receptor antagonists, voltage-gated ion channel blockers, and other molecules considered in the treatment of ischemic stroke, may find utility in the treatment of the active phase of multiple sclerosis relapses. Proteomic profiling of axons loosing their myelin sheaths will help identify putative drug targets that specifically mediate the degenerative events. Genomic and proteomic array technologies may furthermore help identify the molecular determinants of early oligodendrocyte degeneration that has been put forward as the first step of the multiple sclerosis disease mechanisms (Trapp, 2004).

12.1.3 Animal Models and Clinical Development

Multiple sclerosis research relies heavily on the EAE model, which accurately reflects many features of the human disease. Simple forms of the EAE model use myelin fragments or peptides of partial sequences of the myelin proteins, myelin basic protein, and myelin oligodendrocyte glycoprotein, in simple immunization protocols. Demyelination and neurological deficits evolve over several days and resolve gradually. In more complex versions of the EAE model, immunization with specific peptide sequences of myelin proteins and transfer of myelin-reactive T-cells from immunized to naïve animals, elicit rhythmic relapse-remission cycles that more accurately reflect the human disease. The EAE animal model is a good predictor for efficacy of drug candidates interfering with the auto-immune cascade, but it does not replicate early oligodendritic degeneration that may precede the immunological events (Seamons et al., 2003).

Clinical development of drug candidates in multiple sclerosis is greatly facilitated by the use of MRI surrogate markers. Phase II proof-of-concept studies rely on measurements of plaques functionally defined as white matter abnormalities in MRI. The further demonstration of clinical efficacy of drug candidates requires clinical observations of patient disabilities and relapse rates. These phase III trials are lengthy and complex because of the pronounced interindividual variability of multiple sclerosis patients. Trials with several different agents over the past years have established a robust comparative database and validation for the MRI surrogate markers. Despite the intrinsic difficulties, drug development in multiple sclerosis is now possible in a decisive and timely fashion.

Multiple sclerosis illustrates the potential and excitement of modern drug discovery. It has been helped by the easy acceptance of biological therapeutics and the availability of an imaging surrogate marker that predicts therapeutic efficacy. Multiple sclerosis is perhaps the most advanced field of drug discovery in the neurosciences. The creativity and exploratory zest of its investigators may be a paradigmatic example for events yet to occur in other indications.

12.2 HUNTINGTON'S DISEASE AND THE POLYGLUTAMINE DISEASES

Huntington's disease is an inherited autosomal dominant neurological disease that affects about 0.01% of the Caucasian population. The disease typically starts between 20 and 50 years of age with mild motor and emotional disturbances. Gradually it progresses to a state of constant movement and restlessness described by the term chorea, the Greek word for dance. Increasing emotional and cognitive disabilities accompany the worsening motor symptoms, and the disease invariably leads to death within about 20 years from first diagnosis. Postmortem analysis of the brain of Huntington's disease patients reveals neuronal degeneration in several brain areas and most pronounced changes in the basal ganglia. The population of spiny, GABAergic projection neurons, which provides an inhibitory input to globus pallidum and other areas of the extrapyramidal motor system, is completely lost in the brains of people who died of advanced Huntington's disease. The degeneration of these neurons represents the pathological hallmark of the illness, and the loss of their inhibitory influence on motor systems is believed to be the major contributor to the over-activity. Less pronounced degenerative events in other neuronal populations contribute to the generation of the complex behavioral changes in the disease (Vonsattel and DiFiglia, 1998).

Huntington's disease is caused by the expansion of a CAG trinucleotide repeat sequence that encodes the polyglutamine stretch in the protein Huntingtin. Expansion beyond 35 repeats causes pathological changes, and the length of the expansion is the principal determinant of onset and severity of the illness. Repeat lengths increase over subsequent generations, causing earlier onset, anticipation, in the children of carriers. Expansions beyond 70 repeats have not been observed and are most likely lethal at the embryonic stage. Huntington's disease is a member of the polyglutamine repeat disease family, which includes several forms of spino-cerebellar ataxia and spinobulbar muscular atrophy. The diseases share general aspects of neuronal pathology, but the genes carrying the mutation and the neuronal populations affected are distinct in every case (Cummings and Zoghbi, 2000).

12.2.1 Molecular Disease Mechanisms and Target Opportunities

Huntingtin is a large protein that participates in membrane and vesicle trafficking. Mice carrying a null mutation of the gene die at embryonic stages. Huntingtin is widely expressed in the brain in patterns different from the neuropathological changes in the Huntington's disease brain and unable to explain the differential neuronal vulnerability. Huntingtin interacts with many transcription factors, proteins involved in protein trans-port, and with a small number of enzymes. The interactions are determined by amino acids close to the N-terminal of Huntingtin, where also the polyglutamine stretch is located. Expansions of the polyglutamine stretch alter many of the protein–protein interactions, by either enhancing or reducing them. Proteolytic cleavage of the mutated protein generates an N-terminal fragment that includes the polyglutamine stretch. This fragment is able to aggregate as β-sheet in the cytoplasm, the nucleus, and also in axon terminals and to cause novel protein–protein interactions not seen with the normal protein (Li and Li, 2004).

Changes in protein–protein interactions disturb cellular function at many levels (Fig. 12.2). Aberrant contacts with transcriptional regulators create pathological gene expression patterns. Altered interactions with cell traffic protein impede axonal transport and synaptic function. The specific length of the polyglutamine expansion determines the precise nature of the interactions with other proteins and generates patient-specific disease mechanisms that seem to offer little hope for drug discovery. However, common pathological steps present interference points for drugs that might correct at least some of the pathological events (Table 12.2). Huntingtin binds to histone acetyltransferase, an enzyme necessary for histone acetylation during gene expression. Enzyme activity is reduced by the expanded Huntingtin polyglutamine repeats. The balance between histone acetyl-transferase and histone acetylase activity determines histone acetylation, suggesting that

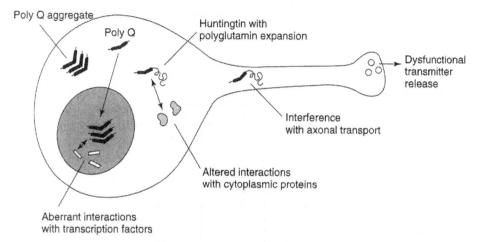

Figure 12.2 Pathological consequences of the polyglutamine expansion in the Huntingtin protein. The polyglutamine expansion alters the interactions of Huntingtin with transcription factors, trafficking proteins and enzymes. Following proteolytic cleavage, the *N*-terminus with the polyglutamine stretch forms β-sheet aggregations in the cytoplasm and nucleus.

Table 12.2 Drug discovery opportunities in Huntington's disease

Polyglutamine aggregation inhibitors
Histone acetylase inhibitors
Glutamate receptor antagonists
Antioxidants
Neurotrophic factor mimetics
Caspase inhibitors

inhibition of the acetylase might correct for the Huntington's disease deficit. Two inhibitors of histone acetylase, butyrate and suberoylanilide hydroxamic acid, have beneficial effects in transgenic animal models of Huntington's disease (Hockley et al., 2003; Ferrante et al., 2003). Histone acetylase inhibitors are explored for cancer treatment, accelerating the parallel drug development for Huntington's disease. An alternative approach to Huntington's disease drug discovery is proved by polyglutamine aggregation inhibitors. These compounds are expected to prevent aberrant binding of cellular regulators to β-sheet aggregates and the steric obstruction of growing polymers. Peptidic inhibitors of polyglutamine aggregation prevent toxicity in cell cultures (Thakur et al., 2004). Brain-penetrant analogs of these compounds are expected to be beneficial in Huntington's disease.

12.2.2 Neuronal Disease Mechanisms

Transgenic animals expressing the mutated *huntingtin* gene delineate the sequence of events from the polyglutamine expansion to the neuropathology and aberrant behavior of Huntington's disease. The most relevant observations are derived from gene knock-in mice where the mutated human gene has been inserted into the genetic frame of the deleted mouse gene. Subtle behavioral changes at early adult stages are the first observable events in these animals. They are followed by various alterations in proteins participating in neurotransmitter functions. The early reduction of enkephalin in the striatum replicates the human pathology where the loss of enkephalin-positive neurons in the striatum precedes the degeneration of other cells. Glutamate receptor expression changes in the transgenic mice with a prominent reduction in levels of presynaptic metabotropic glutamate receptors. Neuronal shrinkage and atrophy become apparent subsequently, together with the formation of polyglutamine aggregates in the cytoplasm. Nuclear aggregates and neuron loss emerge last and are seen at advanced stages of the animal's life span.

The loss of presynaptic metabotropic glutamate receptors is believed to enhance glutamatergic transmission through NMDA receptors and supports speculations that excitotoxic death is a feature of Huntington's disease. Earlier animal models replicated the striatal cell death by injecting of ionotropic glutamate receptor agonists into the striatum of rodents. Similar neuronal degeneration is achieved by injecting the mitochondrial inhibitor 3-nitropropionic acid into the striatum. These findings lend support to speculations that energy failure is a contributor to neuron death in Huntington's disease. The natural mitochondrial antioxidant, coenzyme Q10, and the NMDA receptor antagonist, remacemide, produce beneficial effects in transgenic and neurotoxicity animal models of Huntington's disease but failed to produce significant benefits in the corresponding clinical trials (Ferrante et al., 2002). Similarly the attempts to improve energy metabolism in Huntington's patients with large doses of creatine failed to show beneficial effects (Verbessem et al., 2003). Despite these early setbacks antioxidant and anti-excitotoxity approaches remain conceptually attractive for drug discovery because of the observations in animal models. More specific modulations of glutamate receptor mechanisms and the energy metabolism may be able to provide the desired therapeutic effects in patients.

The molecular mechanisms of neuronal death in Huntington's disease provide additional interference points for drug discovery efforts. The animal model and human postmortem studies depict a complex picture with only a minor contribution of apoptotic steps (Hickey and Chesselet, 2003). Nevertheless, caspases might participate in the disease process since the Huntingtin protein contains a caspase cleavage site and a caspase inhibitor has been effective in an excitotoxicity animal model of the disease (Toulmond et al., 2004). Neuronal loss in these animal models is prevented by several members of the neurotrophin family, including BDNF and the GDNF family of neurotrophic factors (Gratacos et al., 2001). Environmental enrichment elevates the expression of BDNF and has beneficial effects in a transgenic animal model Huntington's disease, suggesting a therapeutic approach with neurotrophic factor mimetics (Spires et al., 2004). Future studies on transgenic animal models will help to identify the most attractive putative drug targets. It seems possible that a detailed picture of sequential events will emerge that ascribes an optimal drug therapy for each stage of the progressing disease.

12.2.3 Animal Models and Clinical Development

Early animal models employed local injections of glutamate receptor agonists or mitochondrial toxins to destroy neurons in the basal ganglia. Kainic acid, quinolinic acid, and 3-nitropropionic acid were the most widely used agents that destroy neuronal cell bodies while spearing afferent axons and local glial cells. The transgenic animals much more closely reflect the human disease process (Menalled and Chesselet, 2002). Early transgenic mice models expressed parts of the mutated human gene on the normal genetic mouse background. Several strains with various lengths of the polyglutamine stretch have been described. The more recently introduced knock-in mice represent almost ideal animal models that appear to replicate most of the human disease. These animal models greatly facilitate drug discovery and make it possible to evaluate many drug candidates for selection to clinical development.

Clinical development in Huntington's disease is comparable to that of Alzheimer's and Parkinson's disease. Symptomatic effects will be easily discerned in short-term behavioral studies. Disease-modifying drugs require observation times of several months but will provide decisive results if sufficiently powered. The recent advances in molecular understanding of the disease mechanisms, the availability of optimal animal models, and the relatively simple clinical trials sustain the hope that effective drugs can be found for this very complex disease.

12.3 CREUTZFELDT-JAKOB DISEASE AND THE PRION DISEASES

Scrapie is a very common prion disease that is epidemic in sheep herds. Related human diseases, including Creutzfeldt-Jakob disease (CJD) and kuru, are very rare and affect only about 0.0001% of the general population. Despite the very small prevalence in humans, the prion diseases have attracted immense attention because of their scientific exceptionality, and the recent spread of scrapie from sheep to bovine herds and possibly to humans. The potential of a massive human epidemic caused by beef consumption has created fear in the general population and triggered corrective governmental action. Indeed, prion diseases have devastating consequences for affected humans. Within a time period of a few months to a few years, they progress to severe dementia, motor deficits, and death. The diseases cause widespread and massive neuron degeneration in the brain. Surviving neurons typically contain large vacuoles, generating a sponge-like (spongiform) appearance. Massive gliosis invades the areas of neuronal loss. There is neither prevention nor treatment for the prion diseases (DeArmon and Prusiner, 2003).

12.3.1 Disease Mechanism

Prion diseases originate from alterations in the prion protein (PrP^C), a membrane-anchored protein that is widely expressed by neurons, lymphocytes, and other cells outside of the nervous system (Aguzzi and Polymenidou, 2004). A protease-resistant version of this protein (PrP^{Sc}), most likely a conformationally changed form of PrP^C, is the causative agent. The insoluble PrP^{Sc} accumulates in the brain and forms amyloid aggregates with similar characteristics as the $A\beta$ aggregates in Alzheimer's disease. Once present, from the very beginning of the disease process, PrP^{Sc} promotes its own generation from PrP^C. The molecular details of this process remain to be elucidated. It has been speculated that the two forms are in a highly asymmetrical equilibrium with each other and that the rarely formed PrP^{Sc} acts as seed for nucleation of the aggregates that shift the equilibrium toward PrP^{Sc}. An alternative hypothesis predicts that PrP^{Sc} acts as an autocatalyst for the conversion of PrP^C to PrP^{Sc}, which then accumulates in the aggregates. Prion disease can occur spontaneously by stochastic conversion, in sporadic CJD (Fig. 12.3). In several forms of familial CJD, the conversion is facilitated by mutations of PrP^C. In acquired CJD, PrP^{Sc} serves as infectious agent that propagates the conversion. Kuru, the now largely extinct disease in parts of New Guinea, was transmitted by cannibalistic practices. Acquired CJD

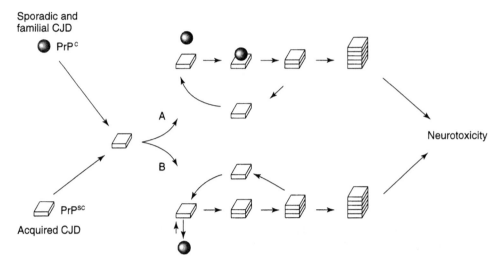

Figure 12.3   Mechanisms of prion diseases. The protease-resistant version of the prion protein (PrP^{Sc}) appears in the brain following inoculation or by spontaneous generation from the native form (PrP^{C}). In the brain, PrP^{Sc} promotes its own formation from PrP^{C}. PrP^{Sc} may act as an autocatalyst (**A**), or the two forms may be in equilibrium with the rare PrP^{Sc} acting as seed for nucleation of aggregates (**B**). The increasing quantities of PrP^{Sc} cause dysfunction and death of neurons.

is able to jump from species to species among mammals with a delay in the appearance of symptoms. Bovine spongiform encephalitis (mad cow disease) is believed to have originated from sheep offal feeding to cows in agriculture, and the newly described form of variant CJD in humans from exposure of humans to infected beef. Very strong evidence supports the view that the infection agent in acquired CJD is exclusively composed of prion (protein only) protein and does not include any viral or other nucleic acids.

12.3.2 Approaches to Drug Discovery

The knowledge of disease mechanisms and the related conjectures offer several appealing prospects for pharmacological interference. Preventing the conversion of PrP^{C} to PrP^{Sc} is achieved with several types of compounds in cell culture assays. Congo red, a compound used for the staining of amyloid aggregates, amphotericin B, an anti-fungal drug, quinacrine, an anti-malaria drug, and curcumin, an ingredient of the Indian spice turmeric, are effective in the culture screening assays (Caughey et al., 2003). While beneficial in culture, quinacrine failed to prevent the progression of the disease in mice carrying acquired CJD, and was toxic to the liver in human trials (Scoazec et al., 2003), pointing to the limited predictive power of the cell culture screening assays. In absence of precise understanding of the biophysical mechanisms controlling the prion protein conversion, it is difficult to assess the significance of the cell culture models for the disease process in the brain. The combination of cell culture screening with testing on animals carrying CJD provides a more powerful approach. Quinoline derivatives have been identified that work in cell cultures, delay the disease progression in CJD mice, and may be safe enough for human trials (Murakami-Kubo et al., 2004).

Intracerebral transfer of tissue extracts or fragments containing PrP^{Sc} is the most effective way for the transmission of acquired CJD. However, acquisition of CJD through transfer to peripheral organs has been documented in animals. Following systemic injection, PrP^{Sc} is transported to lymphoid organs where it promotes the further conversion of PrP^C to PrP^{Sc}. High levels of PrP^{Sc} are detected in the spleen and skeletal muscle. From the lymphoid tissues, PrP^{Sc} spreads to the peripheral nerves and gradually enters the central nervous system to cause the typical CJD progression. The peripheral tissues provide an opportunity for molecular diagnosis of CJD. Early detection of the disease, before the spreading to the brain, may make it possible to attack PrP^{Sc} with biologics unable to cross the blood-brain barrier. Passive immunization with anti-PrP antibodies slows down the progression of PrP^{Sc} formation of mice carrying the disease in peripheral organs (White et al., 2003). Active immunization of humans at risk might prevent the earliest events in the pathological cascade. Theoretically it should be possible to generate an immune response specifically to PrP^{Sc} given the suspected conformational differences to PrP^C. Such antibodies are expected to provide efficacious and safe prevention of systemic CJD transmission.

The behavioral deterioration and death in CJD are caused by the destructive events in the brain. The molecular mechanisms of the neuronal degeneration appear to be complex and await full characterization. PrP^C is necessary for the toxicity of PrP^{Sc}, since transplanted brain tissue of PrP^C knockout mice to wild-type mice carrying CJD remains viable despite the degeneration of the surrounding host tissue (Brandner et al., 1996). Flupirtine, a functional antagonist of NMDA glutamate receptor with unknown receptor site, prevents the destructive effects of PrP^{Sc} on neurons in culture, suggesting the possibility of an excitotoxic contribution to cell death in CJD. Encouraging results with flupirtine have been obtained in exploratory trials with CJD patients in which the cognitive decline was used as endpoint (Otto et al., 2004). Studies on the mechanisms of neural toxicity in CJD will hopefully identify appropriate targets for rational drug discovery.

Several mammalian species succumb to acquired CJD following intracerebral inoculation. They provide adequate models for the disease process and the testing of drug candidates. The ability to modify the disease process with genetic manipulations has made the mouse the preferred species. Inherited forms of CJD have been successfully reproduced in mice by expression of human Pr^P disease genes (Harris et al., 2003). Given the severity and rapid progression of human CJD, it will be possible to conduct decisive clinical trials with the emerging drug candidates.

CJD and the related prion diseases present a scientifically fascinating and medically relevant field for drug discovery. Fears for large human epidemics have not materialized and the patient number remains very low when compared to other nervous system diseases, making it difficult to obtain the economic support for directed drug discovery efforts. However, the availability of highly relevant animal models makes it possible to rapidly test many compounds approved for human use in other indications, thus avoiding the costs of a dedicated medicinal chemistry program. Alternative, antibody-based approaches might provide a further economically justifiable alternative. Hopefully the scientific uniqueness of prion diseases and their devastating nature will sustain the ongoing efforts.

12.4 AMYOTROPHIC LATERAL SCLEROSIS (ALS)

ALS, also known as Lou Gehrig's disease, is a devastating and rapidly progressive degenerative illness of the primary motor neurons that control the skeletal muscles (Rowland and Shneider, 2001). Lou Gehrig was a professional baseball player who succumbed to ALS, which transformed him within a few years from a successful athlete to a paralyzed

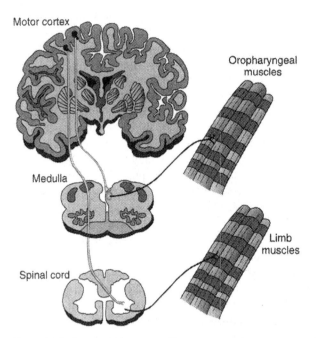

Figure 12.4   Degeneration upper and lower motor neurons cause muscle atrophy and other neurological deficits in ALS. (Reprinted with permission, Rowland and Schneider, 2001)

and disabled person. The name of the disease articulates the two principal pathological events. "Amyotrophic" refers to the atrophy and weakening of the skeletal muscles. "Lateral sclerosis" depicts the hardening of the lateral columns of the spinal cord, a consequence of motor axon degeneration and the resulting gliosis. Both the upper, corticospinal and the lower, spino-muscular motor neurons degenerate in ALS (Fig. 12.4). The loss of the upper motor neurons causes spasticity, hyperreflexia, and the degeneration of the lower motor neurons explains the muscular atrophy. Patients typically progress within five years from first diagnosis to death by respiratory failure. The worldwide prevalence of ALS is approximately 0.005% of the general population. Related to ALS are several forms of rare, typically hereditary, spinal muscular atrophies in which only the lower motor neurons degenerate.

12.4.1 Superoxide Dismutase and Neurofilament Aggregation

Environmental influences are at least contributing factors to ALS, since the disease has been linked to the exposure to food sources and the participation in specific military activities. Approximately 10% of the cases are caused by inherited mutations, 20% of which localized to the gene encoding Cu/Zn superoxide dismutase (SOD). While different mutations cause individual modifications of the standard ALS disease pattern, all familial forms of SOD share the selective motor neuron degeneration and the other pathological features of ALS. The pathology is not caused by the lack of SOD activity, since mice with null mutations of the SOD gene do not show motor neuron degeneration, whereas mice expressing a human SOD disease gene on top of a wild-type mouse genetic background succumb to a murine form of ALS with very similar progressive course as the human disease. The mutations may cause SOD, which normally catalyzes the conversion of superoxide radicals to hydrogen peroxide and oxygen, to generate alternative oxidative species. SOD contains a Cu^{2+} ion at the catalytic site, raising the possibility that diminished binding of this ion may release it for toxic actions on various cell constituents. Detailed understanding of the functions of mutated SOD will be necessary to define the most promising drug discovery strategies (Valentine and Hart, 2003). So far simple antioxidant approaches with vitamin E therapy have failed to show significant effects in the treatment of sporadic ALS (Desnuelle et al., 2001).

Motor neurons of ALS patients and of transgenic mice with SOD disease genes contain aggregated neurofilaments in cell bodies and axons. The neurofilament proteins may have been altered by the products of dysfunctional SOD or by the Cu^{2+} ions released from the mutated enzyme. The motor neuron degeneration of ALS may be a consequence of the various disturbances of cellular functions imposed by the aggregates. Parallel to the situation in Alzheimer's disease, it thus seems reasonable to hypothesize that compounds preventing the neurofilament aggregations will be beneficial for the treatment of ALS. Probably as a consequence of the aggregate formation, heat shock proteins are upregulated in motor neurons of patients and the mutant mice, suggesting the activation of chaperone functions. The disease progression of mutant SOD mice is influenced by genetic manipulations of neurofilament gene expression (Couillard-Despres et al., 1998). Arimoclomol, a compound able to induce heat shock proteins, prolongs the survival of SOD mutant mice (Kieran et al., 2004). These tentative results identify an intriguing approach to drug discovery, which seems justified for a rapidly progressing fatal diseases, despite the many adverse effects anticipated from alterations of chaperone functions that are of general importance for cellular mechanism.

12.4.2 Riluzole and Excitotoxic Neurodegeneration

Circumstantial data point to excitotoxic processes in ALS pathology. Glutamate levels were increased in some ALS patients and riluzole, the only approved and marginally effective drug for the treatment of ALS, inhibits glutamate release at high doses by an unknown mechanism of action. A defect in RNA editing for the GluR2 subunit of the AMPA receptors has been detected in sporadic ALS patients (Kawahara et al., 2004). Selective antagonists of glutamate receptors involved in excitotoxicity may thus have therapeutic utility in ALS, though earlier experiences with nonselective glutamate receptor inhibitors failed to generate supportive clinical data.

As for other neurodegenerative diseases, neurotrophic factors may be able to delay or prevent the atrophy and death of the vulnerable neuronal populations. Motor neurons express receptors for several growth factors. IGF-1, BDNF, and neurotrophin-3 are beneficial in animal models of motor neuron diseases. BNDF and IGF-1 were evaluated in extensive clinical studies and failed to show robust clinical benefits. The negative outcome of these decisive clinical studies strongly diminishes the enthusiasm for related drug discovery approaches, despite more recent data suggesting that improved delivery methods might result in more robust clinical effects (Kaspar et al., 2003).

12.4.3 Animal Models and Clinical Development

The familial form of ALS caused by SOD mutations has been accurately reproduced in transgenic mice. The progression of neurological deficits in the mouse reproduces those of the human disease in a compressed time frame. They are widely used for the testing of drug candidates for ALS. Examples of compounds that improve neurological symptoms and prolong the life span of the mice but fail in clinical trials illustrate the limitation of this animal model (Groeneveld et al., 2003). Several mouse strains with altered neurofilament gene expression exhibit aggregates and motor neuron degeneration, and may represent an alternative model for ALS. Before the availability of the transgenic technologies, several mouse strains with inherited forms of motor neuron degeneration were used for drug discovery. Positive results with growth factors supported clinical trials with negative outcomes, illustrating their limited utility. Better understanding of the ALS disease mechanisms is expected to generate gradually improved transgenic mouse models (Price et al., 1994).

The rapid progression and severity of ALS makes it possible to execute decisive clinical trials with relatively small numbers of patients. The devastating nature of the disease and the discovery of disease genes maintain the enthusiasm of the drug discovery community for this field, despite the setbacks with antioxidant and growth factor therapies.

12.5   PERIPHERAL NEUROPATHIES

The neuropathies of the peripheral nervous system affect a large number of people and represent a major unmet medical need. Approximately 30% of the diabetes patients, or 1% of the general population gradually develop degenerative changes of the peripheral nerves. They experience numbness and various aspects of paresthesia, abnormal sensations of the skin such as tingling, tickling, itching, and burning. Painful sensations, sometimes severe, may accompany the altered sensations. Sensory neuropathy is typically dominant, but in many patients autonomic neuropathic changes impair cardiovascular and visceral functions, leading to hypotension, as well as problems with digestive, urinary, and sexual functions. The neuropathy is a significant contributor to the reduced quality of life of elderly diabetes patients. The behavioral sensations reflect degenerative changes of the peripheral nerves including demyelination and dieing back of the terminal ramifications. At the electrophysiological level the morphological changes manifest themselves as reduced conduction velocity.

There are many forms of hereditary peripheral neuropathy, for which the umbrella term Charcot-Marie-Tooth disease is typically used. The prevalence of this disease has been estimated at approximately 0.05% of the general population. Fourteen genes with several hundred individual mutations have been identified as causes for various forms of this condition (Young and Suter, 2003). They include dominant and recessive mutations in genes coding for proteins linked to myelin sheath functions or to axonal functions of the neurons. Common to all diseases are progressive demyelination and axonal atrophy, but every mutation causes a distinct pathological picture and behavioral form of neuropathy. Among the primary demyelinating forms are those caused by mutations of important components of myelin, the peripheral myelinating protein 22 and the P0 myelin protein. Thinning and loss of myelin sheath causes nerve conduction aberrations as those described for multiple sclerosis in the central nervous system. Among the axonal forms of Charcot-Marie-Tooth disease are mutations in kinesin1B, a protein with an essential role in axonal transport, and the neurofilament light chain, an important structural component of the neuronal cytoskeleton. The neurons with the longest axons are first to succumb to the degenerative processes, explaining why the diseases tend to manifest themselves initially in the distal parts of the limbs.

Drug-induced neuropathies frequently occur as a disturbing adverse effect in cancer chemotherapy (Verstappen et al., 2003). Cytostatic compounds such as paclitaxel and cisplatin interfere with axonal functions and cause the behavioral signs of neuropathy. Sensory abnormalities, those linked to proprioception and gait in particular, tend to dominate, but other sensory and motor functions may be affected too. Fortunately the symptoms typically disappear within a few months of discontinuation, but in many patients the neuropathy limits the duration and maximal dosing of the cancer therapy and thus reduces its efficacy.

12.5.1 Drug Discovery Approaches

Diabetic and drug-induced neuropathies will be prevented by effective treatment of the primary disease or removal of the causative agents. Drug discovery for diabetes focuses on improved correction of the deficits in insulin signaling and prevention of the detrimental consequences of hyperglycemia. Both aspects of the disease mechanisms contribute to the neuropathy (Sima, 2003). Many neurons, including the sensory neurons, express insulin receptors that mediate metabolic and trophic effects of the hormone. Hyperglycemia activates the polyol pathway, by which glucose is converted to sorbitol by aldose reductase and then to fructose by sorbitol dehydrogenase. The elevated levels of intracellular sorbitol and fructose interfere with phosphoinositol signaling and cause multiple metabolic dysfunctions. Increased glucose and fructose concentrations cause excessive conjugation to proteins and accelerate the formation of advanced glycation end products, which accumulate during normal aging in many organs. Drugs that successfully interfere with these metabolic processes are expected to prevent and treat diabetic neuropathy. Diabetes is a dominant medical condition. The discussion of the associated, broad and very intense drug discovery efforts is outside of the frame of this volume.

The various forms of Charcot-Marie-Tooth disease generate a tantalizing problem for drug discovery. In principle, it is possible to elucidate the disease mechanism of every subform and define an optimal interference point and drug receptor site. Future pharmacogenetic therapy would determine the genetic defect of each patient and then select the corresponding treatment that provides specific correction. Practically, it may take a long time to reach this ideal stage of targeted medicine, because most of the mutations affect structural proteins with dysfunctions difficult to correct with drugs and because the small number of patients with a specific mutation makes it tough to justify the always costly drug discovery efforts. Drug discovery thus continues to focus on the common features shared by all neuropathies. Several approaches, discussed in detail in Chapter 15, attempt to relieve the painful sensations that accompany many forms of neuropathy. Neurotrophic factors are pursued with the goal to strengthen the structural integrity of neurons and to improve their resistance to the disease process. Parallel to the drug discovery strategy for multiple sclerosis, it may be possible to stimulate remyelination of the denuded axons of the peripheral nerves.

Neurotrophic factor therapy is a conceptually alluring, general approach to neuropathy, since these growth factors enhance the expression of proteins necessary for signaling functions and regenerative growth (Anand, 2004). In cell culture and animal models they make neurons more resistant to toxins and manipulations that replicate disease processes. Despite substantial efforts over many years, no neurotrophic factor has shown convincing efficacy in decisive clinical trials as yet. NGF was pursued for painful diabetic neuropathy, since the pain-mediating sensory neurons express the corresponding TrkA receptor in adult animals and humans. Regardless of apparently robust effects in animal models of diabetic neuropathy and exploratory human studies, large-scale clinical trials failed to show significant efficacy. The human studies revealed that NGF robustly induces pain following subcutaneous injections and have pushed drug discovery to consider NGF as a mediator of pain, discussed in more detail in Chapter 15. It seems possible that the pain sensation has limited the tolerable dose of NGF to levels below those necessary for the neurotrophic effects. Separation of the receptor mechanisms mediating the neurotrophic from pain-related effects will be necessary to further explore the therapeutic potential of NGF in diabetic neuropathy (Apfel, 2002). The TrkC neurotrophin receptors that mediate the actions of neurotrophin-3 are predominantly expressed by sensory neurons innervating the muscle spindles and providing the brain with proprioceptive information. These neurons are particularly vulnerable to the cytostatic drugs of cancer therapy. Beneficial effects of neurotrophin-3 in an animal model of cisplatin neuropathy support pursuing this growth factor for human therapy (Gao et al., 1995). Most sensory neurons express receptors for members of the GDNF protein family, providing an alternative therapeutic approach to the neurotrophins. Positive findings have been obtained with several other growth factors, including IGF-1, that might improve neuropathy by direct actions on the neurons or by improving the underlying diabetic condition (Zhuang et al., 1997). All the neurotrophic proteins appear to share poor pharmacokinetic properties, making it necessary to introduce stabilizing modifications or find suitable mimetics.

12.5.2 Animal Models and Clinical Development

Two frequently used rat models of diabetes also exhibit neuropathy and serve for the testing of drug candidates to alleviate the neurological condition (Table 12.3). In the first model, diabetes is induced by injections of streptozotocin (STZ), a compound that destroys the insulin-secreting pancreatic β-cells. STZ, a potent alkylating agent, interferes with gene replication and expression in many organs (Bolzan and Bianchi, 2002). The treated animals are very ill with many health issues beyond the diabetes. The additional effects of STZ complicate the interpretation of drug candidate effects on the neuropathy. The second model is provided by the Zucker Diabetic Fatty rats, a strain with a loss of function mutation of the leptin receptor (Schmidt et al., 2003). Diabetes and diabetic neuropathy are secondary to the obesity, making these animals a very useful model for type 2 diabetes and its secondary problems. Neuropathies induced by cytostatic drugs are directly reproduced

Table 12.3   Animal models for peripheral neuropathies

Diabetic Neuropathy
Streptozotocin (STZ) treated rats
Zucker Diabetic Fatty rats

Drug-Induced Neuropathy
Paclitaxel treated rodents
Cisplatin treated rodents
Pyridoxine treated rodents

Charcot-Marie-Tooth Disease
Transgenic rodent models

in rodents to generate adequate models for drug-induced neuropathies. Paclitaxel and cis-platin induce pronounced sensory neuropathy. Pyridoxine, a natural vitamin, induces neuropathy at high doses, and provides a simple animal model of initial evaluations of drug candidates. Several forms of Charcot-Marie-Tooth disease have been replicated in transgenic animals and will enable the drug discovery researchers to evaluate compounds in almost ideal models (Tanaka and Hirokawa, 2002). Reductions in nerve conductance velocity, degenerative changes in the myelin sheath, and loss of axons are the parameters typically measured to quantify the neuropathy.

The experience with NGF illustrates the difficulties of clinical development for anti-neuropathy compounds. The slow development of neuropathies over months and years and the heterogeneity of the patient population mandate large and long trials. Routine clinical examinations of neuropathy focus on neuronal functions at the distal limbs, where regeneration is most difficult to achieve. Experimental medical research aims at defining functional and morphological surrogate markers, such as nerve terminal density in skin biopsies, to directly monitor the regeneration of nerve terminals into denervated skin areas. Validated surrogate markers will greatly facilitate the currently difficult trial design and execution. There is no effective therapy for the treatment of neuropathy at this time. The field is wide open for innovative drug discovery research.

12.6 CONCLUSIONS

Multiple sclerosis, Huntington's disease, ALS, CJD, and the related diseases typically receive limited attention in drug discovery because their prevalence is lower than that of the dominant neurological diseases. Peripheral neuropathies are given secondary consideration in the framework of pain or diabetic disorders. The human suffering inflicted by them, however, mandates dedicated drug discovery efforts.

The causes of multiple sclerosis are poorly understood, but the progressive demyelination clearly involves autoimmune mechanisms against components of the myelin sheath. Current drugs suppress the immune response or prevent the migration of immune cells into the brain. Drug discovery efforts explore chemokines, cytokines, neuropeptides, and enzymes that are upregulated in areas of demyelination in the brain. Stimulation of the remyelinating processes, and prevention of oligodendrocyte and axonal degeneration, are alternative strategies. Multiple sclerosis research relies heavily on animal models of experimental autoimmune encephalitis. Advanced utilization of surrogate markers facilitates the clinical trial design and execution.

Huntington's disease is caused by the expansion of a polyglutamine stretch in the protein Huntingtin, which mediates many aberrant protein–protein interactions and impairs normal cellular functions. Despite the very complex disease mechanisms it seems possible to identify interference points for drugs to correct several of the pathological interactions. Transgenic animals have been created that replicate the human disease and identify excitotoxicity and energy failure as approaches for drug discovery.

CJD and the related prion disease are very rare, but have attracted interest because of their scientific uniqueness and the fear of future epidemics. They are caused by alterations in the normal prion protein (PrP^C), which is transformed to the scrapie version, PrP^{Sc}, by spontaneous events that can be facilitated by mutations, or by the presence of PrP^{Sc} that promotes its own generation. Cell culture and animal models make it possible to test many drug candidates for efficacy. Antibodies against either form of PrP are pursued to prevent the propagation of PrP^{Sc} or its migration into the brain.

ALS, the degeneration of the cortico-spinal and spino-muscular motor neurons, has genetic and environmental causes. The best-studied genetic form, caused by a gain of function mutation of superoxide dismutase, has been reproduced in transgenic animal models that support drug discovery research for all of ALS. The animal studies point to excitotoxic processes as common events. The only approved, and marginally efficacious drug, riluzole, inhibits glutamate release by an unknown mechanism. As for other neurodegenerative diseases, neurotrophic factors may be able to delay or prevent the atrophy and death of the vulnerable neuronal populations.

Peripheral neuropathy is a common consequence of diabetes and a frequent adverse effect of cancer chemotherapy. Charcot-Marie-Tooth disease encompasses many forms of hereditary neuropathies caused by mutations in genes encoding glial and neuronal proteins. Drug discovery focuses on common disease pathways and explores strategies to induce remyelination and axonal regeneration.

The devastating nature of the diseases, the lack of efficacious drugs, and the highly intriguing disease mechanisms generate tantalizing fields of opportunity for drug discovery research.

REFERENCES

Further Reading

AGUZZI, A., and POLYMENIDOU, M. Mammalian prion biology: One century of evolving concepts. *Cell* 116: 313–327, 2004.

ANAND, P. Neurotrophic factors and their receptors in human sensory neuropathies. *Prog. Brain Res.* 146: 477–492, 2004.

COMPSTON, A., and COLES, A. Multiple sclerosis. *Lancet* 359: 1221–1231, 2002.

CUMMINGS, C.J., and ZOGHBI, H.Y. Trinucleotide repeats: mechanisms and pathophysiology. *Annu. Rev. Genomics Hum. Genet.* 1: 281–328, 2000.

DEARMON, S.J., and PRUSINER, S.B. Perspective on prion biology, prion disease pathogenesis, and pharmacologic approaches to treatment. *Clin. Lab. Med.* 23: 1–41, 2003.

LI, S.H., and LI, X.J. Huntingtin–protein interactions and the pathogenesis of Huntington's disease. *Trends Genet.* 20: 146–154, 2004.

MENALLED, L.B., and Chesselet, M.F. Mouse models of Huntington's disease. *Trends Pharmacol. Sci.* 23: 32–39, 2002.

ROWLAND, L.P., and SHNEIDER, N.A. Amyotrophic lateral sclerosis. *N. Eng. J. Med.* 344: 1688–1701, 2001.

SEAMONS, A., PERCHELLET, A., and GOVERMAN, J. Immune tolerance to myelin proteins. *Immunol. Res.* 28: 201–221, 2003.

SIMA, A.A.F. New insights into the metabolic and molecular basis for diabetic neuropathy. *Cell. Mol. Life Sci.* 60: 2445–2464, 2003.

TRAPP, B.D. Pathogenesis of multiple sclerosis: The eyes only see what the mind is prepared to comprehend. *An. Neurol.* 55: 495–497, 2004.

VONSATTEL, J.P., and DIFIGLIA, M. Huntington's disease. *J. Neuropathol. Exp. Neurol.* 57: 369–384, 1998.

YOUNG, P., and SUTER, U. The causes of Charcot-Marie-Tooth disease. *Cell. Mol. Life Sci.* 60: 2547–2560, 2003.

ZAMVIL, S.S., and STEINMAN, L. Diverse targets for intervention during inflammatory and neurodegenerative phases of multiple sclerosis. *Neuron* 38: 685–688, 2003.

Citations

APFEL, S.C. Nerve growth factor for the treatment of diabetic neuropathy: What went wrong, what went right, and what does the future hold? *Int. Rev. Neurobiol.* 50: 393–413, 2002.

BARNETT, M.H., and PRINEAS, J.W. Relapsing and remitting multiple sclerosis: pathology and the newly forming lesion. *An. Neurol.* 55: 458–468, 2004.

BOLZAN, A.D., and BIANCHI, M.S. Genotoxicity of streptozotocin. *Mutat. Res.* 512: 121–134, 2002.

BRANDNER, S., ISENMANN, S., RAEBER, A., FISCHER, M., SAILER, A., KOBAYASHI, Y., MARINO, S., WEISSMANN, C., and AGUZZI, A. Normal host prion necessary for scrapie-induced neurotoxicity. *Nature* 379: 339–343, 1996.

CAUGHEY, B., RAYMOND, L.D., RAYMOND, G.J., MAXSON, L., SILVEIRA, J., and BARON, G.S. Inhibition of protease-resistant prion protein accumulation in vitro by curcumin. *J. Virol.* 77: 5499–5502, 2003.

COULLIARD-DESPRES, S., ZHU, Q., WONG, P.C., PRICE, D.L., CLEVELAND, D.W., and JULIEN, J.P. Protective effect of neurofilament heavy gene overexpression in motor neuron disease induced by mutant superoxide dismutase. *Proc. Natl. Acad. Sci. USA* 95: 9626–9630, 1998.

DESNUELLE, C., DIB, M., GARREL, C., FAVIER, A., and the ALS riluzole-tocopherol Study Group. A double-blind, placebo-controlled randomized clinical trial of alpha-tocopherol (vitamin E) in the treatment of amyotrophic lateral sclerosis. *Amyotroph. Lateral. Scler. Other Motor Neuron Disord.* 2: 9–18, 2001.

FERRANTE, R.J., ANDREASSEN, O.A., DEDEOGLU, A., FERRANTE, K.L., JENKINS, B.G., HERSCH, S.M., and BEAL, M.F. Therapeutic effects of coenzyme Q10 and remacemide in transgenic mouse models of Huntington's disease. *J. Neurosci.* 22: 1592–1599, 2002.

FERRANTE, R.J., KUBILUS, J.K., LEE, J., RYU, H., BEESEN, A., ZUCKER, B., SMITH, K., KOWALL, N.W., RATAN, R.R., LUTHI-CARTER, R., and HERSCH, S.M. Histone deacetylase inhibition by sodium butyrate chemotherapy ameliorates the neurodegenerative phenotype in Huntington's disease mice. *J. Neurosci.* 23: 9418–9427, 2003.

GAO, W.Q., DYBDAL, N., SHINSKY, N., MURNANE, A., SCHMELZER, C., SIEGEL, M., KELLER, G., HEFTI, F., PHILLIPS, H.S., and WINSLOW, J.W. Neurotrophin-3 reverses experimental cisplatin-induced peripheral sensory neuropathy. *An. Neurol.* 38: 30–37, 1995.

GRATACOS, E., PEREZ-NAVARRO, E., TOLOSA, E., ARENAS, E., and ALBERCH, J. Neuroprotection of striatal neurons against kainate excitotoxicity by neurotrophins and GDNF family members. *J. Neurochem.* 78: 1287–1296, 2001.

GROENEVELD, G.J., VELDINK, J.H., VAN DER TWEEL, I., KALMIJN, S., BEIJER, C., DE VISSER, M., WOKKE, J.H., FRANSSEN, H., and VAN DEN BERG, L.H. A randomized sequential trial of creatinine in amyotrophic lateral sclerosis. *An. Neurol.* 53: 437–445, 2003.

HARRIS, D.A., CHIESA, R., DRISALDI, B., QUAGLIO, E., MIGHELI, A., PICCARDO, P., and GHETTI, B. A murine model of a familial prion disease. *Clin. Lab. Med.* 23: 175–186, 2003.

HICKEY, M.A., and CHESSELET, M.F. Apoptosis in Huntington's disease. *Prog. Neuropsychopharmacol. Biol. Psych.* 2: 255–265, 2003.

HOCKLY, E., RICHON, V.M., WOODMAN, B., SMITH, D.L., ZHOU, X., ROSA, E., SATHASIVAM, K., GHAZI-NOORI, S., MAHAL, A., LOWDEN, P.A., STEFFAN, J.S., MARSH, J.L., THOMPSON, L.M., LEWIS, C.M., MARKS, P.A., and BATES, G.P. Suberoylanilide hydroxamic acid, a histone deacetylase inhibitor, ameliorates motor deficits in a mouse model of Huntington's disease. *Proc. Natl. Acad. Sci. USA* 100: 2041–2046, 2003.

KALVYVAS, A., and DAVID, S. Cytosolic phospholipase A2 plays a key role in the pathogenesis of multiple sclerosis-like disease. *Neuron* 41: 323–335, 2204.

KASPAR, B.K., LLADO, J., SHERKAT, N., ROTHSTEIN, J.D., and GAGE, F.H. Retrograde viral delivery of IGF-1 pro-

longs survival in a mouse ALS model. *Science* 301: 839–842, 2003.

KAWAHARA, Y., ITO, K., SUN, H., AIZAWA, H., KANAZAWA, I., and KWAK, S. RNA editing and death of motor neurons. *Nature* 427: 801, 2004.

KIERAN, D., KALMAR, B., DICK, J.R.T., RIDDOCH-CONTRERAS, J., BURNSTOCK, G., and GREENSMITH, L. Treatment with arimoclomol, a coinducer of heat shock proteins, delays disease progression in ALS mice. *Nature Med.* 4: 402–405, 2004.

KOHAMA, I., LANKFORD, K.L., PREININGEROVA, J., WHITE, F.A., VOLLMER, T.L., and KOCSIS, J.D. Transplantation of cryopreserved adult human Schwann cells enhances axonal conduction in demyelinated spinal cord. *J. Neurosci.* 21: 944–950, 2001.

MILLER, D.H., KHAN, O.A., SHEREMATA, W.A., BLUMHARDT, L.D., RICE, G.P., LIBONATI, M.A., WILLMER-HULME, A.J., DALTON, C.M., MISKIEL, K.A., and O'CONNOR, P.W., and International Natalizumab Multiple Sclerosis Trial Group. A controlled trial of natalizumab for relapsing multiple sclerosis. *N. Eng. J. Med.* 348: 15–23, 2003.

MURAKAMI-KUBO, I., DOH-URA, K., ISHIKAWA, K., KAWATAKE, S., SASAKI, K., KIRA, J., OHTA, S., and IWAKI, T. Quinoline derivatives are therapeutic candidates for transmissible spongiform encephalopathies. *J. Virol.* 78: 1281–1288, 2004.

OTTO, M., CEPEK, L., RATZKA, P., DOEHLINGER, S., BOEKHOFF, I., WILTFANG, J., IRLE, E., PERGANDE, G., ELLERS-LENZ, B., WINDL, O., KRETSCHMAR, H.A., POSER, S., and PRANGE, H. Efficacy of flupirtine on cognitive function in patients with CJD: A double-blind study. *Neurology* 62: 714–718, 2004.

PAUL, C., and BOLTON, C. Modulation of blood-brain barrier dysfunction and neurological deficits during acute experimental allergic encephalomyelitis by the *N*-methyl-D-aspartate receptor antagonist memantine. *J. Pharmacol. Exp. Ther.* 302: 50–57, 2002.

PRICE, D.L., CLEVELAND, D.W., and KOLIATSOS, V.E. Motor neurone disease and animal models. *Neurobiol. Disord.* 1: 3–11, 1994.

SCHMIDT, R.E., DORSEY, D.A., BEAUDET, L.N., and PETERSON, R.G. Analysis of the Zucker Diabetic Fatty (ZDF) type 2 diabetic rat model suggests a neurotrophic role for insulin/IGF-I in diabetic autonomic neuropathy. *Am. J. Pathol.* 163: 21–28, 2003.

SPIRES, T.L., GROTE, H.E., VARSHNEY, N.K., CORDERY, P.M., VAN DELLEN, A., BLAKEMORE, C., and HANNAN, A.J. Environmental enrichment rescues protein deficits in a mouse model of Huntington's disease, indicating a possible disease mechanism. *J. Neurochem.* 24: 2270–2276, 2004.

STEINMAN, L., and ZAMVIL, S. Transcriptional analysis of targets in multiple sclerosis. *Nature Rev. Immunol.* 3: 483–492, 2003.

TANAKA, Y., and HIROKAWA, N. Mouse models of Charcot-Marie-Tooth disease. *Trends Genet.* 18: 39–44, 2002.

THAKUR, A.K., YANG, W., and WETZEL, R. Inhibition of polyglutamine aggregate toxicity by a structure-based elongation inhibitor. *FASEB J.* 18: 923–925, 2004.

TOULMOND, S., TANG, K., BUREAU, Y., ASHDOWN, H., DEGEN, S., O'DONNELL, R., TAM, J., HAN, Y., COLUCCI, J., GIROUX, A., ZHU, Y., BOUCHER, M., PIKOUNIS, B., XANTHOUDAKIS, S., ROY, S., RIGBY, M., ZAMBONI, R., ROBERTSON, G.S., NG, G.Y.K., NICHOLSON, D.W., and FLÜCKIGER, J.P. Neuroprotective effects of M826, a reversible caspase-3 inhibitor, in the rat malonate model of Huntington's disease. *Br. J. Pharmacol.* 141: 689–697, 2004.

VALENTINE, J.S., and HART, P.J. Misfolded CuZnSOD and amyotrophic lateral sclerosis. *Proc. Natl. Acad. Sci. USA.* 100: 3617–3622, 2003.

VERBESSEM, P., LEMIERE, J., EIJNDE, B.O., SWINNEN, S., VANHEES, L., VAN LEEMPUTTE, M., HESPEL, P., and DOM R. Creatine supplementation in Huntington's disease: A placebo-controlled pilot trial. *Neurology* 61: 925–930, 2003.

VERSTAPPEN, C.C.P., HEIMANS, J.J., HOEKMAN, K., and POSTMA, T.J. Neurotoxic complications of chemotherapy in patients with cancer: Clinical signs and optimal management. *Drugs* 63: 1549–1563, 2003.

WEINER, J.A., HECHT, J.H., and CHUN, J. Lysophosphatidic acid receptor gene vzg-1/lpA1/edg-2 is expressed by mature oligodendrocytes during myelination in the postnatal murine brain. *J. Comp. Neurol.* 398: 587–598, 1998.

WHITE, A.R., ENEVER, P., TAYEBI, M., MUSHENS, R., LINEHAN, J., BRANDNER, S., ANSTEE, D., COLLINGE, J., and HAWKE, S. Monoclonal antibodies inhibit prion replication and delay the development of prion disease. *Nature* 422: 80–83, 2003.

WILSON, H.C., ONISCHKE, C., and RAINE, C.S. Human oligodendrocyte precursor cells in vitro: Phenotypic analysis and differential response to growth factors. *Glia* 44: 153–165, 2003.

ZHUANG, H.X., WUARIN, L., FEI, Z.J., and ISHII, D.N. Insulin-like growth factor (IGF) gene expression is reduced in neural tissues and liver from rats with non-insulin-dependent diabetes mellitus, and IGF treatment ameliorates diabetic neuropathy. *J. Pharmacol. Exp. Ther.* 283: 366–374, 1997.

Chapter 13

Sleep Disorders

Our lives have a daily rhythmic that evolved in synchrony with the rotation of the planet on which we live. The resting phase, sleep, is a fundamental and important component of human life. Poetic descriptions from the world literature more elegantly convey the essential aspects of sleep and dreams than the dry words of scientific language:

> *Now, blessing light on him who first invented this same sleep! It covers a man all over, thoughts and all, like a cloak; it is food for the hungry, drink for the thirsty, heat for the cold, and cold for the hot. It is the current coin that purchases all the pleasures of the world cheap; and the balance that sets the king and the shepherd, the fool and the wise man, even. There is only one thing which somebody put into my head, that I dislike in sleep; it is, that it resembles death; there is very little difference between a man in his first sleep, and a man in his last sleep.*

Miguel de Cervantes, Don Quixote

> *Sleep has its own world,*
> *A boundary between the things misnamed*
> *Death and existence:*
> *Sleep has its own world,*
> *And a wide realm of wild reality,*
> *And dreams in their development have breath,*
> *And tears and tortures, and the touch of joy.*

George Byron, The Dream

Disorders of sleep are very common. Because of the vital importance of sleep, they influence many aspects of human behavior and function. Insufficient sleep causes tiredness and reduced performance, and elevates the risk for accidents. Chronically disturbed sleep is a risk factor for depression and alcoholism. Frequent travelers and shift workers experience jet-lag and change in circadian rhythms that cause acute and, if sustained over years, chronic insomnia. Sleep disturbance can be caused by obstructions in the airways and respiratory diseases, or by a condition called restless leg syndrome, which generates an urge to move the limbs. Effective and useful drugs are available to treat insomnia in most of these conditions. Among them, the benzodiazepine drugs that activate the GABA-A receptors are the most effective ones and are generally safe when used over brief periods of time. Other drugs that are available without prescription are widely used but much less efficacious. Current drug discovery research aims for highly effective and safe drugs that can be used over long periods of time and for drugs that quickly adjust circadian rhythms for intercontinental travelers.

Drug Discovery for Nervous System Diseases, by Franz F. Hefti
ISBN 0-471-46563-1   Copyright © 2005 by John Wiley & Sons, Inc.

Modern sleep research has little room for dreams and their interpretation. Freudian concepts, that dreams provide a window to brain processes outside of the conscious sphere, are seen as a late manifestation of human speculative thinking before the advent of modern neurobiology. Nevertheless, sleep disorders include conditions characterized by vivid and violent dreams, nightmares, with entirely unclear disease mechanisms. Dreams are comparable to hallucinations experienced by schizophrenics, adding support to the view that mechanisms of dream generation and content are medically relevant. They are the subject of interest and fascination for drug discovery research as well, since they may lead to drugs that improve the subjective perception of sleep quality.

13.1 SLEEP MECHANISMS AND SLEEP DISORDERS

Sleep is a well-defined condition with distinct physiological and behavioral aspects. Voluntary movement and consciousness are absent, but the essential involuntary functions such as respiration, cardiovascular activity, and digestion proceed. The sensation but not the perception of sensory stimuli is unaltered, and intense sensory stimuli trigger awakening. The remaining nervous system control over the motor system is responsible for involuntary movement during sleep. Behavioral and electrophysiological observations distinguish normal sleep from rapid eye movement (REM) sleep. During normal sleep, muscle tone is reduced but not absent, and there are episodes of involuntary movement and change of body posture. Electrophysiological recordings from the scalp (electroencephalography, EEG) show regular waves of high amplitude, whereas the wake state is characterized by low-amplitude irregular EEG activity. Normal sleep is further subdivided into four stages that reflect the magnitude of the changes from the wake state to deep sleep. Stages 3 and 4, the stages of deep sleep, typically occur after several hours of sleep only, and are common during the early morning hours for people who maintain regular daily sleep patterns. REM sleep phases interrupt normal sleep. During REM sleep, EEG readings are more similar to those during the wake state than during sleep. Eyes move rapidly, explaining the term REM. Dreams are common during this phase. The body is completely immobilized, though we might imagine that we move. Figure 13.1 illustrates the sleep phases.

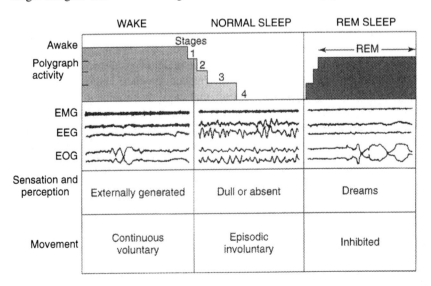

Figure 13.1 Sleep and sleep phases. EMG: electromyogram; EEG: electroencephalogram; EOG: electrooculogram. (Adapted from Hobson and Steriade, 1986)

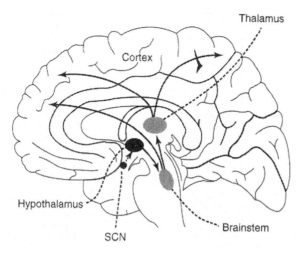

Figure 13.2 Sleep circuits. Neurons in the reticular formation of the brain stem integrate the input from the hypothalamus, which provides information on tiredness, and from the circadian clock of the suprachiasmatic nucleus (SCN). It transmits the regulatory signals for normal sleep and REM sleep to the thalamus where the rhythmic activity patterns typical for sleep are generated. (Reprinted with permission, Mignot et al., 2002)

Many molecular and cellular components of sleep regulation have been discovered, and sufficient information is available to depict a schematic diagram of sleep regulation (Fig. 13.2). Onset, duration, and quality of sleep are determined by tiredness and circadian rhythms. The physiological consequences of tiredness regulate activity patterns of hypothalamic neuronal systems. The brain contains an internal circadian clock, located in the suprachiasmatic nucleus, which is set by the influence of light onto the retina. The hypothalamic systems and the neurons of the suprachiasmatic nucleus project to brainstem areas that integrate the two types of information. The neuronal pathways connecting the suprachiasmatic and hypothalamic neurons to brainstem nuclei are complex and involve many neuropeptide, monoamine, and amino acid transmitters. The brainstem centers project to thalamus and cortex and regulate the activity of the ascending cortical arousal pathways. They initiate the electrophysiological synchronization that characterizes normal sleep as well as the switch from normal to REM sleep.

The suprachiasmatic nucleus is a small structure located at the base of the forebrain, immediately above the chiasm of the optic nerves. The neurons in this nucleus contain a biomolecular oscillator, a biological clock able to measure time and to serve as circadian pacemaker for the brain. The molecular components and mechanism of this clock have been elucidated during recent years with the help of very elegant genetic and molecular biological studies in transgenic flies and mice. Figure 13.3 illustrates the essential aspects of the molecular clock, and its nature as a transcriptional oscillator (Reppert and Weaver, 2002). At the center are several clock genes, *Per*, *Cry*, *Clock*, *Bmal1*, that are expressed in rhythmic circadian patterns. In the nucleus, the transcriptional regulators CLOCK and BMAL1 form heterodimers that activate the transcription of several *Per* and *Cry* genes. Increasing levels of PER and CRY proteins in the cytoplasm cause the phosphorylation of PER by casein kinase1ε and the formation of PER-CRY complexes that translocate back to the nucleus. The PER-CRY complexes prevent the action of CLOCK-BMAL1 dimers and thus turn off their own synthesis. A further nuclear protein, REV-ERBα, is under control of CLOCK-BMAL1 and PER-CRY dimers, and inhibits BMAL1 synthesis. The

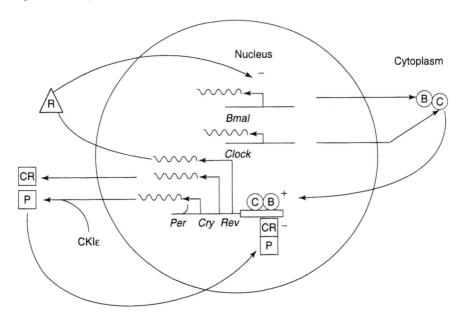

Figure 13.3   Circadian pacemaker of the suprachiasmatic nucleus. The transcriptional regulators CLOCK (C) and BMAL1 (B) form heterodimers that activate the synthesis of PER (P) and CRY (CR). PER is phosphorylated by casein kinase1ε (CK1ε) and forms PER-CRY complexes that translocate back to the nucleus. PER-CRY prevents the action of CLOCK-BMAL1 dimers and turn off their own synthesis. A further protein, REV-ERBα (R), under control of CLOCK-BMAL1 and PER-CRY dimers, inhibits BMAL1 synthesis. The decline of this inhibition restarts the BMAL1 and the cycle. (Adapted from Reppert and Weaver, 2002)

decline of this inhibition restarts the BMAL1 synthesis and the cycle. Knockout mice with null mutations of the major clock genes show pronounced deficits in circadian rhythmic, supporting the view that they are the major components of the molecular clock. However, many detailed aspect remain to be elucidated. The existence of several different *Per* and *Cry* genes and of additional minor players complicate the precise understanding of the transcriptional oscillator.

The circadian pacemaker of the suprachiasmatic neurons maintains an approximately 24 hour rhythm in absence of external input. Without the daily resetting, the transcriptional oscillator drifts and imposes a rhythm out of synchrony with the daily light–dark cycles. Light input to the eye adjusts the rhythm daily. Photosensitive pigments other than those of the rods and cones, and including melanopsin proteins mediate the information to the suprachiasmatic neurons. Neurons containing melanopsin and using glutamate and the pituitary adenylate cyclase-activating polypeptide (PACAP) as transmitters innervate the suprachiasmatic nucleus and form a unique visual pathway that relates information on the duration and quantity of light reaching the retina (Hannibal, 2002). Various efferent pathways from the suprachiasmatic nucleus pass on the information of the circadian clock to the brainstem and other brain areas. Many of these pathways use the neuropeptide prokineticin-2 as transmitter (Cheng et al., 2002). It is not clear whether the suprachiasmatic nucleus is the only structure with an essential pacemaker or whether other brain areas can serve similar roles. Many cells types contain the necessary genes, but lesion studies support the essential role of the suprachiasmatic nucleus. Animals with lesions of this brain structure have similar behavioral deficits as knockout mice lacking the essential clock genes.

The measurement of tiredness is less well understood than the circadian clock. Sleep deprivation is the most powerful trigger for sleep. In absence of stimulatory drugs such as amphetamine, even the most strong-willed efforts cannot prevent a person from falling asleep after an approximately two-day wake period. Sleep deprivation causes multiple metabolic and hormonal changes. The homeostatic systems of the hypothalamus are believed to integrate the various inputs and to provide a measurement of wake time. It remains possible, though, that the brain contains an endogenous molecular or cellular clock that is able to measure the time spent awake and asleep over longer periods of time. The hypothalamic systems known to participate in the regulation of sleep include sleep-promoting GABAergic and galanin-containing neurons and wake-promoting neurons using the peptide orexin as transmitter. These systems project to the various nuclei in the brain stem that initiate and regulate sleep, including the arousal systems of the reticular formation of the pons and the ascending monoaminergic regulatory systems (Mignot et al., 2002).

13.1.1 Insomnia

It has been estimated that more than 10% of the general population experience insomnia, the inability to fall asleep or to sleep for sufficient periods of time. The condition represents a significant medical and societal problem, since it reduces performance and is an important risk factor for many chronic metabolic diseases, depression, and interpersonal relationship problems. Disruption of the daily rhythm causes insomnia by desynchronizing the circadian pacemaker of the suprachiasmatic nucleus from the desired sleep cycle. The transcriptional pacemaker adjusts by approximately one hour per day, and is thus unable to follow the rapid and wide fluctuations imposed by intercontinental travel and shift-working. Insomnia is a common consequence of respiratory disturbances that cause frequent interruptions of sleep. However, many people suffer from reoccurring insomnia in absence of obvious causes or understanding of the disease mechanisms.

Current therapy attempts to correct the behavioral reasons of insomnia when they are known. Many patients respond well to behavioral therapy that reduces the numbers of hours available for sleep and the creation of a facilitating environment during this time interval. Drug therapy relies on benzodiazepine-type GABA-A receptor agonists that are highly effective in inducing and maintaining sleep. Some of the monoamine uptake blocker anti-depressants and other mildly sedative drugs provide frequently used alternatives to treat insomnia. While effective and therapeutically very useful, the existing drugs induce sleep by causing general sedation. They have mild adverse effects and the sleep induced by them is not identical to natural sleep. There is ample room for improvement toward drugs that directly and selectively influence the neuronal pathways controlling sleep.

13.1.2 Hypersomnia and Parasomnias

A relatively small number of people suffer from excessive sleeping. The condition is often a consequence of neurological or metabolic diseases, such as epilepsy and hypothyroidism, and is ameliorated with the treatment of the primary illness. **Narcolepsy** is a rare hypersomnia characterized by sudden attacks of sleep and loss of muscle tone during the day. Genetic studies identified the orexin neurotransmitter system as a principal determinant of narcolepsy in animals (Siegel, 2004). Amphetamine and related stimulatory drugs provide help to patients suffering from hypersomnias. Among them is modafinil, a drug recently approved for the treatment of narcolepsy.

Parasomnias include a number of conditions of abnormal sleep. Most frequent among them is the **restless leg syndrome** that disturbs regular sleep in more than 2% of the population and the elderly in particular. Patients feel a strong urge to move legs and sometimes arms when trying to sleep. Some patients experience muscular jerks during sleep that awaken them. The condition responds to drugs used in Parkinson's disease or pain rather than the typical sleep-inducing drugs, suggesting that the disease mechanisms are related to sensory and motor system dysfunctions. Better understanding of the restless leg syndrome will help to direct drug discovery efforts toward this unpleasant condition that diminishes the quality of life of a significant fraction of the population.

Conditions of abnormal REM sleep and dreaming are included under parasomnias, among them somnambulism, nightmares, and night terrors. Somnambulism with active movement and other complex behaviors during sleep and in absence of consciousness often causes accidents. A small number of patients suffer from regularly reoccurring severe nightmares that may cause fear of sleeping and more general emotional problems. Recent theories on the function of REM sleep and dreams link them to memory processing and consolidation, implying widespread consequences of pathological conditions (Stickgold et al., 2001). Genetics and disease mechanisms of these rare conditions are enigmatic, and there is no effective drug therapy. These sleep disorders together with insomnia represent an important medical need and opportunity for future drug discovery efforts.

13.2 BENZODIAZEPINE RECEPTOR SITE GABA-A AGONISTS

The discovery of the most effective class of drugs for insomnia is closely linked to that of anxiolytic drugs discussed in Chapter 8. The early barbiturates were replaced by benzodiazepine drugs, both of which facilitate the function of the GABA-A receptor ion channels. They increase the influence of the dominant GABAergic inhibitory neuronal systems in the brain and thus induce, at increasing doses, sedation, sleep, and anesthesia. Benzodiazepine drugs that bind to an allosteric receptor site on the heteromeric GABA-A receptors have a much improved adverse effect profile over the barbiturates that cause fatal toxicity at high doses. Diazepam, the first drug of the benzodiazepine drug class, was followed by compounds with short half-lives, more suitable for the treatment of insomnia. A well-known example, triazolam (Halcion) has a time of onset of less than thirty minutes and a half-life of approximately three hours, making it most suitable for the induction of sleep (Fig. 13.4). While very useful, triazolam and similar drugs have undesired effects that include memory disturbances. Detailed studies of sleep EEG furthermore revealed distinct differences between benzodiazepine drug-induced and natural sleep. While sleep duration was the same, the sleep architecture, the distribution of sleep time to the various stages, differed between the two types of sleep.

More recently introduced benzodiazepine receptor ligands take advantage of the existence of several GABA-A receptor subtypes. As discussed in earlier chapters, the sedative actions of benzodiazepine drugs are predominantly mediated by receptors containing the $\alpha 1$ subunit. Knockout mice of the $\alpha 1$ gene have increased susceptibility for seizures supporting the conclusion that GABA-A$\alpha 1$ receptors are general regulators of neuronal excitability in the brain (Kralic et al., 2003). Compounds selectively binding to the benzodiazepine receptor site and facilitating the opening of the GABA-A$\alpha 1$ receptor subtype induce sedation and sleep as effectively as nonselective benzodiazepine receptor agonists. Zolpidem and zaleplon are the first two compounds of this class approved for the treat-

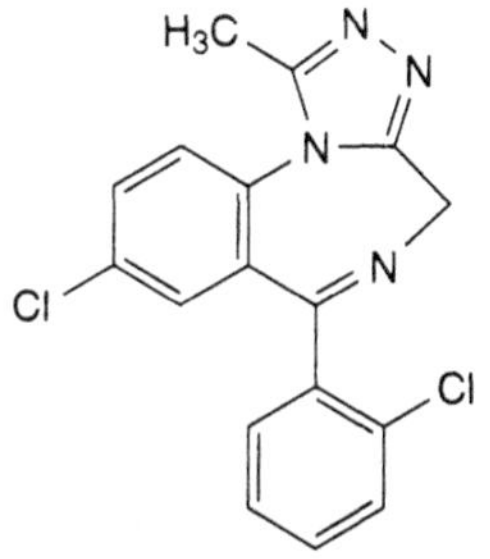

Triazolam

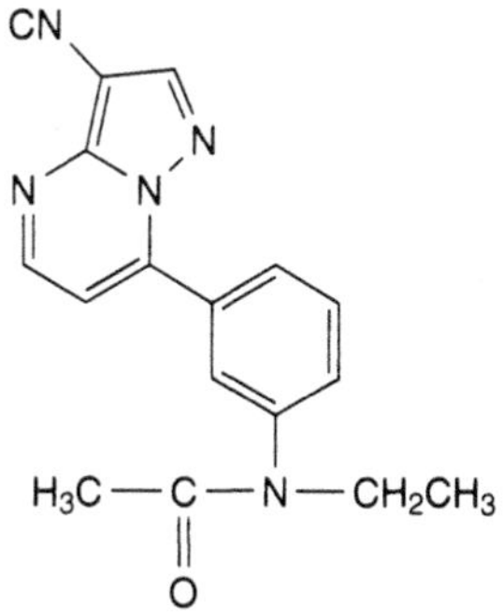

Zaleplon

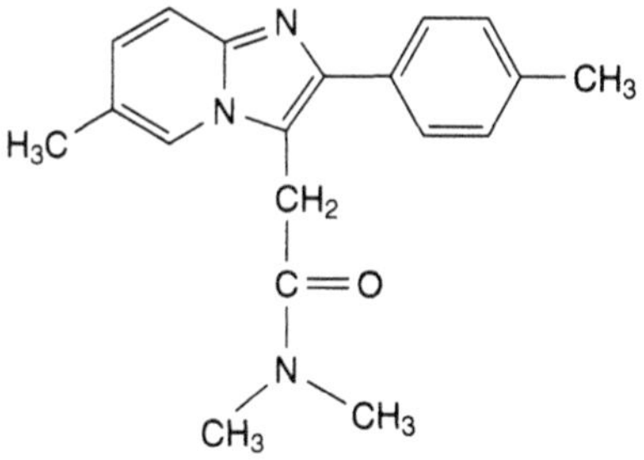

Zolpidem

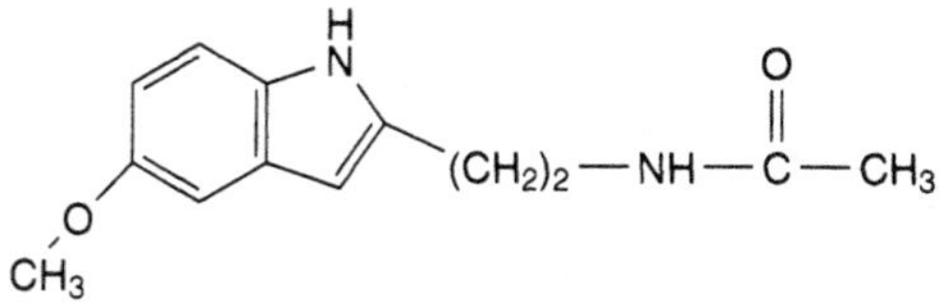

Melatonin

Figure 13.4   Examples of drugs used for the treatment of sleep disorders.

ment of insomnia. Their short half-lives and pharmacokinetic properties are ideal for this therapeutic use. Detailed clinical studies show that these drugs induce and maintain sleep with architecture indistinguishable from normal sleep. They do not seem to cause memory disturbances, nor do they have measurable addictive potential. The GABA-Aα1 benzodiazepine receptor agonists provide highly effective and safe therapy for the insomnia. They seem to be close to ideal drugs, making it difficult to imagine significant improvements that could be achieved with additional drug discovery efforts directed to this receptor group (Schenck et al., 2003). Nevertheless, yet further refinement of the subtype selectivity might bring modest improvements. It may be possible to identify GABA-A receptor subtypes that are selectively expressed by neurons of the sleep circuits in the hypothalamus and brain stem, and to discover GABA-A receptor agonists able to directly suppress activity in the ascending arousal systems.

13.3 ANTIDEPRESSANT DRUGS AND THE REGULATION OF REM SLEEP

Sleep disturbances and insomnia are a common aspect of depressive illness, and antidepressants improve sleep in parallel with the emotional status. Because of this relationship, antidepressant drugs have gradually found acceptance for the treatment of insomnia in absence of clinical trials focused on sleep disorders. Indeed, there is no convincing clinical evidence for a positive effect of antidepressants on insomnia in absence of depression. The various monoamine uptake blocker drugs are perceived as sedative or stimulatory by individual depressed patients with high patient-to-patient variability. SSRIs, the selective serotonin uptake blockers, reduce the percentage of sleep time spent in REM sleep. Contrary to expectations generated by this finding, many patients on antidepressants anecdotally report vivid, colorful dreams.

REM sleep is initiated by a distributed neuronal system in the reticular formation of the pons. Cholinergic input from the population of pedunculopontine neurons, a population with features distinct from the cholinergic neurons of the basal forebrain, facilitates the function of the neurons inducing REM sleep. Serotonergic input from the mesencephalic Raphe nuclei and noradrenergic input from the locus coeruleus inhibit REM sleep. The suppression of REM sleep by SSRIs provides human evidence for the role of the serotonergic neurons. The simple concept of a cholinergic—monoaminergic balance regulating REM sleep reflects the state of the art of neuropharmacology of several decades ago and is being revised by more recent investigations of sleep mechanisms (Pace-Schott and Hobson, 2002). The ongoing delineation of input pathways to the reticular formation and the discovery of transmitter systems with a selective association to sleep pathways are revealing putative drug targets to influence the regulation of REM sleep and sleep architecture. Sleep architecture is believed to be a major determinant of the subjective perception of sleep quality. Most people are able to express an opinion in the morning whether they slept well or poorly, and the perceived sleep quality is often independent of sleep duration. Drugs able to influence sleep architecture are likely to be useful for the treatment of the rare parasomnias, and they might have broader utility in the treatment of the common emotional disorders.

13.4 HISTAMINE RECEPTOR LIGANDS

Clinical observations and neurobiological investigations link histaminergic systems of the brain to sleep and insomnia. Histamine receptor antagonists are widely used for the treatment of allergies, gastric ulcers, and other widespread medical conditions. Early histamine H_1 receptor antagonists such as diphenylhydramine (Benadryl), developed for the treatment of allergy, made many patients drowsy, limiting their day-time use. A second-generation compound designed not to cross the blood-brain barrier retained the desired anti-allergy effect without associated sedation. Neuroanatomical and functional studies revealed the existence of ascending histaminergic projection systems in the brain that originate in the hypothalamus and reticular formation, areas involved in sleep control, and forming divergent projections to most cortical areas. Sleep patterns are altered in mutant mice with a deletion of histidine decarboxylase, the enzyme catalyzing the synthesis of histamine. Drug discovery efforts related to sleep have focused on the H_3 histamine receptor because of its selective expression in the brain. H_3 receptors are located presynaptically on synapses formed by monoaminergic neurons including the histaminergic neurons, where they serve as autoreceptors for histamine. H_3 receptor knockout mice show reduced behavioral activity, whereas pharmacological studies suggest a wake-promoting effect of pharmacological H_3 antagonism (Toyota et al., 2002). Despite these complex results the clinical validation of histamine receptors as drug target for sleep control will keep alive strong interest of drug discovery researchers in histamine mechanisms. It may be possible to selectively influence histaminergic neurons involved in sleep regulation with compounds regulating the synthesis, reuptake, or metabolism of this transmitter.

13.5 MELATONIN

Patient demand and choice rather than formal drug development and approval processes have made melatonin a frequently used over-the-counter drug for insomnia. Melatonin is a natural hormone that is synthesized in the pineal, the dorsal appendix of the diencephalon in the mammalian brain and the evolutionary descendant of a light-sensitive organ in early vertebrates (Fig. 13.5). Melatonin synthesis originates from tryptophan and the enzymatic steps leading to serotonin. Serotonin N-acetyltransferase and hydroxyindole-O-methyltransferase, two enzymes strongly expressed in pineal cells, then convert serotonin to melatonin (5-methoxy-N-acetyltryptamine). The synthesis and activity of both synthetic enzymes levels in the pineal show strong circadian rhythms. There is a sharp raise at the onset of the sleep period and a gradual decline to very low levels at the beginning of the wake period. The circadian rhythm is imposed on the pineal by the pacemaker cells in the suprachiasmatic nucleus and the sympathetic nervous system that relays the information to the pineal. Melatonin is released into the bloodstream and stimulates MT_1 and MT_2 G-protein-coupled receptors expressed in many tissues, including those of the vascular system. Melatonin receptors appear to participate in the regulation of body temperature during sleep. Increased blood flow in distal parts of the skin contributes to the reduction

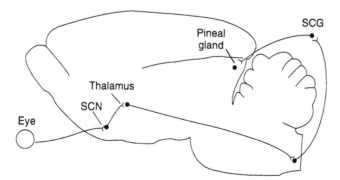

Figure 13.5 Melatonin mechanisms in the pineal. Information on the circadian rhythm from the suprachiasmatic nucleus (SCN) is mediated by the thalamus and sympathetic neurons originating in the upper spinal cord and projecting through the superior cervical ganglion (SCG).

of body temperature during sleep. In some mammalian species melatonin levels integrated over several days reflect the daylight duration and serve as a seasonal clock that determines mating behavior.

Several arguments support the conclusion that the pineal is not a major player in circadian rhythm control in the human brain but that it has retained marginal functions as leftovers of a more powerful role in early vertebrate evolution. Humans unable to synthesize melatonin live normal lives and sleep normally. Adding melatonin during times of peak synthesis and release, at the onset of the circadian sleep phase, has no effect on sleep quality or duration. However, controlled clinical studies have revealed small but statistically significant sleep-promoting effects when melatonin is given during the circadian wake phase (Cajochen et al., 2003). Endogenous melatonin may thus help to reduce jet-lag and the adjustment to a new circadian rhythm, when taken at the time sleep is desired in the new time zone. Melatonin may be useful for blind people who have no light perception and tend to have drifting circadian rhythms.

Somewhat fortuitously, the natural hormone melatonin has adequate pharmacokinetic properties to support oral use. Several companies have active research programs aiming at producing orally active, potent agonists to melatonin receptors, for the effective treatment of conditions where circadian rhythm adjustments are desired. It is not clear which of the two melatonin receptor is the most suitable drug target (von Gall et al., 2002). Melatonin receptor agonists may become particularly useful for the control of jet lag. The relatively narrow spectrum of melatonin actions will limit their effectiveness. Alternative approaches, discussed in the subsequent paragraph, directed at the circadian pacemaker itself, may possibly lead to more powerful drugs.

13.6 DRUGS TO RESET THE CIRCADIAN PACEMAKER

The scientific and clinical findings with melatonin generate optimism that it is possible to treat insomnia by drugs able to reset the circadian clock in the suprachiasmatic nucleus. Receptor sites on the components of the molecular oscillator would provide the most direct approach. Inhibitors or potentiators of the key transcriptional events triggered by the CLOCK-BMAL1 or PER-CRY heteromers would have equal chance to interrupt the existing cycle. However, brain-penetrant and selective transcriptional regulators with appropriate pharmacokinetic properties represent an enormously difficult task for drug discovery, prompting an intense search for more practical alternatives. It might be possible to identify molecules that selectively prevent the formation of the heterodimers. Casein kinase 1ε warrants further exploration, unless this enzyme participates in many other regulatory functions outside of the suprachiasmatic nucleus. Brain-penetrant kinase inhibitors have been produced for other kinases, making the selectivity the major issue for drug discovery efforts.

Rather than attempting to regulate the molecular oscillator itself, it seems possible to influence its input or output pathways. The existence of a dedicated pigment for the measurement of light quantity reaching the retina and of a defined neuronal population transmitting the information to the suprachiasmatic nucleus provides special prospects for drug discovery. The intracellular signaling of the melanopsins may be approachable, and the transmitter mechanisms used by the neurons offer many more traditional drug discovery opportunities. Glutamate and PACAP are the transmitters of the retina-suprachiasmatic neurons. Gene knockout mice unable to synthesize PACAP exhibit altered responses to changes in light–dark rhythms. PACAP acts on three G-protein-coupled receptors, VPAC1,

VPAC2, and PAC1. Knockout mice for the VPAC2 gene have a similar phenotype as mice lacking the neurotransmitter itself. Mice with a null mutation in the gene coding for PAC1 are only marginally affected. The contribution of PACAP to regulation of the suprachiasmatic oscillator may be sufficient to make the optimal receptor agonist of antagonist a useful drug for clock resetting. A more powerful effect is expected from compounds influencing the primary glutamatergic neurotransmitter mechanism. All major groups of ionotropic and metabotropic glutamate receptors exist in the suprachiasmatic nucleus and represent putative drug targets. As for other conditions where glutamatergic transmission plays a role, the selectivity of the contribution of individual receptors represents a significant hurdle for drug discovery. Presynaptic receptors stimulated by modulatory pathways influence transmitter release from the retinal projection to the suprachiasmatic nucleus. The input of the serotonergic neurons from the mesencephalic Raphe nuclei is mediated by 5-HT_7 receptors that represent an intriguing putative drug target because of their relatively selective expression in the brain (Glass et al., 2003).

On the output side of the suprachiasmatic clock, prokineticin 2 receptors (PK2R) have been identified as attractive putative drug target. The neuropeptide prokineticin 2 is selectively expressed in the suprachiasmatic nucleus with a cyclic circadian rhythm. Injections of the peptide into the brain of animals are able to shift the sleep–wake cycle. The receptor for prokineticin 2, PK2R, is expressed in the target areas of the efferent pathways from the suprachiasmatic nucleus. Among them is the paraventricular hypothalamic nucleus, the origin of the projection that regulates the sympathetic nervous system input to the pineal, and other thalamic and hypothalamic nuclei known to participate in sleep regulation (Cheng et al., 2002). PK2R thus appears to be a principal mediator of the output of the circadian pacemaker. Rather than resetting the clock itself, agonists and antagonists to PK2R are expected to override the information of the clock and to induce sleep behavior at desired times.

The circadian pacemaker of the suprachiasmatic nucleus, together with its afferent and efferent pathways, offers many distinct target opportunities with high degrees of experimental justification. It seems likely that one or more of these approaches will lead to drugs that make it possible to adjust the clock's influence on sleep regulation to the desired setting. Compounds able to penetrate into the brain quickly, with very rapid onset of action and very short half-life, will be necessary for optimal therapeutic success. The clinical experience with melatonin, an imperfect molecule from a point of view of theoretical expectations, creates a very optimistic view for drug discovery efforts related to the circadian pacemaker.

13.7 HYPOTHALAMIC REGULATORS OF SLEEP

In addition to the input from the circadian pacemaker, the projections from the hypothalamus provide the second major influence to the brainstem neurons that control sleep. A small population of neurons using the hypocretin/orexin neuropeptides as transmitters has been identified as the most significant player. The preprohypocretin precursor protein gives raise to hypocretin 1 (orexin A) and hypocretin 2 (orexin B), two peptides that stimulate two related G-protein-coupled receptors, hypocretin receptor 1 (orexin receptor 1), and hypocretin receptor 2 (orexin receptor 2). Mice with a null mutation of the preprohypocretin gene have increased periods of sleep during the wake period and abnormal REM sleep patterns. A genetic form of narcolepsy in dogs is caused by a mutation in the hypocretin receptor 2 gene. Hypocretin-secreting neurons show degenerative changes in

Table 13.1   Current and future drugs for the treatment of sleep disorders

---

Current Drugs

Benzodiazepine drugs (GABA-A receptor agonists)
Selective GABA-Aα1 benzodiazepine receptor agonists
Melatonin
NE/5-HT reuptake blockers
Modafinil (for narcolepsy)

Future Drugs

Melatonin receptor agonists
PACAP receptor ligands
5-HT$_7$ receptor ligands
Prokineticin 2 receptor ligands
Hypocretin/orexin receptor ligands

---

humans suffering from narcolepsy. Intracerebral administration of hypocretins reverses narcolepsy in animals. These findings identify the hypocretins as powerful players in the regulation of sleep patterns and the sleep–wake cycle (Siegel, 2004).

The hypocretin-containing neurons are able to exert these powerful effects through direct excitatory projections to the major monoaminergic and cholinergic modulatory neuron systems. They innervate and stimulate histaminergic neurons of the hypothalamus, dopaminergic neurons of the substantia nigra, serotonergic neurons of the mesencephalic Raphe nuclei, noradrenergic neurons of the locus coeruleus, and the cholinergic neurons of the pons as well as the basal forebrain. These highly targeted projection systems make it likely that the hypocretin-containing neurons provide the key output pathway of the hypothalamic circuits that integrate metabolic changes reflecting sleep deprivation. Modafinil, the only currently approved drug for the treatment of narcolepsy, may be effective because it mimics the excitatory effects of the hypocretins on the monoaminergic neurons. The direct projection of the hypocretin-containing neurons to the reticular system of the pons is likely to mediate the influence of these peptides on REM sleep patterns.

The robust effects of the orexins on sleep regulation have prompted drug discovery efforts in several biopharmaceutical companies. Agonists to the hypocretin receptors are expected to provide treatment for narcolepsy. Antagonists may be useful to induce sleep. It may be possible to generate highly specific effects on sleep patterns and mechanisms by exploring drugs that selectively influence the subtypes of the hypocretin receptors. Besides the hypocretins, other hypothalamic peptides participate in the regulation of sleep and may provide future drug targets. The advanced knowledge on the hypocretins supports the view that the hypothalamic control circuits of sleep provide ample opportunity for drug discovery research.

13.8   ANIMAL MODELS AND CLINICAL EVALUATION

Sleep is a common behavioral feature of all higher vertebrates. The architecture of sleep is rather uniform among the mammalian species. While there are variations in the distribution of sleep periods over the day and the fraction of sleep time allocated to different sleep stages, the typical stages of normal sleep and REM sleep are common for the mam-

Table 13.2 Animal models

Rodent Assays
Mice/rat spontaneous activity
Mice/rat circadian rhythmic activity in constant light or dark

Monkey Assays
EEG recordings

malian species used in animal experimentation. In contrast to other neuroscience areas, drug discovery for sleep disorders can rely on established and predictive animal models (Table 13.2). Rodent activity assays are the simplest animal test systems. Spontaneous motor activity, measured, for example, as wheel-running activity, is monitored over several days. Sleep-inducing compounds decrease activity during the active phase and prolong the inactive phase. If the animals are kept in constant dark or light, the circadian pacemaker continues to impose a rhythm that gradually shifts away from the actual daily cycle. Compounds able to reset the circadian pacemaker cause abrupt changes in the regular cycle. Compounds jamming the circadian clock are expected to completely disrupt the rhythms as it occurs following lesions of the suprachiasmatic nucleus (Fig. 13.6).

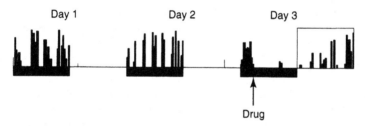

Figure 13.6 Rodent activity patterns. The normal activity pattern is disrupted by the injection of a molecule able to reset the circadian clock. (Adapted from Cheng et al., 2002)

EEG recordings provide direct monitoring of sleep and the quantitative analysis of sleep architecture. Modern microelectronic telemetric devices make it possible to record sleep in mice and rats automatically and without interfering with the animals' normal activities. Cats have been the traditional laboratory species for sleep research because of their natural propensity to sleep for long periods of time. Most of the sleep pathways have been initially defined in cats. The possibility to record EEG in mice, the advent of transgenic technologies, and the animal rights concerns for the typical pet species have brought a substantial shift of research to the rodents. For example, the spontaneous dog model for narcolepsy, caused by a mutant of the hypocretin receptor 2 gene, has been replicated in transgenic mice (Willie et al., 2003).

Monkeys are the most useful models for human sleep studies, since sleep duration and architecture can be measured by EEG in the same way human sleep is formally assessed in clinical settings. Comparative studies identified the rhesus monkeys as the most suitable experimental species for comparison with human sleep (Balzamo et al., 1977). As humans, rhesus monkeys are diurnal animals, removing a complication associated with the nocturnal rodent species. The cycles of the circadian pacemaker and output of the clock appear to be the same in diurnal and nocturnal animals. For example, melatonin release in nocturnal animals also occurs in the dark phase. Not surprisingly, melatonin has therefore been shown to induce sleep in monkeys and humans but not in rodents (Huber et al., 1998). Drug effects observed in rodents cannot be directly extrapolated to humans, making monkey studies an essential component of a sleep drug discovery program.

Clinical trials for drugs to treat insomnia are based on the broad experience with benzodiazepine drugs. Formal analysis of sleep duration and architecture is carried out with volunteers or patients in sleep clinics equipped for the recording of EEG and other vital functions. Larges studies with out-patients rely on questionnaires in which patients record sleep onset, sleep duration, and the perceived quality of sleep. Key issues for drug approval are the addictive potential of a drug candidate and the safety with long-term use. For the differentiation of future drugs for sleep disorders, experimental medicine approaches will be useful in attempts to define the relationship between subjectively perceived sleep quality and sleep architecture. Patterns and duration of sleep change during development and aging, and there are significant interindividual variations in the number of hours needed of sleep to feel rested. Emphasis on the differential aspects of sleep will help future drug candidates to outperform the currently available drugs.

13.9   CONCLUSIONS

Sleep disorders, insomnia in particular, are very common human conditions with significant impact on the quality of life. Insomnia can be caused by disturbances in the daily rhythm, and it frequently accompanies depression and aging. Normal sleep is a well-defined behavioral condition subdivided into four stages of normal sleep and REM sleep, during which dreams occur. Sleep is induced and controlled by ascending neurons from the reticular formation in the pons, which provide broad innervation to the thalamus and cortex. A first regulatory influence to these cells is provided by hypothalamic neurons, which transmit information on metabolic changes associated with sleep deprivation and tiredness. The second input relays the data from the internal circadian clock located in the suprachiasmatic nucleus. Retinal projection neurons to this nucleus synchronize the internal pacemaker with the external day–night cycle.

Currently available drugs provide effective treatment for insomnia. They include the benzodiazepine anxiolytics, which are allosteric agonists for the GABA-A receptors, and the more recently approved selective benzodiazepine receptor agonists for the GABA-Aα1 receptor subtype. The latter drugs induce and maintain sleep with similar characteristics as natural sleep and very few, if any, adverse effects when used occasionally or over short periods of time. Monoamine uptake blocker antidepressants are useful in the treatment of sleep disorders linked to depression. Melatonin, a natural hormone secreted by the pineal, has mild efficacy for insomnia caused by jet lag.

Recent sleep research has identified several opportunities for future drugs that induce natural sleep and correct for shifts in the circadian rhythm. The internal clock is a transcriptional oscillator with specific regulatory proteins that suggest, albeit difficult, approaches for drug discovery efforts. The retinal afferent pathway, which uses glutamate and the neuropeptide PACAP as transmitters, is likely to be more approachable in the search for compounds to re-set the clock. Prokineticin 2, the neuropeptide transmitter of the output pathway from the suprachiasmatic, and its receptor offer a highly attractive putative target for drugs able to override the input from the pacemaker to the sleep circuits in the pons. The hypothalamic input to the sleep pathways uses hypocretin/orexins peptides as transmitter substances. They are powerful regulators of sleep, since disruption of their mechanisms causes narcolepsy, transient attacks of sleep during the wake cycle.

The elucidation of the molecular circadian pacemaker and the discovery of transmitter systems that selectively regulate the sleep pathways directly identify approaches to discover drugs to prevent or induce natural sleep whenever desired.

Mammalian species utilize similar sleep mechanisms, despite the variations in wake–sleep behavior. Simple observations of circadian activity rhythms in rodents provide a useful initial animal assay to test drug candidates. Detailed EEG recordings generate more precise information on sleep patterns and architecture. Extrapolation of rodent data to humans is complicated by the nocturnal activity patterns of mice and rats. EEG analysis in monkeys provides the best animal model to predict efficacy of test compounds in human sleep disorders. The monkey assays directly replicate in-patient human sleep studies with EEG recordings. Large-scale human sleep studies rely on self-evaluation of sleep duration and quality by the participants. Experimental medicine studies attempting to correlate sleep architecture with the subjective perception of sleep quality will facilitate the discovery of drugs superior to the current GABA-Aα1 agonists that induce general sedation. The recent discoveries of sleep mechanisms, together with the persistent need for drugs that reset the internal clock and induce natural sleep, make drug discovery research for sleep disorders a very attractive endeavor.

REFERENCES

Further Reading

HANNIBAL, J. Neurotransmitters of the retino-hypothalamic tract. *Cell Tissue Res.* 309: 73–88, 2002.

MIGNOT, E., TAHERI, S., and NISHINO, S. Sleeping with the hypothalamus: Emerging therapeutic targets for sleep disorders. *Nature Neurosci.* (suppl.) 5: 1071–1075, 2002.

PACE-SCHOTT, E.F., and HOBSON, J.A. The neurobiology of sleep: Genetics, cellular physiology and subcortical networks. *Nature Rev. Neurosci.* 3: 591–605, 2002.

REPPERT, S.M., and WEAVER, D.R. Coordination of circadian timing in mammals. *Nature* 418: 935–941, 2002.

SCHENCK, C.H., MAHOWALD, M.W., and SACK, R.J. Assessment and management of insomnia. *J. Am. Med. Assoc.* 289: 2475–2479, 2003.

SIEGEL, J.M. Hypocretin (orexin): Role in normal behavior and neuropathology. *An. Rev. Psychol.* 55: 125–148, 2004.

STICKGOLD, R., HOBSON, J.A., FOSSE, R., and FOSSE, M. Sleep, learning, and dreams: off-line memory processing. *Science* 294: 1052–1057, 2001.

Citations

BALZAMO, E., SANTUCCI, V., SERI, B., and VUILLON-CACCIUTTOLO, B.J. Nonhuman primates: Laboratory animals of choice for neurophysiologic studies of sleep. *Lab. Anim. Sci.* 5: 879–886, 1977.

CAJOCHEN, C., KRÄUCHI, K., and WIRZ-JUSTICE, A. Role of melatonin in the regulation of human circadian rhythms and sleep. *J. Neuroendocrin.* 15: 432–437, 2003.

CHENG, M.Y., BULLOCK, C.M., LI, C., LEE, A.G., BERMAK, J.C., BELLUZZI, J., WEAVER, D.R., LESLIE, F.M., and ZHOU, Q.Y. Prokineticin 2 transmits the behavioural circadian rhythm of the suprachiasmatic nucleus. *Nature* 417: 405–410, 2002.

GLASS, J.D., GROSSMAN, G.H., FARNBAUCH, L., and DINARDO, L. Midbrain raphe modulation of nonphotic circadian clock resetting and 5-HT release in the mammalian suprachiasmatic nucleus. *J. Neurosci.* 23: 7451–7460, 2003.

HOBSON, A.J., and STERIADE, M. The neuronal basis of behavioral state control. In: *Handbook of Physiology.* F.E. Bloom, ed. American Physiological Society, Bethesda, MD. Sect. 1, vol. 4, pp. 701–823, 1986.

HUBER, R., DEBOER, T., SCHWIREIN, B., and TOBLER, I. Effect of melatonin on sleep and brain temperature in the Djungarian hamster and the rat. *Physiol. Behav.* 65: 77–82, 1998.

KRALIC, J.E., KORPI, E.R., O'BUCKLEY, T.K., HOMANICS, G.E., and MORROW, A.L. Molecular and pharmacological characterization of GABA(A) receptor alpha1 subunit knockout mice. *J. Pharmacol. Exp. Ther.* 302: 1037–1045, 2002.

TOYOTA, H., DUGOVIC, C., KOEHL, M., LAPOSKY, A.D., WEBER, C., NGO, K., WU, Y., LEE, D.H., YANAI, K., SAKURAI, E., WATANABE, T., LIU, C., CHEN, J., BARBIER, A.J., TUREK, F.W., FUNG-LEUNG, W.P., and LOVENBERG, T.W. Behavioral characterization of mice lacking histamine H(3) receptors. *Mol. Pharmacol.* 62: 389–763, 2002.

VON GALL, C., STEHLE, J.H., and WEAVER, D.R. Mammalian melatonin receptors: Molecular biology and signal transduction. *Cell Tissue Res.* 309: 151–162, 2002.

WILLIE, J.T., CHEMELLI, R.M., SINTON, C.M., TOKITA, S., WILLIAMS, S.C., KISANUKI, Y.Y., MARCUS, J.N., LEE, C., ELMQUIST, J.K., KOHLMEIER, K.A., LEONARD, C.S., RICHARDSON, J.A., HAMMER, R.E., and YANAGISAWA, M. Distinct narcolepsy syndromes in orexin receptor-2 and orexin null mice: molecular genetic dissection of non-REM and REM sleep regulatory processes. *Neuron* 38: 715–730, 2003.

Chapter 14

Epilepsy

In epilepsy, spontaneous and excessive neuronal activity in the brain overrides a person's normal behavior. The term epilepsy originates from the Greek verb for take over or seize an object. Epilepsy is a very common neurological condition that has accompanied humankind since early history. Febrile convulsions were an ordinary experience before the advent of antipyretic drugs. Descriptions of spontaneous, intense seizures are found in the world literature. In his tragedy *Julius Caesar,* Shakespeare describes that *"Caesar . . . fell down . . . , and foamed at the mouth, and was speechless."* Many creative artists, including the writers Moliere and Dostoyevsky, and the painter van Gogh suffered from epilepsy, supporting the frequently vocalized belief that seizures favor prolific human activity. However, no formal studies have been conducted in support of this intuitively appealing idea.

The seizure described in Shakespeare's play is readily recognizable as a generalized seizure. Temporal paralysis and loss of consciousness are caused by rhythmic, high-amplitude neuronal discharges in both cerebral hemispheres, which are easily identified with EEG analysis (Fig. 14.1). Generalized seizures represent a serious medical condition that interferes with many aspects of normal human life. Humans susceptible to spontaneous generalized seizure attacks are prevented from driving a car and operating critical machinery. Generalized seizures have a strong genetic component and often occur as part of a complex symptomatic picture of inherited neurological conditions. Partial seizures are typically less impairing than generalized epilepsy. They may manifest themselves as short-lasting disturbances of movement or of intellectual ability. Absence seizures entail the loss of consciousness during a brief period of time. In EEG analysis, partial seizures are recognizable as focal rhythmic discharges that are typically restricted to one side of the brain. Brain injury rather than genetic defects is believed to be the typical cause of partial seizures.

Many effective drugs are available for the treatment of epilepsy. The majority of them have been discovered because of their beneficial effects in animal models of epilepsy. Seizures are induced easily in animals by a variety of stimulatory drugs, and they occur spontaneously in genetic animal models. The easiness and availability of animal models has made it possible to discover drugs based on the behavioral effects alone. Drug discovery research in epilepsy has been successful in absence of precise understanding of the molecular nature receptor sites and drug targets. In consequence the mechanism of action of many of the drugs is poorly understood and several of them appear to act on more than one receptor site. None of the existing drugs is ideal, and they all suffer from various adverse effects. The treatment of chronic epilepsy typically proceeds through the sequen-

Drug Discovery for Nervous System Diseases, by Franz F. Hefti
ISBN 0-471-46563-1   Copyright © 2005 by John Wiley & Sons, Inc.

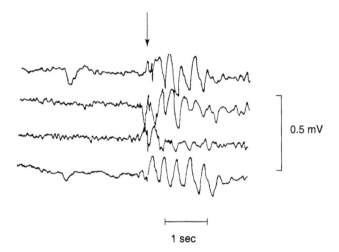

0.5 mV

1 sec

Figure 14.1   EEG pattern of a standard generalized seizure. Four parallel recordings were taken at different positions on the surface of the head.

tial assessment of the various compounds, and each of them is titrated up to a dose where adverse effects are still tolerated. Thus, despite a broad palette of existing drugs for epilepsy, there remains a strong medical need for new and better drugs. Recent discoveries on the molecular biology of neuronal ion channels and on genetic mutants causing epilepsy support the renewed enthusiasm for this field.

14.1   DISEASE MECHANISMS

Epilepsy affects approximately 0.5% of the population, and about 3% of the people have at least one seizure episode during their life span. Complex seizure classifications divide epilepsy into subforms based on the developmental stage of the patient, the behavioral symptoms, and the EEG characteristics. Partial and generalized seizures represent two general categories with many subtypes (Chang et al., 2003).

The generalized seizures include childhood absence epilepsy characterized by short but frequent episodes of loss of attention and activity. The mechanism underlying these seizures is believed to involve part of the thalamic circuitry that regulates sleep. During non-REM sleep the thalamo-cortical neurons impose a rhythmic EEG activity onto the cortical neurons. During absence seizure episodes, the thalamic neurons generate sleep-like rhythm with increased amplitude and lower frequency. As in sleep, the patients are unconscious, and they do not recall the episode. Mutations in the $Ca_v3.2$ Ca^{2+} channel subtype have been identified as the cause of absence seizure disorders in several patients (Chen et al., 2003).

The more severe forms of generalized epilepsy are life-threatening conditions because of the danger for injury during the fall and because of cellular damage caused by the excessive neuronal activity in the brain. Most episodes of generalized seizures last for several minutes only, but sustained general seizures, called status epilepticus, require emergency medical intervention (Lowenstein and Alldredge, 1998). Most types of reoccurring generalized epilepsy have a genetic basis. Well-characterized familial forms with sufficiently large pedigrees have led to the discovery of the disease genes listed in Table 14.1. They include Na^+ channels, K^+-channels, and ionotropic nicotinic and GABAergic transmitter

Table 14.1   Channel mutations causing generalized seizures

Na⁺ Channels
SCN1A (α subunit of Na$_v$1.1 channels)
SCN2A (α subunit of Na$_v$1.2 channels)
SCN1B (β subunit of various channels)

K⁺ Channels
KCNQ2 (K$_v$7.2 channel subunit)
KCNQ3 (K$_v$7.3 channel subunit)

Ca²⁺ Channels
CACNA1H (α_1 subunit of Ca$_v$3.2 channels)

Nicotinic Acetylcholine Receptors
α4 nicotinic subunit
β2 nicotinic subunit

Ionotropic GABA-A Receptors
GABA-A γ2 subunit
GABA-A α1 subunit

receptor channels (Fisher, 2004; Leppert and Singh, 1999; Lossin et al., 2003; Steinlein, 2002). While the precise mechanisms by which these individual mutations cause generalized seizures remain to be elucidated, the discoveries are consistent with the view that all mutations lower the threshold for neuronal activation. Mutations increasing Na⁺ influx or decreasing K⁺ efflux during an action potential prolong the duration of the depolarization and are able to induce repetitive firing of a neuron. Mutations that increase the action of the excitatory nicotinic receptors or decrease the action of inhibitory GABA-A receptors will depolarize the postsynaptic neurons and thus increase the probability of action potential generation. The term hyperexcitability is sometimes used to describe the increased probability of action potential generation and repetitive neuronal firing. The discovery of epilepsy disease mutations in ion channels makes the generalized seizures a member of the channelopathies disease group, which also include familial forms of migraine, ataxia, as well as cardiac disorders.

Partial seizures are a frequent consequence of brain injury caused by traumatic events, ischemic infarcts, or by the growth of intracranial tumors, but they can occur in absence of an identified event. EEG analysis provides the definitive diagnosis. During partial seizures the rhythmic discharges originate in defined brain areas, the epileptic foci, from which they spread over wider regions, sometimes over the entire cerebral hemisphere. The temporal cortex, hippocampus, and the amygdala are the most common foci. In some patients, the seizures start spontaneously, in others, they are triggered by external events, such as light, intense sound, and specific social interactions. It is sometimes possible to precisely define the triggering stimuli and to provide simple behavioral therapy by avoiding them. Surgical removal of the brain area containing the epilepsy focus is an often employed successful therapeutic strategy. For many patients, however, drug therapy represents the only option to treat reoccurring partial seizures. Effective pharmacotherapy reduces the probability that the seizures are initiated at the foci and limits the propagation into the adjacent brain areas.

Experimental induction of seizures in animals causes complex changes in gene expression and cellular plasticity. Distinct and novel patterns of gene transcripts and

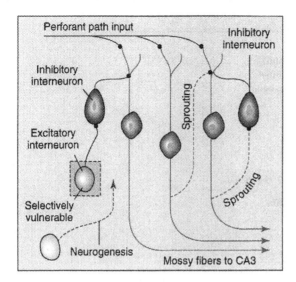

Figure 14.2   Hippocampal plasticity in response to reoccurring seizures. Sprouting of the pyramidal cells of the dentate gyrus and neurogenesis form aberrant, new connections. (Reprinted with permission, Chang and Lowenstein, 2003)

proteins are created by the massive induction of many genes. Many growth factors, including the neurotrophins and their Trk receptors, are among the induced genes and provide the basis for molecular hypotheses to explain plastic changes in the brain (Fig. 14.2). In the hippocampus, seizures lead to the degeneration of pyramidal neurons and interneurons and the growth of axons to areas beyond their normal projection areas. Aberrant sprouting of the mossy fibers of the dentate gyrus pyramidal cells to adjacent neurons is a prominent feature among these events (Zappone and Sloviter, 2004). Hippocampal seizures in animals furthermore increase the rate of neurogenesis in the dentate gyrus, providing an additional mechanism for seizure-induced neuroplasticity.

The analysis of postmortem tissue from epileptic patients supplies strong evidence for similar events in the human brain. Neuronal degeneration and glial cell proliferation in the hippocampus cause hardening and shrinkage of this brain structure, a phenomenon described as hippocampal sclerosis. Mossy fiber sprouting has been documented in human epileptic tissue (Babb et al., 1991). The plastic changes in the hippocampus are believed to be irreversible and to contribute to the hyperexcitability of the hippocampal circuits, and to perpetuate and gradually worsen the epileptic condition. Effective prevention of seizures by drugs will stall these detrimental changes. It seems reasonable to speculate that future drugs able to regulate neuroplasticity and neurogenesis may be able to reverse them.

14.2 CURRENT DRUGS

Physicians treating epileptic patients have at their disposal a variety of drugs with different efficacy and adverse effects profiles (Fig. 14.3). Decision-making charts guide them through the selection, taking into account the type and severity of the seizures, the previous history of treatment, the age of the patient, and drug–drug interaction issues. Some of the anti-epileptic compounds generally depress neuronal activity by increasing the function of the inhibitory GABAergic neurons. These compounds belong to the same drug classes used in the treatment of anxiety and sleep disorders. The mechanisms of action of

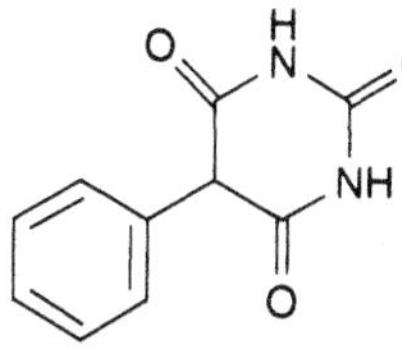

Phenobarbital

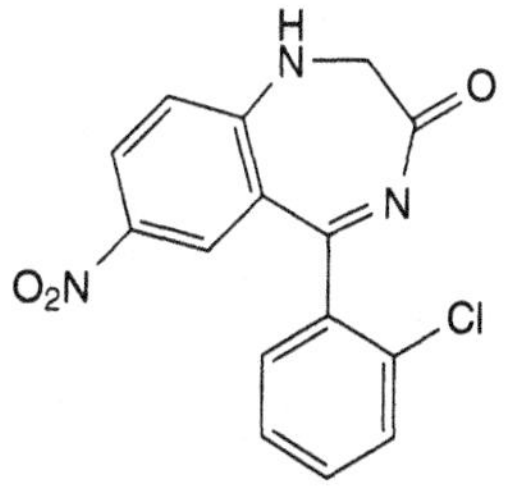

Clonazepam

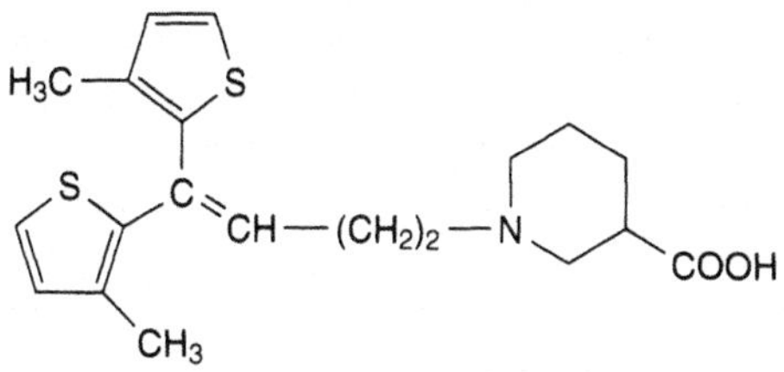

Tiagabine

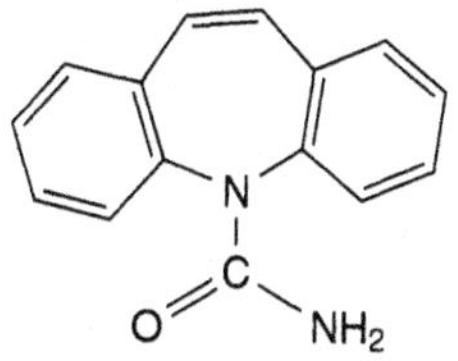

Carbamazepine

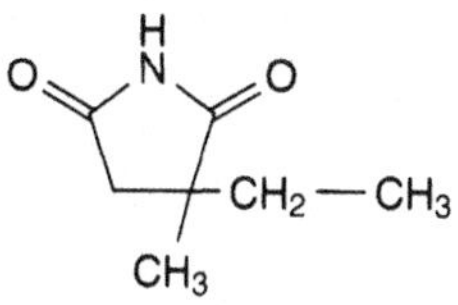

Ethosoximide

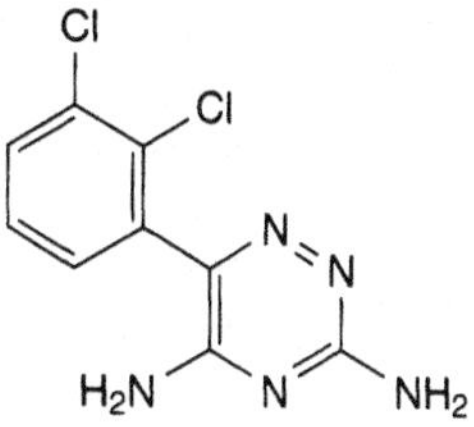

Lamotrigine

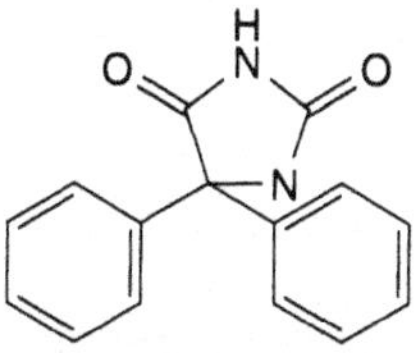

Phenytoin

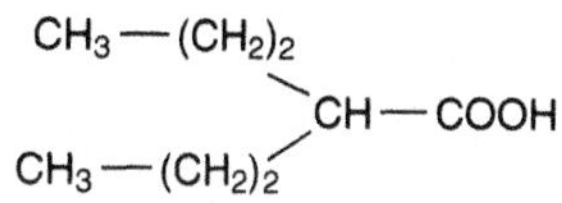

Valproic acid

Figure 14.3 Examples of currently available anti-epileptic drugs.

the other drugs is less well understood, but tentative evidence links many of them to ion channel functions.

14.2.1 Drugs Enhancing GABAergic Inhibition

Phenobarbital was the first clinically effective anti-epileptic drug and has remained useful up to this day (Brodie and Dichter, 1996). As described in earlier chapters, phenobarbital binds to the barbiturate binding sites on GABA-A receptors and potentiates the actions of

GABA on this anion channel, thus hyperpolarizing the neuronal membrane and decreasing the general excitability of the nervous system. It effectively suppresses all types of seizures. Since barbiturates generally reduce GABAergic inhibition and have served as anxiolytics and sleep-inducing drugs, it is not surprising that sedation is a typical adverse effect in the treatment of seizures. Additional toxicities further reduce the utility of phenobarbital.

Several benzodiazepine GABA-A receptor agonists, including diazepam and clonazepam, have been approved as safer alternatives to phenobarbital. While individual compounds are preferred for specific types of seizures, the benzodiazepine drug class covers the entire spectrum of seizures. Sedation and lethargy with long-term use are the most significant side effects. All benzodiazepines used for epilepsy belong to the group of nonselective GABA-A receptor agonists. Similar to the reverse pharmacology efforts in anxiety and sleep research, it may be possible to define GABA-A receptor subtypes that are particularly useful as targets for anti-epileptic drugs. Partial seizures originating in the hippocampus may respond well to agonists selectively acting on GABA-Aα5 containing receptors, since this subunit is preferentially expressed there. However, the possible role of this receptor in memory processes suggests the GABA-Aα5 selective agonists might interfere with cognitive functions. The evaluation in seizure models of mutant mice with null mutations of various GABA-A receptor subunits might help to identify the optimal drug targets for this class of compounds.

The clinical success with GABA-A receptor agonists has triggered drug discovery efforts for alternative strategies to increase GABAergic transmission. Two approved compounds, tiagabine and gabapentin, have resulted from these endeavors, though the clinical efficacy of tiagabine alone can be ascribed with confidence to GABAergic mechanisms. Gabapentin, which will be further discussed in Chapter 15 on pain, is a structural analogue of GABA and an effective drug for the treatment of partial seizures. Its mechanism of action is not understood but does not appear to involve GABAergic mechanisms. Tiagabine inhibits GAT-1, one of the GABA transporters responsible for the reuptake of GABA following synaptic release (Braestrup et al., 1990). It is clinically used for the treatment of partial seizures, though the efficacy is modest when compared to other drugs. Various neurological side effects further limit the use. The other subtypes of GABA transporters, GAT-2, GAT-3, and BGT-1, represent attractive alternative targets for future drugs and remain to be fully explored (Dalby, 2003).

14.2.2 Drugs with Multiple or Unclear Mechanisms

Carbamazepine, ethosuximide, felbamate, lamotrigine, levetiracetam, phenytoin, topimarate, valproic acid, and zonisamide are highly effective anti-epileptic drugs that have been approved for the treatment of partial and generalized seizures, with few exceptions that are useful in one type of seizure only (Dichter and Brodie, 1996; LaRoche and Helmers, 2004). Adverse effects limit the utility of all these drugs. The undesired effects vary from compound to compound but often include neurological and gastrointestinal disturbances. The earlier drugs, carbamazepine, felbamate, phenytoin, and valproic acid, are often used in monotherapy, whereas the other, more recently developed drugs can often be prescribed in combination with older drugs only. The existence of several effective anti-epileptic drugs poses a difficult problem for the development of new compounds. Ethical considerations make it impossible to expose epilepsy patients in clinical trials to new drugs without the known benefits of older drugs. The initial clinical trials thus attempt to show superiority of a drug combination over monotherapy with an earlier drug, and complex, additional studies are later necessary to demonstrate efficacy of the new drug alone.

The mechanism of action of this group of drugs is believed to involve voltage-gated Na^+-, K^+-, and Ca^{2+}-channels, since they all inhibit some of the corresponding electrical currents in electrophysiological studies in vitro (Taylor, 1999). However, for many of the drugs additional evidence links them to ionotropic glutamate receptors. It is believed that the combination of various effects on voltage-gated and glutamate-gated ion channels determines the clinical utility. The identification of the specific, clinically relevant receptors sites appears to be very difficult, however. Most of the drugs require high doses for clinical efficacy. A gram or more of a compound per day and blood concentration in the high μM range are typical. The dose–effect relationship suggests that the drugs bind with relatively low affinity to their receptor sites only, making their characterization a very difficult to impossible task. While reverse pharmacology with clinically effective anti-epileptic drugs is conceptually attractive, it may not succeed for these technical reasons. Alternative approaches, discussed below, seem more attractive than reverse pharmacology to utilize the existing knowledge on voltage-gated ion channels.

14.3 DISCOVERY OF NEW DRUGS

Behavioral screening has yielded several useful drugs and remains an attractive approach because of its simplicity. Rapidly growing information on the compound collections held by the pharmaceutical companies will make it possible to select populations without toxicity, acceptable pharmacokinetic properties, and the ability to penetrate the blood-brain barrier. Compounds with these properties are then rapidly assessed in high-throughput animal models of epilepsy. However, the lack of understanding of the receptor site and the mechanism of action is an impediment for further chemical diversification, and modern drug discovery scientists desire to make decisions based on molecular data, reducing the enthusiasm for the blind approach. The GABAergic mechanisms discussed above continue to provide a persuasive alternative, given the detailed molecular knowledge of the participating receptors and transporters, the existing, efficacious drugs that enhance GABAergic inhibition, and disease-causing mutations in GABA-A receptors. Equally appealing are the drug discovery efforts directed to voltage-gated ion channels, because the various disease genes discovered recently identify them as the primary event in the pathophysiology of many forms of epilepsy (Table 14.2).

Table 14.2   Current and future anti-epileptic drugs

Current Drugs
Drugs Enhancing GABAergic Functions
GABA-A receptor agonists (phenobarbital, clonazepam, diazepam)
GABA uptake inhibitor (tiagabine)

Drugs with Complex Actions on Voltage-Gated and Glutamate-Gated Ion Channels
Carbamazepine, ethosuximide, felbamate, lamotrigine, levetiracetam, phenytoin, topimarate, valproic acid, and zonisamide

Future Drugs
Use-dependent inhibitors of voltage-gated Na^+- and Ca^{2+}-channels
Specific inhibitors for disease-related ion channels

14.3.1 Voltage-Gated Ion Channels

Several biopharmaceutical companies have active drug discovery programs for inhibitors of voltage-gated Na^+-, K^+-, and Ca^{2+}-channels. The medicinal chemistry efforts rely on known inhibitors as starting point or expand on new compounds identified in assays that measure the function of the channel. The critical path on the biology side typically consists of a binding assay, followed by in vitro function testing with electrophysiology or an ion flux assay, and in vivo studies in epilepsy animal models. A large number of attractive chemical series and compounds with high potency and efficacy have been reported. Among them are channel subtype selective compounds as well as compounds with dual, Na^+- and Ca^{2+}-channel antagonism (Cosford et al., 2002). The large number of subtypes and combinatorial possibilities creates a difficult selection problem that can only be solved by better understanding of disease.

Rather than attempting to select the most appropriate ion channel subtype as target, drug discovery research may possibly concentrate on disease-relevant properties shared by all voltage-gated ion channels. During seizures the voltage-gated ion channels open repeatedly, at high frequency, and over prolonged periods of time. The channels are able to sustain rapid activity for limited periods of time only. They carry less and less current at repeated openings, a phenomenon referred to as **use dependence** and illustrated in Figure 14.4. A mutation in the $Na_v1.1$ channel causing generalized epilepsy changes the use dependence properties of the channel (Stampanato et al., 2001). This feature is likely to underlie the excessive neuronal activity during the seizures. Some of the existing antiepileptic drugs appear to preferentially suppress channel function at high frequency. Compounds able to increase the use dependence of voltage-gated ion channels thus emerge as the most attractive drug targets. Even in absence of precise understanding of the molecular basis of use dependence, it is possible to select drug candidates in relatively simple in vitro electrophysiological test systems. Comparing the effects of test compounds on channels stimulated at low and high frequency will identify those selectively able to alter use dependence. Compounds able to increase use dependence of subgroups of voltage-gated ion channels are expected to be clinically useful for many forms of seizures based on these considerations.

14.3.2 Pharmacogenetics of Inherited Epilepsy

The considerations on use dependence of ion channels, together with the discovery of several disease-causing mutations in ion channels, evoke an ideal scenario of future epilepsy drug therapy. Every newly diagnosed seizure patient will undergo genetic testing with sequence analysis of the neuronal ion channels. In many cases, in particular, the generalized seizure disorders, a specific mutation will be found in one of the channels. Expression of the mutated channel and functional analysis will then reveal the nature of the channel dysfunction, most often a change in use dependence properties. Based on this information, a drug previously approved for clinical use will be chosen from a battery of compounds. It will be selective for the mutated ion channel and will correct the aberrant properties. Diagnostic and therapeutic efforts will be closely linked in this concept of future pharmacotherapy (Glauser, 2002). The concept and the tools are available to generate this utopian world of targeted medicine for seizure disorders. In contrast to other nervous system diseases with a strong genetic component, the disease-causing mutations in epilepsy occur in easily drugable molecules, the ion channels. The combination of

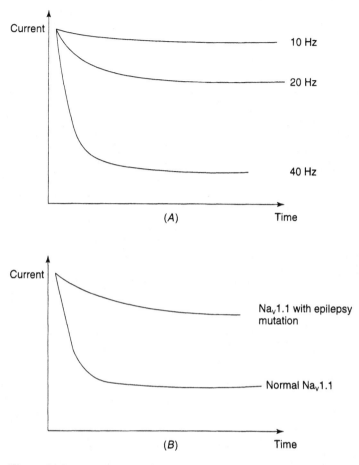

Figure 14.4 Use dependence of the Na$_v$1.1 voltage-gated sodium channel in epilepsy. The channel protein is expressed in frog oocytes and is activated by short burst of electrical stimulation at various frequencies. The resulting current is measured with electrophysiological methods. (**A**) At the low frequency, the channel sustains constant current over extended periods of time. At higher frequencies, the currents rapidly decline to much lower levels. (**B**) A point mutation in the voltage-sensing domain of the Na$_v$1.1 channel reduces the use dependence of the channel and causes a form of generalized seizure disorder. (Adapted from Stampanato et al., 2001)

pharmacogenetics with channel molecular biology embodies a highly attractive approach for epilepsy drug discovery.

14.4 ANIMAL MODELS AND CLINICAL EVALUATION

Animal models to evaluate epilepsy drug candidates include a basic set of routinely employed rodent assays as well as a large number of modifications and less widely used tests (Table 14.3). The basic assays are relatively simple, allowing investigators to rapidly assess many compounds. They are broadly grouped into electrical stimulation models, chemical stimulation models, and genetic models of human epilepsy (Sarkisian, 2001; White, 2003).

Table 14.3   Animal models

Electrical Stimulation Models
General Seizures
Maximal electrical stimulation (MES) model

Partial Seizures
Kindling models (hippocampus, amygdala, cortex stimulation)

Chemical Stimulation Models
Generalized Seizures
Pentylenetetrazole (PTZ) model
Glutamate receptor agonist-induced seizures

Partial Seizures
Intracerebral injections of GABA-A antagonists or glutamate receptor agonists

Genetic Models
Spontaneous mutations with generalized reoccurring seizures (e.g., *tottering*, *rocker*, *ducky*,
   stargazer, *lethargic* mice)
Transgenic mice expressing human disease gene

Seizures can be induced in rodents by brief electrical stimulation of the brain or associated organs. In the maximal electrical stimulation (MES) model, short stimulatory electrical pulses of a few seconds are applied to the corneas. They elicit prolonged, generalized
seizures that are quantified using EEG recordings or standardized behavioral scoring.
Phenytoin was identified with the MES assay, whereas tiagabine is ineffective in this test,
limiting its predictive power as a standard model for generalized human epilepsy. Focal
stimulation of specific brain areas generates animal models for partial seizures. Typically
electrodes are implanted unilaterally into the hippocampus or the amygdala. With repeated
stimulations over several days, the sensitivity to the electrical pulses increases over time.
An initially subconvulsant current induces seizures over repeated test sessions. This
process is referred to as kindling, and the kindling model has become a standard model
of human partial epilepsy. It is more labor intensive than the MES model but has an excellent record as predictor of efficacy in humans.

Chemical seizure models are a frequently used alternative to the electrical stimulation assays. In the pentylenetetrazole (PTZ) model, generalized seizures are induced by
systemic injections of PTZ, an antagonist to the GABA-A receptors. The hyperexcitability induced by suppressing GABAergic inhibition causes seizures of various duration and
intensity, dependent on the PTZ dose. The PTZ model is responsive to most clinical useful
anti-epileptic drugs, and it serves as useful first step in the evaluation of anti-seizure activity of drug candidates. PTZ does not respond to lamotrigine, however, which points out
that it cannot be considered an absolutely reliable predictor of human efficacy. In a variant
of the test, often used in safety evaluations of drug candidates, subthreshold doses of PTZ
are injected, and the ability of other drugs to induce seizures under these conditions is
measured to assess the danger of proconvulsant effects in humans. Many other compounds
besides PTZ are able to elicit generalized seizures, among them many glutamate receptor
agonists such as the most widely used kainic acid. Partial seizures can be chemically
induced by local injections into the brain of PTZ and many other agents, glutamate agonists and GABA-A receptor antagonists in particular. Many variants of the partial chem-

ical epilepsy models have been reported in the literature, making comparison of results and compound effects often difficult.

Many rodent strains with inherited seizure disorders have been identified by chance observations and provide genetic epilepsy models. Most of them exhibit unique forms of spontaneously occurring generalized seizures. The most commonly used strains, the *tottering, rocker, ducky, stargazer, and lethargic* mice, have all been linked to mutations in voltage-gated Ca^{2+} channels (Felix, 2002). While useful for the evaluation of drug candidates, these mice strains will gradually be replaced by transgenic mice reproducing the human disease mutations. In the example of the Na$_v$1.2 channel, mutations of the SCN2A gene cause seizure disorders in both mice and humans (Kearney et al., 2001; Kamiya et al., 2004). Mutant mice with a null mutation of the mouse gene and an inserted mutant human transgene will represent a true animal model of the human form of inherited epilepsy. These animal models will directly predict efficacy of drug candidates in the corresponding form of human epilepsy.

The clinical development of anti-epileptic drugs is conceptually simple. Reduction of seizure frequency and duration are the medically relevant endpoints, and they can be measured reliably. In practice, the existence of many effective drugs makes clinical trial design very complex. Studies with new drug candidates have to establish equivalence of efficacy with the existing drugs. To avoid taking patients off the effective drugs, a new drug is typically tested as an add-on to the existing therapy. For this reason only a few of the newer drugs have been approved for monotherapy as yet. Long-term studies are needed to assess the adverse effect profiles of the new drugs. It is anticipated that future drug candidates, ones that directly correct the molecular deficit of a hereditary form of epilepsy and are devoid of adverse effects, will receive faster approval than the current norm. The characterization of disease genes and the discovery of specific drugs for each mutation will fragment epilepsy into precisely defined subforms with specific drug therapy.

14.5 CONCLUSIONS

Epilepsy is a difficult and common neurological disorder with genetic and environmental causes. Generalized seizures involving both hemispheres of the brain are often caused by mutations in genes encoding neuronal ion channels. Partial seizures typically have a focal origin generated by local brain injury and remain confined to a single hemisphere. Ion channel dysfunctions or aberrant neuronal connections generate a status of hyperexcitability of neuronal systems that leads to rhythmic excessive discharges during seizures. Several drugs provide effective seizure control. They differ in efficacy for specific subtypes of seizures and in their adverse effect profiles. Because of the side effects, there remains a strong need for more specific anti-epileptic drugs.

The current drugs include benzodiazepine and barbiturate agonists for the GABA-A receptor and an inhibitor of GABA uptake, which decrease hyperexcitability by global enhancement of GABAergic inhibition. Similar to the situation in anxiety and sleep disorders, the molecular variety of GABAergic mechanisms offers many opportunities for further drug discovery in epilepsy.

Most of the other currently approved drugs lack a clearly defined mechanism of action and may exert their beneficial effects by binding to several different receptor sites. Some of the drugs inhibit voltage-gated Na$^+$ or Ca^{2+} channels, and this suggests, together with the discovery of disease-causing mutations, that these channels may be optimal drug targets. Compounds able to selectively suppress repeated openings of the channels, able to increase the use dependence of the channels, appear to be ideal for therapeutic use.

Genetic epilepsy offers an unrivaled occasion for a new, pharmacogenetic approach to drug discovery. In contrast to the situation in other inherited nervous system diseases, the epilepsy disease genes encode directly drugable protein targets. It is feasible to generate an optimal drug for every form of hereditary seizure disorder, bridging diagnostics and therapeutics in future treatment.

Epilepsy drug discovery is facilitated by several relative simple animal models with good predictive power for human efficacy. They include electrical and chemical stimulation assays as well as several genetic models. Transgenic mice replicating the human ion channel mutations are expected to provide the most relevant future animal models.

Clinical development of anti-epilepsy drugs relies on well-tested trial designs with seizure frequency and severity as endpoints. The existence of effective drugs necessitates comparative studies that complicate and prolong the development programs.

Despite the existence of several effective and useful drugs, epilepsy is a highly attractive and timely field for new drug discovery. The recent advances in ion channel molecular biology and in disease genes discovery create an unprecedented opportunity to find ideal drugs that selectively target the various subforms of epilepsy.

REFERENCES

Further Reading

BRODIE, M.J., and DICHTER, M.A. Antiepileptic drugs. *N. Eng. J. Med.* 334: 168–175, 1996.

CHANG, B.S., and LOWENSTEIN, D.H. Epilepsy. *N. Eng. J. Med.* 349: 1257–1266, 2003.

DALBY, N.O. Inhibition of gamma-aminobutyric acid uptake: Anatomy, physiology and effects against epileptic seizures. *Eur. J. Pharmacol.* 479: 127–137, 2003.

DICHTER, M.A., and BRODIE, M.J. New antiepileptic drugs. *N. Eng. J. Med.* 334: 1583–1590, 1996.

GLAUSER, T.A. Advancing the medical management of epilepsy: Disease modification and pharmacogenetics. *J. Child Neurol.* (suppl. 1) 17: S85–93, 2002.

LAROCHE, S.M., and HELMERS, S.L. The new antiepileptic drugs. *J. Am. Med. Assoc.* 291: 605–614, 2004.

LEPPERT, M.F., and SINGH, N. Susceptibility genes in human epilepsy. *Semin. Neurol.* 19: 397–405, 1999.

LOWENSTEIN, D.H., and ALLDREDGE, B.K. Status epilepticus. *N. Eng. J. Med.* 338: 970–976, 1998.

SARKISIAN, M.R. Overview of the current animal models for human seizure and epileptic disorders. *Epilepsy Behav.* 2: 201–216, 2001.

STEINLEIN, O.K. Nicotinic acetylcholine receptors and epilepsy. *Curr. Drug Targ. CNS Neurol. Disord.* 1: 443–448, 2002.

TAYLOR, C.P. Mechanisms of new antiepileptic drugs. *Adv. Neurol.* 79: 1011–1026, 1999.

WHITE, H.S. Preclinical development of antiepileptic drugs: Past, present, and future directions. *Epilepsia* 44: 2–8, 2003.

References

BABB, T.L., KUPFER, W.R., PRETORIOUS, J.K., CRADALL, P.H., and LEVESQUE, M.F. Synaptic reorganization by mossy fibers in human epileptic fascia dentate. *Neuroscience* 42: 351–363, 2001.

BRAESTRUP, C., NIELSEN, E.B., SONNEWALD, U., KNUTSEN, L.J., ANDERSEN, K.E., JANSEN, J.A., FREDERIKSEN, K., ANDERSEN, P.H., MORTENSEN, A., and SUZDAK, P.D. (R)-N-[4,4-*bis*(3-methyl-2-thienyl)but-3-en-1-yl]nipecotic acid binds with high affinity to the brain gamma-aminobutyric acid uptake carrier. *J. Neurochem.* 54: 639–647, 1990.

CHEN, Y., LU, J., PAN, H., ZHANG, Y., WU, H., XU, K., LIU, X, JIANG, Y. BAO, X., YAO, Z., DING, K., LO, W.H., QIANG, B., CHAN, P., SHEN, Y., and WU. X. Association between genetic variation of CACNA1H and childhood absence epilepsy. *An. Neurol.* 54: 239–243, 2003.

COSFORD, N.D.P., MEINKE, P.T., STAUDERMAN, A., and HESS, S.D. Recent advances in the modulation of voltage-gated ion channels for the treatment of epilepsy. *Curr. Drug Targ. CNS Neurol. Disord.* 1: 81–104, 2002.

FELIX, R. Insights from mouse models of absence epilepsy into Ca^{2-} channel physiology and disease etiology. *Cell. Mol. Neurobiol.* 22: 103–120, 2002.

FISHER, J.L. A mutation in the GABA(A) receptor alpha1 subunit linked to human epilepsy affects channel gating properties. *Neuropharmacology* 46: 629–637, 2004.

HUANG, R.Q., BELL-HORNER, C.L., DIBAS, M.I., COVEY, D.F., DREWE, J.A., and DILLON, G.H. Pentylenetetrazole-induced inhibition of recombinant gamma-aminobutyric acid type A (GABA(A)) receptors: mechanism and site of action. *J. Pharmacol. Exp. Ther.* 298: 986–995, 2001.

KAMIYA, K., KANEDA, M., SUGAWARA, T., MAZAKI, E., OKAMURA, N., MONTAL, M., MAKITA, N., TANAKA, M., FUKUSHIMA, K., FUJIWARA, T., INOUE, Y., and YAMAKAWA, K. A nonsense mutation of the sodium channel gene SCN2A in a patient with intractable epilepsy and mental decline. *J. Neurosci.* 24: 2690–2698, 2004.

LOSSIN, C., WANG, D.W., RHODES, T.H., VANOYE, C.G., and GEORGE, A.L., Jr. Molecular basis of inherited epilepsy. *Neuron* 34: 877–884, 2002.

SPAMPANATO, J., ESCAYG, A., MEISLER, M.H., and GOLDIN, A.L. Functional effects of two voltage-gated sodium channel mutations that cause generalized epilepsy with febrile seizures plus type 2. *J. Neurosci.* 21: 7481–7490, 2001.

ZAPPONE, C.A., and SLOVITER, R.S. Translamellar disinhibition in the rat hippocampal dentate gyrus after seizure-induced degeneration of vulnerable hilar neurons. *J. Neurosci.* 24: 853–864, 2004.

Chapter 15

Pain

"What a pain!" the exclamation used habitually for unpleasant and undesired events and situations must be one of the most common human expressions. Physical and emotional pain is a frequent, but regrettably accepted part of daily life. The explanation truly refers to suffering, whereas the medical definition of pain is limited to the sensation and perception of physical pain. Simple physical pain is not a disease. It evolved as protective mechanism that alerts an organism to an injury or to destructive overuse of a muscle, joint, or other part of the sensorymotor system.

Given the protective nature of pain, why suppress it? When the injury has been recognized and receives proper medical attention, the pain is no longer necessary and becomes a disturbance. Suppression of pain is beneficial for the transport of an injured person to the hospital, for a soldier wounded and awaiting evacuation in the battlefield, and for a patient who is recovering from elective surgery. Many chronic diseases are associated with pain. It makes sense to suppress the pain during the time of healing or when no treatment is available. Age-related degenerative diseases such as osteoarthritis and some forms of cancer are chronic diseases with pain as a significant component.

Pain is a subjective perception. Physical pain starts with a sensation in the skin, muscle, or other internal organs, where it is initiated by specific receptors on sensory nerve endings. The signal is transmitted to the brain, the site of the perception. Sensation and perception are only loosely coupled, and many sensory and emotional processes influence the translation. The severe physical pain of childbirth is perceived as less unpleasant than pain caused by an accident. Strong attention to another event can completely suppress the perception of pain. While the sensation of pain is not memorized, the fear of its reoccurrence and the memory of the associated events can become major burdens for victims of crime and torture. Pain is thus a complex and multifaceted aspect of human life that influences and is influenced by other sensations and emotions.

Drugs to treat physical pain are among the most widely used drugs in the modern world. The two principal classes are the nonsteroidal anti-inflammatory drugs (NSAIDs) and the opiate drugs, both of which were discovered many centuries ago from natural products and have been diversified to many variations. In addition there are more recently discovered drugs for chronic pain and for migraine. None of the existing drugs are without problems. NSAIDs are not fully effective in severe pain conditions and cause gastrointestinal adverse effects. Opiates, while highly effective, have a strong potential to cause dependence and addiction in addition to multiple adverse effects. The migraine drugs are effective only in a fraction of the people. The search for new and better pain medication thus addresses a very significant medical need. Fortunately recent breakthrough dis-

Drug Discovery for Nervous System Diseases, by Franz F. Hefti
ISBN 0-471-46563-1   Copyright © 2005 by John Wiley & Sons, Inc.

coveries in the molecular understanding of pain sensation have opened new avenues of investigation in drug discovery. There are many new and exciting approaches and putative pain targets with a high probability of future success.

15.1   PAIN MECHANISMS

Pain relievers are the most frequently used type of drugs. Approximately one-quarter of the population takes advantage of them during a given year. Pain is ubiquitous and exists in various forms. Transient pain, for example, caused by intense physical contact not causing injury, is frequent, typically mild, and easily tolerated without pain medication. Acute pain associated with tissue injury is reasonably well remedied with existing drugs, when mild to moderate. Severe pain following burns, massive injury, or significant surgery continues to create a challenge for drug therapy. Chronic pain represents the most significant medical need, whether mild, moderate, or severe. Persistent inflammation and tissue injury are a cause of chronic pain. Alterations of pain-mediating neurons often generate chronic pain conditions that are referred to as neuropathic pain. Migraine is a distinct pathological entity that involves acute, often severe pain but also other sensory disturbances. From point of view of drug discovery, development, and regulatory approval, the distinctions among mild, moderate, and severe pain and between acute and chronic pain are important because they are used for the definition of drug categories (Loeser and Melzack, 1999).

The sensation of pain is initiated by specific receptor proteins located on bare nerve endings of sensory neurons (Figs. 15.1, 15.2, 15.3). In contrast to the sensory axons that mediate touch or tension, the terminals of the pain-mediating axons are not encapsulated and they lack any anatomical specialization. Earlier electrophysiological studies characterized mechanical nociceptors, polymodal nociceptors, and thermoreceptors. More recent progress, however, has started to elucidate the molecular nature of the primary receptors and to initiate the true molecular definition of pain sensation. A central role is played by the transient receptor potential (TRP) ion channels (see Fig. 4.15). TRPV1, TRPV2, TRPV3, TRPV4, TRPM8, and TRPA1 (also called ANKTM1) respond in individual and specific ways to changes in temperature, changes in the ionic environment, and specific chemical stimuli. These complex response patterns allow the TRP channels to mediate the early responses to mechanical and thermal pain as well as some of the secondary responses caused by changes in the cellular environment. Several G-protein-coupled receptors participate in the sensation of molecular mediators of pain such as prostaglandins, bradykinin, substance P, and other neuropeptides. Tyrosine kinase receptors convey the actions of nerve growth factor (NGF) and other growth factors that are able to regulate pain in addition to their neurotrophic roles. The molecular mediators of pain are released from tissue following injury or inflammation. The release can be direct from injured cells or indirect through release from mast cells, which are a repository of inflammatory mediators. Multiple interactions between the various receptor proteins generate a complicated picture of molecular pain sensation that does not sustain the view of a clear separation between mechanical, thermal, and chemical modalities. The molecular receptors of pain stimulate ion channels in the sensory axons by direct molecular associations or intracellular mediators. These interactions, which are yet to be fully understood, initiate the flow of action potentials in the sensory axons and transmit the pain information to the spinal cord (Hunt and Mantyh, 2001).

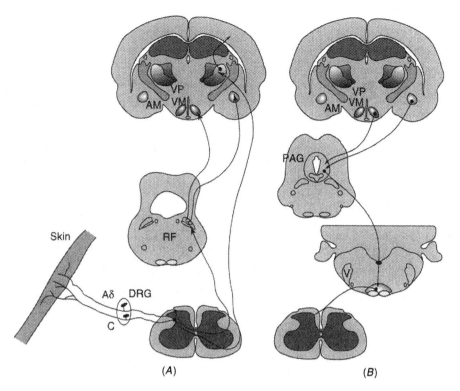

Figure 15.1 Major pain pathways. (**A**) Ascending pain pathways originate in the skin and other pain-sensitive organs. Aδ- and C-fibers provided by the sensory neurons in the dorsal root ganglia transmit the information to the spinal cord. Two ascending pathways relate the information to the brain, the spinothalamic and spinoreticular pathways. Several other minor pathways contribute. (**B**) Descending pathways able to control the flow of pain information originate in the amygdala and hypothalamus and relay in the periaqueductal gray to descending neurons. AM: amygdala; DRG: dorsal root ganglion; PAG: periaqueductual gray; RF: reticular formation of the pons; VM: ventromedial thalamus; VP: ventral posterior thalamus. (Reprinted with permission, Hunt and Mantyh, 2001)

Sensory axons mediating pain innervate all tissues except the central nervous system itself. They originate in the dorsal root ganglia adjacent to the spinal cord. Each sensory neuron sends out a short axon that splits into two branches just at the exit from the ganglion. One branch projects to the target tissue of pain sensation, and the other to the dorsal horn of the spinal cord. Sensory neurons thus provide a direct point-to-point cable link between the site of pain sensation and the spinal cord. Two types of sensory axons mediate pain: first, a small population of rapidly conducting myelinated axons, the Aδ-fibers, and, second, a larger population of slowly conducting unmyelinated axons, the C-fibers. The Aδ fibers typically fire short bursts of action potentials at the onset of pain sensation, providing a rapidly adapting response. They are responsible for the initial sharp pain caused by an injury, and they mediate the withdrawal reflex through a direct link to motor neurons in the spinal cord. The C-fibers tend to fire over longer periods of time and provide a slowly adopting response. They convey the continuing deep and burning pain. Various subpopulations of C-fibers have been defined based on selective expression of ion channels and neurotransmitter receptors, or neurotrophic factor dependency during early development. This research area is rapidly evolving and highly important from a drug discovery

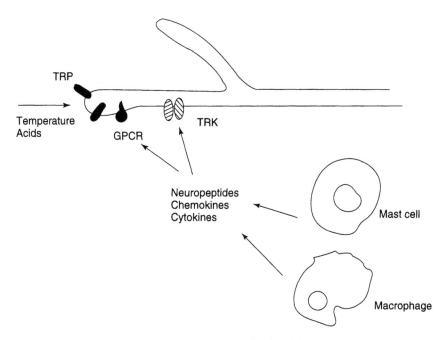

Figure 15.2 Pain sensation at the sensory nerve ending. TRP channels, various G-protein-coupled receptors and tyrosine kinase receptors sense and mediate the effects of physical and molecular mediators of pain. GPCR: G-protein-coupled receptor; TRP: transient receptor potential and related channels; TRK: tyrosine kinase receptors.

point of view. Any receptor or ion channel that is selectively expressed by a subpopulation of pain-mediating sensory neurons may lead to drugs able to precisely regulate the various components of pain.

In the spinal cord the sensory axons relay the pain information to the dendrites and cell bodies of neurons for the transmission to the brain and the generation of the motor withdrawal reflex. Synapses on interneurons and motor neurons mediate the involuntary motor reflex that withdraws an extended limb from the site of injury. Pain transmission engages direct and indirect pathways. The Aδ-fibers form synapses onto neurons of lamina I, the outermost layer of the dorsal horn, which provide the brain with precise information on the location and intensity of pain. The information from the C-fibers to these neurons is relayed indirectly, via interneurons located in lamina II of the dorsal horn that synapse onto the projection neurons in lamina I. In the spinal cord the pain information is mixed with information on other sensory modalities transmitted by sensory axons other than Aδ- and C-fibers. Thus at least some of the ascending pathways transport information of mixed sensory modality. The **gate control hypothesis** provides a simple concept for the suppression of pain by other sensory modalities. The interneurons in the spinal cord receive inhibitory input from C-fibers and excitatory input from fibers carrying sensory modalities other than pain. Since the interneurons are inhibitory on projection neurons, strong sensory input from other modalities can suppress pain transmission from Aδ- and C-fibers.

Many neurotransmitters and receptors participate in the synaptic transmission of pain information in the spinal cord (Besson, 1999). Glutamate is the primary transmitter of

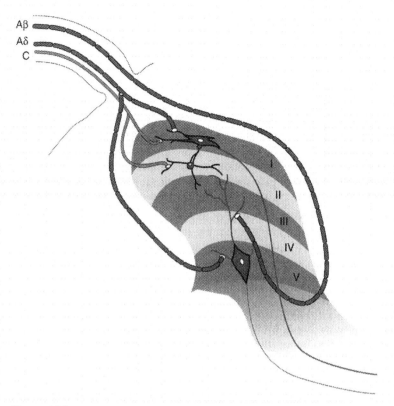

Figure 15.3 Pain transmission in the spinal cord. Specific pain information is transmitted by Aδ- and C-fibers to lamina I of the dorsal horn. Neurons in lamina II and V integrate the pain information with other sensory modalities transmitted by Aβ-fibers. (Adapted from Fields, 1987)

the sensory neurons, and the dorsal horn contains many subtypes of ionotropic and metabotropic glutamate receptors. The sensory neurons also release neuropeptides, substance P, and calcitonin gene-related peptide (CGRP) in particular. Interneurons utilize the inhibitory transmitters, GABA, and glycine but co-release neuropeptides such as enkephalins and galanin. The multitude of neurotransmitters and receptors in the spinal cord offers a rich area of opportunity for drug discovery. Many neurotransmitter receptor ligands effectively block pain, but they have multiple other effects because the same receptors participate in the transmission of other sensory modalities. The loss of the clear anatomical distinction of pain from other sensory modalities in the spinal cord creates a most significant hurdle for drug discovery.

The projections neurons of the dorsal horn build several distinct pathways to the brain. Most axons cross over to the other side of the spinal cord at the level of origin and ascend within the anterolateral white matter, constituting the **anterolateral system**. Some of these axons form the spinothalamic pathway. They innervate directly the lateral thalamic nuclei from which a further thalamo-cortical projection relays the pain information to the somatosensory cortex. The spinoreticular tract is built by axons projecting to the reticular formation of the pons where many sensory modalities are integrated. Several other ramifications form minor additional pain pathways, including the spinomesencephalic pathway projecting to the periaqueductal gray matter of the midbrain. Neurons of the anterolateral system utilize glutamate as their primary transmitter, but their synapses in the projection areas are influenced by many other transmitters and neuropeptides. Neurons from the mesencephalic area and the pons build direct or indirect connections to the lateral thalamus, the somatosensory cortex, and other areas of cortical integration. The cortical areas are the seat of the perception of pain and the integration with other aspects of conscious perception and decision making. Imaging studies implicate strong influences of pain sensation on the anterior cingulated cortex, an area linked to emotional feelings, and the prefrontal cortex, the area associated with higher cognitive functions.

The brain is not a just a final station for pain information, it is able to influence the sensation and transmission of pain through descending pathways. Noradrenergic neurons of the locus coeruleus and serotonergic neurons from the nucleus Raphe magnus in the medulla descend in the dorsolateral gray matter of the spinal cord and innervate both interneurons and projecting neurons that are part of the pain systems. The descending neurons receive regulatory inputs from many forebrain areas and a major direct input from the periaqueductal gray matter in the midbrain. The descending pathways further compli- cate the picture of pain transmission, but they offer additional opportunity to influence pain sensation and perception by drugs.

In its simplest form, pain is a transient and direct transmission of information about a noxious event to the brain. Most forms of pain, the medically relevant ones in particu- lar, are more complex. Inflammation, sustained injury, and healing processes modify the quality and duration of pain. They are able to alter the threshold for pain sensation, causing a normally mild stimulus to be a painful one. This phenomenon is called **hyperalgesia** and is commonly experienced during fever. A related but distinct phenomenon is called **allodynia**, where stimuli not normally causing pain become painful. For example, a light touch not causing any pain in normal skin is perceived as very painful on burned skin. The intensity and duration of pain sensations influence the nature of future ones. Many molecular and cellular processes underlie the changes of pain sensation and perception. Inflamed tissues release secondary pain mediators such as bradykinin and prostaglandins. Repeated painful stimulation alters the patterns of gene expression in the sensory neurons and enhances the synthesis of ion channels and neurotransmitter-related proteins for sig- naling. The resulting changes in synaptic strength enable functional plasticity in all pain pathways. Prolonged stimulation tends to increase the efficacy of the pain pathways, a phenomenon referred to as **wind-up** of pain transmission. Patients typically do not become tolerant to pain but perceive it as gradually worse, a further reason for strong drug discovery efforts on chronic pain.

Given the complex nature of pain mechanisms and the many participating molecular components, it is perhaps surprising that only a few types of drugs are available for the treatment of pain (Fig. 15.4). The NSAIDs prevent the formation of prostaglandins, one of the secondary mediators of pain sensation. Opiates suppress pain transmission in the spinal cord and pain perception in the brain. Serotonin 5-$HT_{1B/D}$ agonists are effective in aborting migraine attacks by modifying signaling from cerebral blood vessels. Gabapentin and tricyclic antidepressant drugs have found use in the treatment of chronic neuropathy despite relatively modest efficacy and poorly understood mechanisms of action. The com- plexity of pain systems suggests many more approaches and putative drug targets (Table 15.1).

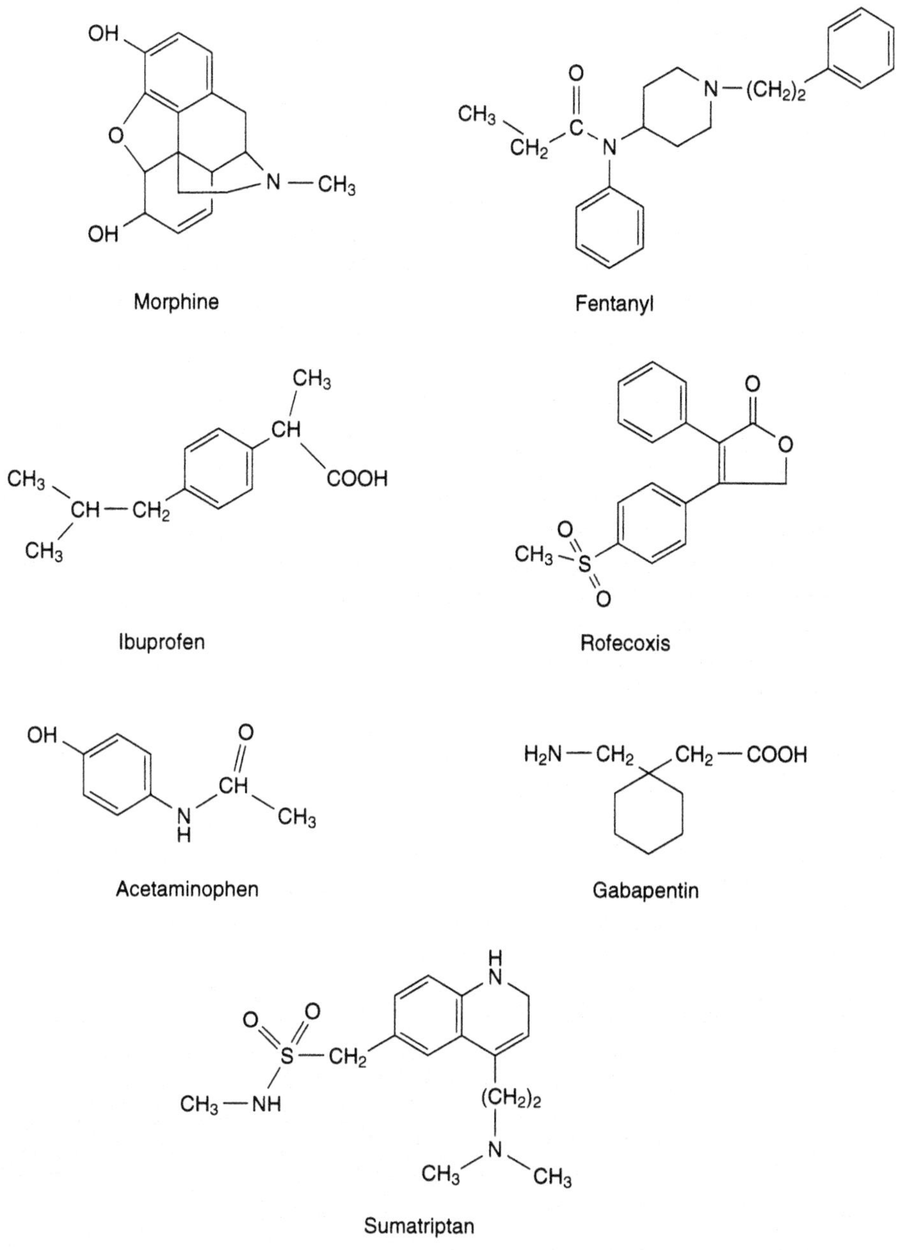

Morphine

Fentanyl

Ibuprofen

Rofecoxis

Acetaminophen

Gabapentin

Sumatriptan

Figure 15.4 Examples of currently available drugs for pain.

Table 15.1 Current and future drugs for pain

Current Drugs
Morphine and opioid receptor agonists
NSAIDs (nonselective Cox inhibitors)
Cox-2 inhibitors
Acetaminophen
Gabapentin
Triptans (5-HT$_{1B/D}$ agonists, migraine)

Future Drugs and Targets
Prostaglandin Mechanisms
Inhibitors of Cox-2 induction
Prostanoid synthase inhibitors
Prostaglandin receptor antagonists

TRP Channels Mechanisms
TRPV1 antagonists
TRPV4 antagonists
TRPA1 (ANKTM1) antagonists

Neuropeptides, Cytokines, and Chemokines
Bradykinin B1 and B2 receptor antagonists
Interleukin antagonists
Chemokine receptor antagonists
TrkA NGF receptor antagonists
p38 Map kinase inhibitors
CGRP receptor antagonists (migraine)

Sensory Neuron-Specific Channels
Na$_v$1.8 Na$^+$ channel antagonists
Na$_v$1.9 Na$^+$ channel antagonists
P2X$_{2/3}$ antagonists
ASIC3 antagonists

15.2 NSAIDs AND PROSTAGLANDIN INHIBITORS

Aspirin, the first NSAID was introduced into clinical practice more than a century ago. The compound, acetylsalicylic acid, is a derivative of an active ingredient extracted from the bark of the willow, which was recognized much earlier to have beneficial effects on fever and pain. Acetylsalicylic acid and all subsequent NSAIDs, such as ibuprofen, inhibit the formation of prostaglandins (Fig. 15.5). Prostaglandin synthesis is initiated by the cleavage of arachidonic acid from phospholipids of the cell membrane by phospholipase A$_2$. Thirteen isoforms of this ubiquitous enzyme are known that differ in expression patterns, substrate specificity, and catalytic activity. Arachidonic acid is converted in two steps by cyclooxygenases (Cox): first, to prostaglandin G$_2$ and, second, to prostaglandin H$_2$. Isomerases (prostandoid synthases) then convert prostaglandin H$_2$ to prostaglandins D$_2$, E$_2$, F$_2$, prostacyclin I$_2$, and thromboxane A$_2$. The prostaglandins activate corresponding G-protein-coupled receptors, called DP, EP, FP, IP, and TP receptors. They influence pain signaling by intracellular interactions with TRP channels, sodium channels, and other proteins involved in the sensation and transmission of pain (Samand et al., 2002).

Cox exists in two isoforms, Cox-1 and Cox-2. Both are membrane-bound enzymes that share a high degree of sequence and structure homology but differ in expression

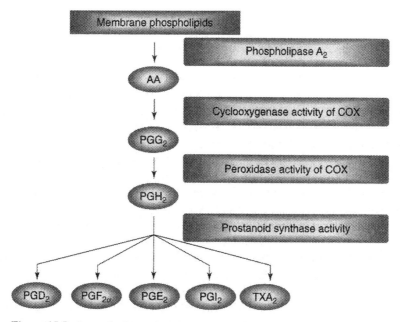

Figure 15.5   Prostaglandin synthesis. AA: arachidonic acid; COX: cyclooxygenase: PG: prostaglandin. (Reprinted with permission, Samad et al., 2002, Elsevier)

patterns and regulation. Cox-1 is constitutively expressed in most tissue, including those of the nervous, vesicular, and gastrointestinal systems. It generates prostaglandins, for their role as short-lived, local regulators of cellular functions. Cox-2 levels are normally low, but this enzyme is strongly induced following tissue injury or inflammation, for the production of prostaglandins that mediate the local pain response.

Traditional NSAIDs, including most of the widely available "over-the-counter pain killers," inhibit both Cox-1 and Cox-2. The inhibition of Cox-2 provides the most significant contribution to pain relief, whereas inhibition of Cox-1 is responsible for the most significant adverse effects of these compounds. The damage of the gastrointestinal mucosa and the resulting risk for bleeding and ulcer formation is attributed to the inhibition of Cox-1. The recognition of these relationships suggested that a reverse pharmacology approach toward selective Cox-2 inhibitors would generate drugs able to relieve pain without reduced adverse effect risk. The first selective Cox-2 inhibitors, rofecoxib and celecoxib, were introduced into clinical practice a few years ago. They are as effective as the nonselective NSAIDs and are less likely to induce gastrointestinal disturbances. While providing a significant advantage over classical NSAIDs for chronic use in particular, they are not ideal drugs. The concept that Cox-1 and Cox-2 are constitutive and inducible enzymes, respectively, is not true in an absolute way. Some forms of injury stimulate the expression of Cox-1, and Cox-2 serves an important constitutive function in the kidney. Further improvements are thus possible in the discovery of drugs that inhibit the prostaglandin contribution to pain (Fitzgerald, 2003).

The pathways of synthesis of prostaglandins and the mechanism of action offer ample maneuvering room for further drug discovery. Inhibition of phospholipase A$_2$ or prostandoid synthase activities is expected to produce the same effects as inhibition of Cox. The existence of many isoforms with different specificities and expression patterns provides an opportunity to selectively influence the synthesis of the pain-mediating prostaglandins. Detailed studies of expression patterns during normal conditions and pain states will help in the selection of the most promising target. Gene or protein array techniques appear particularly attractive to approach this problem. Rather than inhibiting the enzymes of the biosynthetic pathway, it may be possible to suppress the induction of enzymes during injury and inflammation. Upstream regulators of Cox-2 induction include interleukin-1 and other cytokines. Inhibitors of cytokine synthesis, antibodies against them, or selective antagonists to their receptors are conceptually equivalent approaches. The G-protein-coupled receptors mediating the action of the prostaglandin themselves appear to be the most direct way to new drugs. Selective inhibitors to the receptors mediating the pain sensation are expected to be as effective for pain control as the NSAIDs. Several companies have active programs on prostaglandin receptor inhibitors, but no attractive compounds have emerged from them as yet.

The beneficial effects of NSAIDs are not limited to pain. They attenuate the inflammatory response following tissue injury and are able to normalize body temperature during fever. The combination of these effects makes the NSAIDs particularly useful for the treatment of influenza and other conditions characterized by pain as well as inflammation. Prostaglandins are engaged in complex regulatory interactions with cytokines during an inflammatory process. The success of recently introduced drugs for rheumatoid arthritis such as inhibitors of tumor necrosis factor-α (TNF-α) illustrates the rapid progress in understanding of inflammation mechanisms. Understanding the molecular basis of the relationship between inflammation and pain may turn out to be a successful general strategy to find new pain medication.

The picture of the prostaglandins is yet further complicated by the discovery that they modulate pain transmission in the spinal cord and the brain (Dirig and Yaksh, 1999). In addition to their important role as signaling molecules at the site of injury and inflammation, they are part of the synaptic transmission machinery that transmits pain sensation from the sensory axon to the neurons of the anterolateral systems in the spinal cord and then to the brain. Prostaglandins are produced and released from spinal cord and brain tissue. The expression of the synthetic enzymes, Cox in particular, is influenced by disease processes, including Alzheimer's disease. Prostaglandin receptors are located pre- and postsynaptically in the spinal cord and the brain. The prostaglandins appear to provide a positive feedback loop enabling more effective synaptic transmission. They may thus contribute to the sensitization and wind-up of chronic pain perception in the central nervous system. It may be possible to design prostaglandin inhibitors that regulate the central components in a preferential way by making them extremely brain penetrant. Blood-brain barrier penetration of NSAIDs has received little attention in the past but may represent a most fruitful approach to improved pain medication. Despite the long tradition and the very detailed understanding of prostaglandin mechanisms, this area continues to look very attractive for pain drug discovery.

Acetaminophen, also called paracetamol, is one of the most frequently used medications for the control of pain and fever and is often discussed together with the NSAIDs. In contrast to the NSAIDs, however, acetaminophen is only a poor inhibitor of the Cox enzymes, and it does not suppress tissue inflammation. Its mechanism of action remains an enigma. The adverse effect profile of acetaminophen is superior to that of the NSAIDs, but at high doses it can cause fatal liver toxicity. Recent drug discovery efforts have revealed an efficacious and potent derivative of acetaminophen with the ability to release nitric oxide. This nitroacetaminophen is effective in animal models of pain without causing liver toxicity. Tentative evidence suggests the involvement of caspases and the transcription factor NF-κB in the mechanism of action of this intriguing compound (Moore and Marshall, 2003).

15.3   TRP CHANNELS

Inhibition of primary nociceptors—the molecules that sense extreme pressure, extreme temperatures, noxious chemicals, and the compounds released from injured tissue—is conceptually the most effective way to drugs for acute pain. Some of the TRP channels belong to this group, and TRPV1 appears to play a primary role. It is selectively expressed in the small sensory neurons of the dorsal root ganglion that send out the pain transmitting C-fibers. TRPV1 channels respond to temperatures above 43°C, to capsaicin, the active ingredient of hot peppers, to H^+, to anandamide, a natural cannabinoid receptor ligand, and also to adenosine that may act as an endogenous inhibitor. Sensation of H^+ is useful because tissue injury quickly causes acidosis in the extracellular fluid. The receptor specificity of TRPV1 provides a direct molecular explanation for the perception of peppers as hot. Capsaicin stimulation of TRPV1 in the mouth activates the same systems that respond to heat and activate sweat glands on the scalp. The TRPV1 receptors are influenced indirectly by other mediators of acute and inflammatory pain. Bradykinin receptors and the TrkA NGF receptors contribute to the activation of TRPV1 though intracellular phosphoinositol signaling mechanisms. The ability to respond to multiple direct and indirect activators allows the TRPV1 channels to integrate the inputs of many mediators of pain.

Experiments with TRPV1 knockout animals and with specific antagonists document its essential and selective contribution to normal pain sensation. Mice with a null mutation of the TRPV1 gene are normal, except for a much reduced response to painful stimuli (Caterina et al., 2000). Capsaicin is an agonist for TRPV1 and causes acute and burning pain when administered to the skin. The response rapidly desensitizes, at least in part because the sensory neurons are depleted of secondary transmitter mediators such as substance P and CGRP. Antagonists for the capsaicin receptor site were produced even before the molecular characterization of TRPV1. Among them is capsazepine, a close structural analogue that suppresses pain in animals, but it was not further developed as a drug most likely because of poor pharmacokinetic properties. The discovery of TRPV1 has reinvigorated these efforts and the first drug candidates have emerged. The new, selective TRPV1 antagonists are highly effective in animal models of acute inflammatory and chronic pain (Pomonis et al., 2003), sustaining the expectation that TRPV1 antagonists may become clinically useful drugs for the treatment of pain.

TRP channels other than TRPV1 may have utility as drug targets by themselves or for drugs that enhance the effects of selective TRPV1 antagonists (Clapham, 2003). TRPV2 channels are activated by higher temperatures (>52°C), and they are expressed by sensory neurons but also several tissues outside of the nervous system. TRPV4 is active at temperatures above 24°C, and it is activated by pressure as well as several chemical mediators including prostaglandin derivatives. It is located in many sensory neurons including pain-mediating C-fibers and also in many nonneuronal tissues. Reducing the expression of TRPV4 has beneficial effects in an animal model of painful neuropathy (Alessandri-Haber et al., 2004). TRPM8 responds to cold, is activated by temperatures below 26°C, and is expressed predominantly in sensory neurons. The channel harbors the receptor site for menthol, a chemical inducing cold sensation, which provides a natural starting point for a medicinal chemistry program. TRPA1 (ANKTM1) is activated by yet lower temperatures (<18°C) and is also the receptor site for allyl isothiocyanate, mustard oil, the active ingredient of horseradish, wasabi, and mustard. In addition it is influenced by cannabinol and bradykinin. TRPA1 is highly expressed by small sensory neurons and often co-localizes with TRPV1 (Story et al., 2003; Jordt et al., 2004). Extreme cold is perceived as painful, and cold skin is more sensitive to pressure stimuli, suggesting that inhibitors of TRPA1 might be beneficial for pain relief. As for the other TRP channels, the receptor site for natural ligands offers a convenient starting point for drug discovery efforts.

The TRP channels provide a most fascinating illustration of the complexity and beauty of terrestrial life and the opportunity for pharmacological exploitation. A single protein is able to sense changes in temperature and ionic environment. Evolution has provided plants with protective chemicals that cause a painful response in herbivores by directly activating the same sensory receptors. Humans have found culinary use of these plants to enhance sensory perception at the edge of painful sensation. The active ingredients identify receptor sites and chemical starting points for drug discovery programs. Most intriguing is the responsiveness of TRPV1 and TRPA1 to cannabinoids, identifying them as ionotropic cannabinoid receptors besides the metabotropic G-protein-coupled cannabinoid receptors. It is intriguing to speculate that effects on the TRP channels may mediate some of the enhancement of sensory perception described by cannabis consumers. The pharmacology of cannabinoid receptors may reveal medical utility for psychiatric diseases associated with altered sensory perception in addition to that for pain. Taken together, these considerations identify the TRP receptor area as one of the most interesting playing fields for future drug discovery.

15.4 OTHER PERIPHERAL MEDIATORS OF ACUTE PAIN

Tissue injury and inflammation induce the local synthesis and release of several mediators that directly or indirectly activate the $A\delta$- and C-sensory nerve fibers. The term "inflammatory soup" is sometimes used as a vague descriptor for this group of molecules. It includes prostaglandins, the monoamines serotonin and histamine, peptides such as bradykinin, protein-signaling factors such as interleukins, chemokines, TNF-α, and NGF, and additionally, ATP and protons. Tissue-specific cells, keratinocytes, fibroblasts, and muscle cells, contribute to the production of these mediators, as well as invading mast cells, macrophages, and granulocytes. Antagonists for any of the mediators are potentially useful to suppress acute pain, and their receptors represent putative drug targets of high interest. The prostaglandins and their receptors have been discussed above. The role of serotonin receptors will be addressed in the section on migraine. Histamine receptors are widely expressed outside of the pain pathways, reducing their attraction for pain drug discovery efforts. The other mediators and their receptors are discussed in the following paragraphs.

15.4.1 Bradykinin

Among the molecules causing pain when injected into the skin, bradykinin stands out as one of the most potent ones. It increases the vascular permeability and causes plasma extravasation at the site of injury, thereby enhancing the inflammatory response. It directly stimulates bradykinin B_1 and B_2 receptors on sensory fibers, which contribute to the activation TRPV1 channels (Shin et al., 2002). Both receptors appear suitable as drug targets. The B_2 receptors are constitutively expressed at high levels and inflammatory hyperalgesia is reduced in mice with null mutations of this receptor. The B_1 receptor is expressed at low levels normally but is induced in chronic pain states and inflammation, making it a putative target for drugs to control pain associated with chronic inflammation. B_1 receptor knockout mice respond only weakly to inflammatory pain. Selective B_1 antagonists suppress nociceptive reflexes in the spinal cord of animals with peripheral inflammation but not in normal animals (Mason et al., 2002). Both bradykinin receptors also exist in the spinal cord and the brain, complicating the simple picture of bradykinin as a peripheral pain mediator. Additional information on the expression of bradykinin receptors under normal conditions and disease states will help to determine the optimal receptor specificity and brain penetration for a drug candidate with highest chance to suppress pain in humans.

15.4.2 Cytokines

Several interleukins and chemokines induce strong pain sensations when injected into the skin. The sensory neurons of the dorsal root ganglia express many of the corresponding receptors in support of the view that the cytokines elicit a direct pain response (Oh et al., 2001). The findings blur the simple picture of clearly separated inflammatory and pain processes and opens up a new field of opportunity for drug discovery. Initial findings suggest that antagonists to IL-1 have analgesic potential (Wolf et al., 2003). A large number of putative drug targets await exploration, creating a difficult problem of prioritization. It will be necessary to identify the most potent mediators of pain and to assess the ability of a selective antagonist to make a meaningful contribution to pain in humans. Despite these difficulties the cytokine receptors are very appealing putative targets for future pain drugs. Small molecules selectively inhibiting the receptor sites of the cytokine receptor proteins as well as biological molecules able to capture the ligands are feasible as effective drugs.

15.4.3 Nerve Growth Factor

Nerve growth factor (NGF) is a perhaps surprising member of the pain mediator group. NGF is well-known as the first neurotrophic factor that drove the conceptualization of this research field. As with other neurotrophic factors, NGF regulates survival and maturation of neurons during early development. Mice with knockout mutations of NGF or its TrkA receptor are born with defective sensory and sympathetic nervous systems. In the adult peripheral nervous system NGF serves a new and unique role as potent mediator of the initial pain response. Normally developed sensory and sympathetic neurons no longer require NGF and are even able to regenerate in absence of NGF. In the adult organism the majority of $A\delta$- and C-fibers express TrkA receptors. Injections of NGF into normal skin causes prolonged pain sensation.

Tissue injury and inflammation strongly upregulate the synthesis and release of NGF from keratinocytes, fibroblasts, and muscle cells. NGF stimulates pain transmission by the sensory neurons through three complementary mechanisms. First, NGF directly activates TrkA receptors on sensory neurons. The TrkA receptors modify the function of TRPV1 channels and axonal sodium channels for signal transmission. Second, the released NGF stimulates TrkA receptors located on mast cells, causing the release of other pain mediators, including prostaglandins, serotonin, and bradykinin, that further enhance the pain response. Third, the stimulation of TrkA receptors by NGF on sensory neurons results in retrograde signaling to the cell body of the sensory neurons located in the dorsal root ganglia. This signal enhances the synthesis of the neurotransmitters substance P and CGRP, and ion channels that mediate pain sensation as well as signal propagation in the sensory axons and synaptic transmission to neurons in the spinal cord (Ji et al., 2002).

Biological antagonists against NGF are effective in animal models of acute inflammatory pain as well as chronic neuropathic pain (McMahon et al., 1995). Selective antagonists to TrkA receptors or biologicals able to capture NGF are thus expected to have beneficial effects in various pain conditions.

15.4.4   ATP and P2X Receptors

ATP released from injured cells is recognized by a family of specific cationic ion channels, the P2X receptors. They respond most robustly to ATP but also bind related purine derivatives and are part of a large purine receptor group that includes ion channels as well as G-protein-coupled receptors (Burnstock, 2000). Besides being a mediator of pain and the principal source of chemical energy in the cells, ATP serves as neurotransmitter in purinergic synapses. Seven related genes encode the proteins that form the functional $P2X_{1-7}$ receptors. Most of them are widely expressed in the nervous system, with the exception of $P2X_2$ and $P2X_3$ (which exist predominantly in small sensory neurons of the dorsal root ganglia), in subpopulations of sensory neurons that lack substance P and CGRP. The P2X containing neurons are responsive to glial cell-derived neurotrophic factor (GDNF) rather than NGF during early development, thus defining an interesting subpopulation of sensory neurons with potentially unique functions in pain sensation. In the sensory neurons the $P2X_2$ and $P2X_3$ form homo- and heteromeric channels. Gene knockout mice lacking the $P2X_3$ form show diminished responses to some forms of painful stimuli. A selective antagonist to $P2X_3$ and $P2X_{2/3}$ receptors blunts the response of rats to inflammatory pain but not other forms of acute pain, and is very effective in a model of chronic neuropathic pain (Jarvis et al., 2002). These findings are compatible with the view that ATP plays a role in the generation of inflammatory pain and a yet more important role in the development of chronic pain states. Indeed, intrathecal injection of the antagonist was more effective than local injection at the peripheral nerve, supporting the view that synaptic functions of ATP make an important contributor to chronic pain transmission.

15.4.5   H⁺ and the ASIC Channels

Acidosis, a feature of injured tissue, is recognized by TRPV1 but also a family of more specialized acid-sensing ionic channels (ASICs). Four genes encoding ASIC1-4 with several splicing variants have been characterized. They form homo- or heterotetrameric cation channels that are activated by low pH. They are widely expressed in the nervous system, but ASIC3 is abundant in sensory neurons where it co-localizes with CGRP. This channel appears to sense cardiac acidosis and to contribute to the sensation of chest pain. Mutant mice with null mutations of the ASIC3 channel respond abnormally to painful stimuli. Some of the direct responses are enhanced, whereas the development of chronic pain states is impaired. It has been speculated that the primary role of the ASICs is not in the direct sensation of pain but in the detection of fluctuations in microcirculation in nervous system and other tissues. In addition they appear to play a role in synaptic transmission, since knockout mice have deficits in synaptic plasticity. In the dorsal root ganglia, the expression of ASIC3 is regulated by NGF, compatible with the view that the channel is able to modify the pain response (Krishtal, 2003).

Many of the primary pain mediators and their receptors have the potential to lead to new, efficacious and selective pain drugs. Many of them participate in pain transmission in the spinal cord and the brain in addition to their role in pain sensation. These multiple roles increase the potential efficacy for drugs interfering with their actions, but they also increase the likelihood of effects unrelated to pain sensation.

15.5 SENSORY NEURON-SPECIFIC Na⁺ CHANNELS

Local anesthetics such as lidocaine are widely used to block well-defined regional pain. Injections onto the dental nerve prevent pain sensation during dental surgery. Epidural injections minimize pain during childbirth. Lidocaine is a general and potent inhibitor of voltage-gated sodium channels and prevents the propagation of axon potentials in all axons exposed to pharmacologically active concentrations. Systemic use of general Na⁺ channel antagonists would result in severe, life-threatening consequences, since these channels support essential functions in the nervous and cardiovascular system. Therapeutic utility could be obtained with compounds that specifically inhibit sodium channels in neurons participating in pain transmission. The sensory neurons of the dorsal root ganglia express the sodium channels, $Na_v1.1$ and $Na_v1.6$–$Na_v1.9$. The expression of channels $Na_v1.8$ and $Na_v1.9$ is restricted to the small sensory neurons that provide Aδ- and C-fibers for pain transmission. As an exception to the typical response of voltage-gated Na⁺ channels, these two channels are not inhibited by tetradotoxin and are responsible for tetradotoxin-resistant currents in sensory axons. Tetradotoxin-resistant currents were recognized for their special role in pain functions before the cloning of the channel proteins. They are enhanced during inflammatory pain, suggesting that blocking $Na_v1.8$ and $Na_v1.9$ channels may have beneficial effects in established pain states.

Drug discovery research has focused on $Na_v1.8$ because of its abundant expression in small sensory neurons. Studies on gene knockout mice point to a very special function in pain. $Na_v1.8$ knockout mice are normal except for impaired sensitivity to painful stimuli. The initial response to acute painful stimuli is only marginally affected, but these mice fail to develop hyperalgesia to prolonged painful stimulation (Laird et al., 2002). Suppression of $Na_v1.8$ channels may thus be particularly beneficial for treating pain during inflammation and protracted healing processes after injury. The $Na_v1.8$ channels are indubitably one of the most enticing novel drug targets in the pain area, and several biopharmaceutical companies are actively pursuing them. Local anesthetics, which bind to sites responsible for voltage-gating, offer a starting point for small-molecule drug discovery programs. Several natural toxins of peptidic nature bind to various parts of the channel protein and identify additional receptor sites (Table 15.2). Blockers of Na⁺ channels are used by many predatory animals to paralyze the victims, as illustrated by scorpion toxins, conotoxins derived from snails, and pompilidodotoxin from wasps. Since the drug target

Table 15.2 Toxins and drugs for voltage-gated Na⁺ channels

Drugs and Toxins	Mechanism of Action
Local anesthetics	Bind to inner surface of channel pore; produce use-dependent blocks
α-Scorpion toxin, β-scorpion toxin, β-pompilidotoxin	Immobilize voltage sensor
Tetrodotoxin, saxitonin, μ-conotoxins	Occlude channel pore
Veratridine, batrachotoxin, brevetoxins	Shift voltage dependence

is outside of the blood-brain barrier, peptide derivatives and other large biological molecules are not disadvantaged and may provide a rapid approach to drug discovery.

Despite the strong rationale for $Na_v1.8$, it would be wrong the neglect the other voltage-gated Na^+ channels. Because of its restricted expression and secondary role, $Na_v1.9$ may permit mild modulatory effects on pain transmission that could be useful for chronic, but not disabling pain states. $Na_v1.1$ and $Na_v1.6$ are nervous system specific, and it may be possible to exclude the central nervous system component by generating antagonists that do not cross the blood-brain barrier. The activity of the Na^+ channels determines the pharmacological effects of some of the inhibitors. Their efficacy and potency is enhanced during periods of high channel opening frequency. Activity-dependent antagonists may be able to suppress pain without blocking normal sensation, since channels open more frequently during pain transmission. The molecular complexity makes the voltage-dependent Na^+ channels a scientifically particularly interesting topic for drug discovery (Clare et al., 2000).

15.6   PAIN TRANSMISSION IN SPINAL CORD AND ASCENDING PATHWAYS

The first synaptic transmission of pain information takes places in the dorsal horn of the spinal cord. Effective pain relief is expected from any agent able to prevent neurotransmitter release from the sensory afferents or block the neurotransmitter receptors on postsynaptic neurons. Additional target opportunities are provided by the local interneurons and their neurotransmitter mechanisms. While conceptually very attractive, inhibition of pain transmission in the spinal cord encounters several difficulties. There appears to be no selective pain neurotransmitter nor pain transmission mechanism. Additional, undesired effects are thus likely for inhibitors of spinal cord pain transmission. The spinal cord synapses are within the blood barrier, enforcing more rigorous structural constraints on drug candidates than on those inhibiting pain mechanisms at the distal terminal of the sensory axons. Biological drugs have to be given by invasive procedures to be effective. Despite these caveats, several strategies have emerged that may lead to clinically effective and useful inhibitors of pain transmission.

15.6.1   Ziconotide and Ca^{2+} Channel Blockers

Voltage-gated Ca^{2+} channels of the $Ca_v2.2$ subtype, also called N-type Ca^{2+} channels, are expressed by small sensory neurons and are abundant in the dorsal horn of the spinal cord. They co-localize with substance P, a co-transmitter of the sensory neurons, and are the likely mediators of neurotransmitter release from sensory nerve endings. $Ca_v2.2$ channels are inhibited by ω-conopeptide, a toxin produced by a predatory marine snail. Intrathecal infusions of ω-conopeptide to rats blunt their response to painful stimuli. The selectivity of $Ca_v2.2$ channels is provided by the $\alpha1B$ subunit, which forms functional channels together with β and $\alpha2\delta$ subunits. Mice with null mutations of $\alpha1B$ have diminished pain sensitivity (Saegusa et al., 2001). Experimental chronic pain in animals causes massive upregulation of this subunit. Ziconotide, a synthetic derivate of ω-conotoxin, has been developed as drug and shown good efficacy in human studies when given intrathecally to patients with severe cancer pain. Cardiovascular functions of $Ca_v2.2$ preclude systemic administration of ziconotide. Adverse effects were common even with intrathecal administration. Ziconotide and related $Ca_v2.2$ blockers are thus likely to find a role in the treatment of severe opioid-resistant pain as it occurs in certain forms of cancer. More general use seems feasible for drugs with a higher degree of selectivity than ziconotide. Various β subunits may characterize subtypes of the $Ca_v2.2$ receptors and provide opportunity for specific inhibitors. As argued for the voltage-gated Na^+ channels, it may be possible to design activity-dependent inhibitors of $Ca_v2.2$ blocking only those channels that are hyperactive in pain conditions.

15.6.2 Glutamate Receptor Antagonists

Pain-mediating Aδ- and C-fibers release glutamate as their primary transmitter that stimulates various pre- and postsynaptic ionotropic and metabotropic glutamate receptors. Inhibitors of the NMDA subtypes are effective in animal pain assays. Ketamine, one of the NMDA antagonists, is frequently used to control pain in veterinary medicine and, occasionally, for treatment of severe opiate-resistant pain in humans. As discussed in Chapter 11 on ischemic stroke, NMDA antagonists cause a broad array of effects, including psychotic symptoms, which make impossible their use as general drugs. The problem may be overcome with subtype-selective compounds. NMDA receptors are composed of the NMDAR1 subunit that associates with additional NMDAR2A–2D subunits. The dorsal horn is enriched in NR2B subunits, suggesting that selective inhibition of NMDA receptors with this subtype may provide effective pain control with minimal adverse effects. Several companies have reported the synthesis of selective inhibitors of NR2B-containing NMDA receptors that are effective in animal models of pain and do not show obvious adverse effects in tests of other behavioral functions (Clairborne et al., 2003). Further explorative studies will hopefully confirm that this attractive profile is maintained in humans.

Ionotropic glutamate receptors other than NMDA receptors, and metabotropic glutamate receptors are widely expressed in pain pathways and contribute to the synaptic regulation of pain transmission. Intrathecal administration of AMPA and kainate receptor antagonists attenuates the pain responses in experimental animals. Chronic pain conditions alter the expression levels of specific subunits of AMPA and kainate receptors in the spinal cord and the brain stem (Guo et al., 2002). Among the metabotropic glutamate receptors, the $mGluR_1$ subtype has been most strongly linked to spinal and subcortical pain pathways. Selective antagonists are highly effective in various animal models (Varney and Gereau, 2002). All these receptors participate in many neuronal functions other than pain, making the therapeutic window between desired and adverse effects the major issue for drug discovery programs. Those receptors with highest relative expression in pain pathways and those that are upregulated during chronic pain states will provide the most promising putative drug targets. Unfortunately, none of the glutamate receptor subtypes appears to be uniquely limited to pain pathways, thus limiting the expectations for these drug discovery approaches.

15.6.3 Neuropeptide Transmitters

Neuropeptides are produced and released as co-transmitters by sensory neurons, interneurons in the spinal cord, and many neurons that influence pain transmission in the ascending pathways. Substance P stands out among them, both from a historical and biological perspective. The majority of pain-conducting sensory neurons contain substance P, and this peptide was the first histochemical marker for sensory cells and axons. Substance P was the first transmitter linked to pain transmission, and it was hypothesized several decades ago that antagonists for substance P receptors might have utility as drugs for pain treatment. The NK_1 neurokinin receptor subtype dominates in the spinal cord where it mediates the actions of substance P on postsynaptic neurons. Knockout mice with deletions of the NK_1 receptor gene or the gene coding for preprotachykinin, the precursor protein from which substance P is cleaved, show a blunted response to painful stimuli. Selective NK_1 receptor antagonists attenuate the response to painful stimuli in various animal models. Despite the convincing animal data and the high expectations generated by them, aprepritant, a selective NK_1 antagonist approved for the control of emesis in humans, failed to show any efficacy in clinical studies of acute and chronic pain (Hill, 2000). It is possible that further clinical studies will reveal utility of this compound for special pain conditions. However, the disconnect between animal and human data remains astonishing. Incomplete evolutionary conservation of peptide expression offers a speculative explanation for the discrepancy.

Important other peptides in pain transmission include CGRP and the enkephalins. As substance P, CGRP is contained in a large fraction of the small sensory neurons and their pain-conducting axons. Similar arguments for CGRP receptors as target for new pain drugs can be made as those for the NK_1 receptor. The most attractive utility for CGRP antagonists appears to be for the control of migraine pain. Enkephalins, further discussed in the section on opioids, are abundant as co-transmitters in spinal cord interneurons and act on presynaptic opioid receptors on the terminals of the sensory axons. In addition to the opioid receptors, sensory neurons express orphan G-protein-coupled receptors that may mediate the actions of yet to be discovered neuropeptides. The family of *mas*-related genes (Mrgs) contains several G-protein-coupled receptors that are selectively expressed by the small sensory neurons. They are activated by peptides of the RF-amide group (peptides with an arginin-phenylalanin-amide motive at the *C*-terminal), but the precise ligands of the sensory-neuron specific Mrgs remain to be identified. Their unique expression patterns have prompted the exploration of utility as drug targets (Zylka et al., 2003). Significant species differences complicate this evaluation, and add weight to the view that neuropeptide mechanisms have elevated evolutionary variability.

15.6.4 Adenosine Receptor Antagonists

Adenosine is a ubiquitous metabolite and signaling molecule that activates the G-protein-coupled adenosine receptors A_1, A_{2A}, A_{2B}, and A_3. These receptors are widely expressed within and outside of the nervous system and mediate many physiological functions. The interest in these receptors from the pain perspective reflects anecdotal evidence for beneficial effects of caffeine. Many of the generally available remedies for pain and cold contain caffeine, in absence of robust medical evidence for efficacy. Adenosine is contained in sensory neurons and released in the spinal cord, where it is able to influence the activity of postsynaptic neurons. Selective antagonists for the A_{2B} receptor subtype blunted the response to painful stimuli in animal models of acute pain, suggesting that this receptor might provide a target for pain drugs (Abo-Salem et al., 2004). At least some of the actions of adenosine may reflect direct actions on the TRPV1 channel protein (Puntembekar et al., 2004).

15.6.5 Cannabinoid Receptor Agonists

The analgesic effects of cannabis have been heralded by patient advocates who suffer from cancer, AIDS, and other chronic diseases with a pain component. The drug indubitably improves the well-being of the patients, although it is not clear whether analgesic or psychogenic effects make the dominant contribution. The active ingredient of cannabis, tetrahydrocannabinol activates two types of G-protein-coupled receptors, the CB_1 and CB_2 receptors. Most behavioral effects are mediated by the CB_1 subtype, which is expressed abundantly in the spinal cord and the brain, whereas the CB_2 subtype dominates in non-neuronal tissues. Both receptors respond to cannabinol derivatives and to endogenous ligands, including anandamide. Mice with null mutations of the CB_1 gene respond normally to direct painful stimuli. Agonists of both receptors show diminished hyperalgesia following inflammation. However, the CB_1 receptors are among the regulators of appetite and food intake, making it likely that weight gain will be an adverse effect of such drugs. CB_1 reverse agonists, believed to suppress constitutively active receptors, are in clinical development for the treatment of obesity. Despite these caveats the pharmacology of cannabinoid receptor sites offers unique potential because binding sites not only exist on CB_1 and CB_2 receptors but also on TRPV1 and TRPA1 temperature-sensitive channels (Iversen, 2003). Compounds with agonistic effects on CB_1 and antagonistic effects on the channels, while difficult to produce, might have uniquely beneficial action in the treatment of pain.

15.7 OPIATES AND PAIN PERCEPTION

To this day morphine remains one of the most useful drugs and a true marvel of natural pharmacology. For intolerable, severe pain morphine and other opiates are the only drugs with satisfactory efficacy. The spectrum and pattern of opiate actions is very complex. They affect pain sensation, but their beneficial actions mainly reflect their ability to alter the transmission and perception of pain. Patients on opiate medication may say that they still feel the pain but no longer care about it. The medical benefits of morphine and opiates are limited by a complex array of additional and adverse effects. These compounds generate intellectual confusion, they immobilize the gastrointestinal system, and they cause respiratory depression that is fatal at high doses. First-time users typically experience sedation, nausea, and vomiting. With repeated use, pleasant sensations tend to take over. Recurring use of opiates is associated with a general feeling of well-being and sometimes euphoria. Over the millennia of its use in many cultures, opium with its active ingredient morphine has been consumed for recreational purpose. Praise for the beneficial effects are abundant in poetry and belletristic literature, as illustrated by a quote from the English author Thomas de Quincey written in 1821:

> The opium eater . . . feels that the diviner part of his nature is paramount; that is, the moral affections are in a state of cloudless serenity; and over all is the great light of majestic intellect . . .

The abundance of purified morphine and its frequent use from the mid nineteenth century on, however, have revealed in bright light the ugly consequences of chronic opiate use, addiction and dependence. Morphine addiction is a known but well-contained problem in the medical community. Much more significant is the problem generated by the abuse of morphine derivatives such as heroin that destroys the emotional and economic basis of many human lives. Most large cities have a subculture of opiate addicts with links to criminal activities.

Opiate actions are mediated by G-protein-coupled receptors, the μ, δ, and κ opioid receptors. The medical community has started to adopt the corresponding, easier acronyms MOR, DOR, and KOR. Several neuropeptides function as naturally occurring ligands for these receptors. These endogenous opioid peptides include leu- and met-enkephalins, dynorphin-A and -B, and several variants of endorphin. The peptides are cleavage products of precursor polypeptides with multiple functions. Proenkephalin contains the sequences for the two enkephalins. Proopiomelanocortin is the precursor of melanocyte-stimulating hormone (MSH), adrenocorticotropin (ACTH), and β-endorphin. The two dynorphins and an endorphin are cleaved from prodynorphin. Two endogenous opioid peptides composed of only four amino acids, endomorphin-1 and endomorphin-2, activate selectively the μ receptor subtype (Zadina, 2002). They are abundant in nervous system areas containing this receptor subtype. The synthetic pathway generating these peptides in vivo remains to be characterized. All endogenous opioids are widely distributed and are participants in many physiological processes, and the complex expression and cleavage patterns tend to complicate the study of opioid mechanism.

Agonistic stimulation of μ receptors is responsible for most analgesic effects of the opiates. This receptor subtype is abundant in neuronal pathways of pain sensation and transmission. It is expressed by small sensory neurons of the dorsal root ganglia from which it is transported to the peripheral pain-sensing nerve endings and the terminals in the spinal cord that transmit information to interneurons and ascending neurons. Many interneurons in the dorsal horn contain opioid peptides that modify the release of sensory neuron transmitters through presynaptic receptors and postsynaptic receptors on ascending projection neurons. The spinal cord functions support the view that endogenous opioids suppress neuronal activity in absence of pain sensation and that exogenous opiate drugs enhance these naturally occurring actions. However, the inability of opioid receptor antagonists to produce significant behavioral effects in normal animals minimizes the significance of these physiological processes. Opioid-containing interneurons in the spinal cord are innervated by the descending serotonergic and noradrenergic neurons and mediate their descending regulatory influence in pain transmission. In the brain, μ receptors and endogenous opioids are abundant in areas linked to pain control, including the thalamus and the periaqueductal gray. The receptors and their ligands are also plentiful in areas linked to emotional control, the amygdala, hippocampus, and locus coeruleus, in subcortical motor areas, as well as in many cortical areas. The wide distribution patterns explain the complexity of behavioral effects produced by opiate drugs (Kieffer and Gaveriaux-Ruff, 2002).

Drug discovery efforts over more than a century have yielded many opiate drugs with different potency and pharmacokinetic profiles. Methadone is used as less potent substitute to heroin in the treatment of drug addicts. Naloxone, an opioid receptor antagonist, is used to stop detrimental effects of opiate overdosing. Fentanyl is a highly potent, frequently used compound that selectively activates the μ receptor subtype. Its spectrum of action and addictive potential is very similar to that of morphine and other nonselective opioid receptor agonists, supporting the conclusion that δ and κ receptors do not significantly contribute to analgesic and the adverse effects of opiates. It remains possible that μ agonists with specific antagonistic or agonistic contributions by the δ and κ receptors will have superior profiles, but the long history of failed efforts tends to diminish the enthusiasm for this approach. Despite many claims it has not been possible to adequately separate the desired analgesic effects of opiates from their multiple adverse effects and addictive potential (Ballantyne and Mao, 2003).

Progress in opioid receptor drug discovery opioid is achievable when separating the peripheral from central effects. Several research groups are exploring the therapeutic potential of opiate agonists that do not cross the blood-brain barrier. These compounds activate receptors on peripheral endings of the sensory nerve terminals that mediate the actions of opioid peptides released in response to tissue injury and inflammation. In animal models local injections of opiate drugs at the site of inflammation suppress some of the pain responses. In the clinical setting opiates are given locally for pain control following knee surgery. Local opiate therapy is not as effective as systemic therapy, however, and clinical trials have failed with an opiate unable to cross into the brain. Compounds with different receptor activity profiles may show better efficacy in the future. The κ receptors in particular are believed to be key mediators of peripheral opiate sensation (Stein et al., 2003).

Utilization of blood-brain barrier selectivity provides the basis for an approach to improve the adverse effect profile of existing opiate drugs. From a practical perspective, gastrointestinal immobility is the dominant adverse effect in pain control following surgery with hospitalization. Patients can only be released from the hospital when gastrointestinal functions have returned to normal. While perhaps of secondary medical importance, this adverse effect of opiates is a major determinant of hospitalization costs and medical expenditure for the entire society. The gastrointestinal effects of opiates are predominantly mediated by μ receptors located outside of the blood-brain barrier. Since the analgesic opiate effects in severe pain are primarily mediated by receptors in the spinal cord and the brain, it is possible to suppress in a selective way the effects on gastrointestinal functions with μ antagonists unable to cross the blood-brain barrier. A first drug candidate of this kind, alvimopan, reduced the hospitalization stay following surgery in a clinical study (Taguchi et al., 2001). It seems likely that this and similar drugs will improve the quality of post-operative pain control. The peripheral opiate receptor antagonists provide only a partial success, though, since the medically most relevant adverse effects of opiates, respiratory depression, and addiction are mediated by receptors within the brain.

15.8 CHRONIC NEUROPATHIC PAIN

Many patients suffer from chronic pain in absence of external painful stimuli. Neuropathic, the term used to describe this condition, reflects the concept that pathological changes in the nervous system itself are responsible for the erroneous pain signal transmission. Painful neuropathy is often experienced by patients who suffered traumatic nervous system injury at an earlier time. Compression of a peripheral nerve because of a ruptured vertebral disk and transection of a nerve during severe limb injury are examples. Neuropathic pain is a frequent consequence of diabetes. Acute viral infections by herpes or HIV often leave behind neuropathic pain as a disturbing reminder of the primary pathological process. Painful neuropathy can be initiated by demyelization in multiple sclerosis or by mutations in genes encoding myelin components and causing hereditary neuropathy. Drug-induced neuropathies are common in cancer treatment and occur as a consequence of alcohol abuse. The various forms of neuropathies present distinct clinical features but share the pain component.

The molecular mechanisms responsible for the pain sensation are yet to be clarified in detail, but three principal components have emerged. First, past injury to sensory neurons leaves them with increased propensity to generate action potentials in absence of pain stimuli. In absence of a molecular guidance toward the natural target, transected sensory axons tend to sprout locally and form aberrant connections or a local axon ball where pain transmission is being generated. Spontaneous activity often originates at the site of nerve compression or demyelination, thus generating ectopic discharges. Phantom pain following limb amputation may be caused by such spontaneous pain transmission. The redistribution of ion channels, including $Na_v1.8$, is believed to contribute to the generation of ectopic discharges.

Spinal sensitization is a second major contributor to neuropathic pain. Many mediators of pain, NGF in particular, increase the expression in the dorsal root sensory ganglia of molecular components for axonal and synaptic transmission. Ion channels, neurotransmitters, and neurotransmitter receptors become more abundant and increase pain transmission to the ascending pathways. Activation of p38 Map kinase in spinal cord glial cells contributes to spinal sensitization (Tsuda et al., 2004). It appears that many molecular players, which are gradually being discovered by modern pain research, participate in the complex mechanisms of spinal cord synaptic plasticity. The third contributor to neuropathic pain, plasticity in the brain, is the least understood. Imaging studies in patients point to considerable rearrangements in the cortical areas activated during pain perception. Functional as well as morphological plasticity of pain systems in the spinal cord and the brain contribute to the wind-up of chronic pain perception.

The current therapy for neuropathic pain is highly unsatisfactory (Mendell and Sahenk, 2003). NSAIDs show little or no efficacy. Opiates reduce neuropathic pain, but high doses with considerable adverse effects are required for meaningful efficacy. In absence of truly efficacious drugs, clinical experimentation has led to the introduction of many compounds with partial efficacy into the pharmacotherapy of painful neuropathies. Several anti-epileptic drugs are among them, including gabapentin, a widely prescribed and commercially very successful compound. Gabapentin requires very high doses for meaningful clinical efficacy, and adverse effects, even though mild, are common at these drug levels. The compound is a structural derivative of the inhibitory neurotransmitter GABA, but there is no convincing evidence that it stimulates any of the GABAergic mechanisms. It binds with relatively high affinity to the $\alpha_2\delta$ auxiliary subunit of voltage-gated Ca^{2+} channels, suggesting that its mechanism of action is related to the regulation of neurotransmitter release. Reverse pharmacology approaches may identify more potent and efficacious gabapentin derivatives. Besides gabapentin, antidepressant monoamine uptake inhibitors are frequently prescribed for the treatment of neuropathy. Early tricyclics appear to be more efficacious than selective serotonin uptake blockers, but few comparative studies have been carried out. For these drugs it is difficult to separate primary effects on neuropathic pain from antidepressant effects, and no distinct mechanism of action for the analgesic effect has been identified.

The current knowledge on neuropathic pain mechanisms provides tentative guidance for target selection and drug discovery efforts. Development and clinical trials of $Na_v1.8$ blockers seem to be an obvious goal because of their selective expression in pain-conducting sensory neurons and involvement in ectopic action potential generation. Components of synaptic mechanisms that are upregulated following chronic pain sensation appear to be attractive, since they might be targets for drugs to counteract spinal sensitization. Several neuropeptides, including galanin, neuropeptide Y, and cholecystokinin, fall into this category. Using gene array technologies, a number of research groups have initiated the broad search for genes that are upregulated in tissues from animal models of neuropathic pain. Extension of these studies to proteomic techniques and to spinal cord tissue from humans with neuropathic pain is likely to identify a number of crucial regulators of synaptic wind-up. Neurotrophic factors have been considered as biological therapeutics for neuropathy because of their ability to promote regeneration of axons, but they may also restore normal patterns of protein expression and so re-establish a pain-free state. Artemin, a member of the glial cell-derived neurotrophic factor (GDNF) protein family, effectively reverses hyperalgesia in an animal model of neuropathic pain (Sah et al., 2003). The significant medical need, the complex and scientifically very interesting mechanisms of neuropathic pain, and the recently emerged opportunities are likely to generate strong drug discovery efforts in this area.

15.9 MIGRAINE

Migraine is the most prevalent painful condition and the most significant one from a socioeconomic point of perspective, measured as days lost at work. Epidemiological studies revealed that 5% of the general population experience more than 15 migraine days per year. The disease is most prevalent between adolescence and middle age and affects women more often than men. Migraine is a unique pathophysiological condition that involves the visual, nervous, cardiovascular, and gastrointestinal systems (Fig. 15.6; Goadsby et al., 2002). The mechanisms generating the painful sensation are fairly well understood. Far less is known about the underlying causes and the triggering and initial events of a migraine attack. Rare familial forms have been associated with a missense

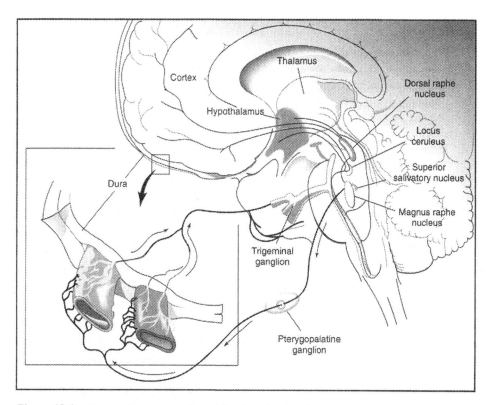

Figure 15.6 Migraine disease mechanisms. Dilatation of the blood vessels in the dura activates the trigeminal sensory neurons and mediate pain information to the brain. The input is modulated by neurons of the Raphe nuclei and the locus coeruleus. A reflex loop is provided by the the parasympathetic system through the pterygopalatine ganglion. (Reprinted with permission. Goatsby et al., 2002)

mutation in the α_1 subunit of the $Ca_v2.1$ voltage-gated Ca^{2+} channel and in the ATP1A2 subunit of Na^+/K^+ ATPase. Most events appear to be caused by a combination of environmental and multiple genetic influences. Migraine attacks are believed to initiate in the brain stem and to involve waves of neuronal activation that slowly propagate from the brain stem generator into wider brain areas, similar to the phenomenon of spreading depression that can be experimentally induced in animals. The concept of propagating wave is able to explain the gradually evolving visual sensations and the frequent nausea at the beginning of the attack. It receives strong experimental support from transgenic animals expressing the human proteins associated with familial migraine where increased susceptibility for cortical spreading depression has been demonstrated (van den Maagdenberg et al., 2004).

The pain sensation during migraine is thought to be a secondary event in the cardiovascular and peripheral nervous system. The brain tissue itself does not contain any pain sensors, and the "headache" is caused by cellular changes at the surface. Axons of sensory neurons from the trigeminal ganglion accompany the large cranial vessels, surface vessels, and meningeal blood vessels. The proximal axonal branches of these sensory neurons synapse in the brainstem onto ascending neurons to the thalamus and other forebrain areas. They also form a reflex connection to the parasympathetic neurons that project through the petrygopalatine ganglion back to the cranial blood vessel. This trigeminal-autonomic reflex loop is believed to be hyperactive in migraine. Release of neuropeptides, including CGRP, and other mediators cause dilatation of the cranial blood vessels. The widening of the blood vessels stimulates pain receptors on trigeminal sensory fibers that mediate the sensation of pain.

Efficacious medications for migraine are available that minimize the disturbances and the pain of migraine. NSAIDs and Cox-2 inhibitors are useful for the treatment of the prolonged headache pain, but they are unable to prevent or abort migraine attacks. Opiates are only very rarely used because of the evident adverse effects at doses to control acute, severe headache pain. Some patients benefit from the use of ergotamine drugs, despite lack of convincing evidence for efficacy in controlled clinical studies. The ergot derivatives bind to various monoamine receptors, increasing the probability of substantial interindividual variations in efficacy. The most effective drugs for migraine therapy are the triptans, agonists for 5-HT$_{1B}$ and 5-HT$_{1D}$ receptors. These receptors mediate vasoconstriction of cerebral blood vessels, making it possible to stop a crucial component of the trigeminal-autonomic reflect loop. Sumatriptan and more recently introduced drugs of the triptan class benefit about a third of the migraine patients in very substantial ways. Their efficacy and safety has been documented in multiple well-designed clinical trials. Many patients, however, respond not at all or to insufficient degrees to the triptans. Thus migraine continues to represent a very significant medical need and area of interest for drug discovery.

Recent drug discovery efforts have concentrated on subtype selective serotonin receptors and on peptide mediators of vasodilatation. Selective 5-HT$_{1D}$ agonists have been pursued because this subtype is selectively located on trigeminal nerve endings, whereas the 5-HT$_{1B}$ receptors are more widely distributed and might mediate adverse effects able to limit dosing of the mixed 5-HT$_{1B/D}$ agonist triptan drugs. 5-HT$_7$ receptors expressed in the brain stem have been the target for drug discovery efforts based on positive observations with agonistic drugs in animal models of migraine. No convincing clinical data have emerged as yet from these efforts. Good progress has been made with the efforts on CGRP, a significant mediator of cerebral vasodilatation. Activity in the trigeminal-autonomic reflex loop causes the release of CGRP from the sensory ending into the local blood stream.

Potent vasodilatory actions of CGRP are mediated by receptors on the vascular cells. A peptidic antagonists to the CGRP receptors, which has to be given by intravenous administration, has been found effective in a double-blinded clinical study with migraine patients, thus providing initial clinical validation for this drug target (Doods et al., 2000). Selective antagonists to the CGRP receptors in the cranial vessels with appropriate pharmacokinetic properties will hopefully provide effective drugs for the treatment of migraine and able to complement the triptans.

15.10 ANIMAL MODELS AND EXPERIMENTAL MEDICINE

A large number of animal models are available for drug testing in the pain area. In their vast majority these are rodent assays, since the justified animal welfare concerns prevent us to expose higher species and monkeys to experimental painful conditions. Several of the models have found general acceptance in the pain field. They provide the backbone for many drug discovery programs. Many variations have been introduced over the years by individual researchers, rendering comparisons of data across laboratories often difficult (Le Bars et al., 2001). The predictive power of the animal models is best in pain conditions with well-understood disease mechanisms, inflammatory pain for example. Animal models for complex conditions such as migraine or neuropathic pain are less well validated. Efficacy of drug candidates in specific animal models often defines the path forward in clinical experimentation. A small number of well-defined conditions are widely used to establish clinical efficacy and to define areas of medical utility. Table 15.3 illustrates some of the feasible pathways from animal model studies to clinical pain conditions.

15.10.1 Acute Pain

Models for acute thermal pain rely on the spinal withdrawal reflex in response to direct heat sensation. In the hot-plate test, rodents are put on a heated surface, and the time interval until they begin to lift and lick their feet is measured to quantify the pain response. In variations of this test, a heat-inducing laser beam is directed to the foot surface, or the paws are immersed into heated water. In the tail-flick assay, the heat source is directed to the tail. Opiate drugs work well in these assays because they increase inhibitory transmission in the spinal cord, whereas the NSAIDs are not effective. The tests have limited value in the prediction of the therapeutic utility of drug candidates, since acute thermal pain is not a necessary component of medically important pain conditions.

Animal assays with pain caused by tissue damage or injury reproduce the events of many medically relevant conditions. In assays for incision pain, small wounds are inflicted in the skin and skeletal muscle. In other injury models, tissue damage is induced by injections of formalin or other noxious agents under the skin, or by burns to the skin. Local injections of immunogens, such as carrageenan or Freund's complete adjuvant, cause pronounced inflammatory pain. Incision, burn, chemical, and inflammatory damage is typically inflicted to the paws of the animals, making it possible to use foot withdrawal as readout for analgesic efficacy. Exposure to heat and touch, measured several days after the injury, is used to assess thermal and mechanical allodynia, respectively. The latency of the response, and the threshold of stimulus intensity causing a response, provide equally valuable measurements. A series of filaments of increasing thickness, the so-called van Frey filaments, are used to define mechanical sensitivity. Water bath or heated surfaces with temperature gradients are used to define the thermal sensitivity threshold.

Table 15.3 Pathways from animal models to clinical indications

Animal Models	Initial Clinical Studies	Medical Condition
Acute Pain		
Incisions pain	Dental impaction	Postoperative pain
Formalin tissue damage	Dental extraction	Injury-induced pain
Experimental inflammatory pain	Bunionectomy	
Burn pain	Joint-replacement surgery	
Chronic Pain		
Chronic Freund's adjuvant-	Osteoarthritis pain	Arthritis pain
induced arthritis	Postherpetic neuralgia	Cancer pain
Cancer pain		Lower back pain
Nerve ligation pain		Phantom limb pain
Dorsal root transection pain		Painful diabetic
Spinal cord injury pain		neuropathy
Visceral Pain		
Turpentine bladder hyperreactivity	Cystitis pain	General visceral pain
Mustard oil colonic pain	Irritable bowel syndrome	
Acetic acid peritoneal pain	Prostatitis pain	
Migraine		
Neurogenic vasodilatation	Familial or frequent	General migraineurs
	migraineurs	and headache patients

Opiates and NSAIDs are effective in the animal models of injury pain and provide positive controls for drug candidates with other mechanisms of action. The assays are directly relevant for human conditions where pain is caused by involuntary tissue damage following accidents or voluntary surgical procedures. Experimental medical tests to establish initial proof-of principle include several postsurgical conditions. Dental impaction pain is the most widely used and simplest clinical trial. Dental extraction, bunionectomy (removal of excessive bone from the foot), knee and hip replacement surgery, arthroscopy, and menstrual pain provide good alternatives. Efficacy in any of these models is a reliable predictor for clinical efficacy in a broad spectrum of medical situations with pain caused by tissue damage.

15.10.2 Chronic Pain

Chronic pain is caused by sustained disease processes that provide ongoing stimulation of pain sensors on the innervating nerves or, alternatively, by pathological processes in the nervous system itself. Animal models of chronic arthritis or cancer pain are examples for assays based on sustained generation of pain stimuli in the periphery. In an animal model for chronic arthritis pain, Freund's complete adjuvant is injected systemically to cause a bodywide inflammatory reaction and significant arthritic degeneration of the joints. To assess the pain, the intensity of vocalization of the animals during forced movement of the ankle joint is measured. Positive results in this model of chronic arthritic pain are often followed by clinical studies in osteoarthritis and subsequent broad evaluation in a variety of arthritic conditions. In models of cancer pain, tumor cells are transplanted to initiate a process of gradual tissue destruction. The predictive power of the models are closely linked to the specific nature of the cancer studied. Morphine provides the gold standard in all animal models of sustained pain. NSAIDs are effective in models with a strong inflammatory component. Detailed comparative studies on inflammatory and cancer pain models have revealed substantial differences in the nature of the pain and the response to drugs (Luger et al., 2002). They remind the investigators of the significant heterogeneity among chronic pain conditions and the need to develop animal models that more precisely reflect the human condition.

In the models of neuropathic pain, surgical procedures on the nervous system itself are performed to induce a painful condition. The most widely used assays are the chronic construction injury model and the dorsal root transection model. A tight ligation of the sciatic nerve produces hyperalgesia and allodynia of the paw in the chronic constriction injury model. A comparable behavioral endpoint is achieved in the dorsal root injury model by transecting some, but not all, of the sensory nerve roots that connect sciatic nerve sensory axons to the spinal cord. In a third type of model, hyperalgesia and allodynia are produced by partial transections of the spinal cord. Morphine, but not NSAIDs, effectively suppresses the pain response in these animals. Gabapentin, a drug used frequently to treat chronic pain, is partially effective, providing substantial validation for these animal models as predictors of clinical efficacy. Initial clinical studies typically use a well-defined clinical condition, for example, postherpetic neuralgia, persistent pain that follows the viral infection of a sensory nerve. Efficacy in such a trial is believed to predict utility in broader conditions including nerve compression pain, phantom limb pain, and painful diabetic neuropathy.

15.10.3 Visceral Pain

Several chronic painful conditions of the viscera are comparable to chronic inflammatory pain, since both are caused by sustained activation of peripheral sensory receptors. They deserve special consideration because of the unique nature and organ-specificity of the corresponding animal models. Turpentine injections into the bladder generate a model for bladder pain and hyperreactivity, which is believed to predict efficacy in painful chronic cystitis, a difficult and harmful disease. Colonic pain is reproduced in animals by injecting mustard oil or trinitrobenzene sulfate into the colon. Acetic acid injections into the peritoneal cavity cause distributed visceral pain. In these animal assays, behavioral signs of discomfort such as abdominal contractions serve as simple readouts for pain. They are often complemented by more precise measurements of pain induced by forced distension of intestinal organs. As for all animal models of pain, the opiates are effective in these animal models and provide a positive control for testing drug candidates with novel mechanisms. Clinical trials for intestinal pain are less well standardized than those for other forms of pain. Painful chronic cystitis and irritable bowel syndrome are often used as initial indications to establish efficacy.

15.10.4 Migraine Pain

There are no established and convincing animal models that replicate the human migraine pathophysiology. Drug discovery programs have relied on animal assays that reproduce the dilatation of blood vessels at the surface of the brain, the process believed to generate the headache pain. In vitro assays, in which rings of human cerebral blood vessels are attached to a pressure transducer, make it possible to directly measure the vasodilatory potential of drug candidates. In an elegant in vivo model, the dilatation is measured directly at the surface of the brain with an intravital microscopy technique (Williamson et al., 1997). The surface of the brain is exposed in anesthetized animals, and electrical stimulation is applied to the dura. The electrical activity causes neurogenic vasodilatation that can be directly observed and quantified. The ability of drug candidates to reduce the vessel expansion serves as predictor of clinical efficacy. Triptan 5-HT$_{1B/D}$ agonists as well as CGRP antagonists are effective in this animal model and will serve as positive controls in the search of future drugs. Transgenic mice replicating the rare forms of familial migraine are being generated by several research groups and will provide valuable tools for the investigation of disease mechanisms as well as utility in drug evaluations.

15.11   CONCLUSIONS

Pain is both an important protective mechanism for the body and the most prevalent medical condition. Many molecular and cellular contributors to pain sensation and perception are known and well understood, but important aspects related to integration of signals and plasticity of the pathways remain to be fully explored. Pain sensation starts with the stimulation of receptor proteins located on the distal axons of sensory neurons that innervate most tissues. The receptors include channels and G-protein-coupled receptors that respond to changes in temperature, pressure, and chemical environment caused by tissue injury and damage. A complex array of primary and secondary mediators provide multiple and partially overlapping stimulatory influences to the pain sensors. Sensory axons originating in neurons of the dorsal root ganglia connect the pain sensors to the spinal cord and transmit the information to interneurons and projection neurons in the dorsal horn. Ascending projections through the brainstem and the thalamus link pain sensation to the cortical areas of pain perception. Enhanced transmission and plasticity in these pathways is a common consequence of sustained pain sensation. Spinal sensitization and wind-up of cerebral circuits are contributors to chronic painful conditions.

The pain pathways offer a wide variety of potential drug targets. Somewhat surprisingly, the current drugs utilize only a small fraction of them. Morphine and opiates, the most effective drugs, act at peripheral receptors, spinal cord synaptic mechanisms and pain circuits in the brain. They provide the gold standard for efficacy of any future pain medications, but their use is limited by significant adverse effects and a high addictive potential. NSAIDs and the more selective Cox-2 inhibitors diminish the actions of prostandoid compounds, a group of important secondary mediators of pain. The mechanisms of action of acetaminophen and gabapentin, widely used for treating, respectively, acute and chronic pain conditions, remain to be discovered. Despite clinical use over more than a century, the opiates and NSAID fields remain fields of opportunity for further improvements.

Current drug discovery efforts exploit an abundance of attractive target opportunities. Among the primary sensor proteins, specific members of the TRP and other channel families make it possible to directly suppress the initial step of pain sensation. Antagonists against the secondary mediators may be equally effective. Interference with bradykinin, NGF, and specific cytokines appears to be among the most promising approaches. Effective drugs may be found among compounds that interfere with the actions of ion channels that are selectively expressed by the pain-conducting sensory neurons. Subtypes of voltage-gated Na^+ and Ca^{2+} channels are targets of encouraging drug discovery efforts. Synaptic mechanisms of spinal cord and ascending pathways use the same molecular components as other central pathways, making it difficult to identify suitable drug targets. Many mechanisms have been identified that lead to powerful blockage of pain transmission, but their clinical utility is questionable because of the expected adverse effects.

An abundant number of animal models support the drug discovery projects in the pain area. For most forms of acute and chronic pain there are established pathways from animal studies, to initial investigations of experimental medicine, and to broader studies in the most prevalent medical conditions. Chronic neuropathic pain, caused by dysfunctions in the nervous system rather than sustained tissue damage, and migraine are special conditions with unique treatment and drug discovery efforts.

The pain area is a highly attractive and promising field for drug discovery. The detailed knowledge and the recent discovery of primary sensors offer ample opportunities as well as scientific challenges for the investigators.

REFERENCES

Further Reading

BALLANTYNE, J.C., and MAO, J. Opioid therapy for chronic pain. *N. Eng. J. Med.* 349: 1943–1953, 2003.

BESSON, J.M. The neurobiology of pain. *Lancet* 353: 1610–1615, 1999.

BURNSTOCK, G. P2X receptors in sensory neurons. *Br. J. Anesth.* 84: 476–488, 2000.

CLAPHAM, D.E. TRP channels as cellular sensors. *Nature* 426: 517–524, 2003.

FIELDS, H.L. *Pain.* McGraw-Hill, New York, 1987.

FITZGERALD, G.A. Cox-2 and beyond: Approaches to prostaglandin inhibition in human disease. *Nature Rev. Drug Disc.* 2: 879–890, 2003.

GOADSBY, P.J., LIPTON, R.B., and FERRARI, M.D. Migraine—Current understanding and treatment. *N. Eng. J. Med.* 346: 257–270, 2002.

HUNT, S.P., and MANTYH, P.W. The molecular dynamics of pain control. *Nature Rev. Neurosci.* 2: 83–91, 2001.

IVERSEN, L.L. Cannabis and the brain. *Brain* 126: 1252–1270, 2003.

KIEFFER, B.L., and GAVERIAUX-RUFF, C. Exploring the opioid system by gene knockout. *Prog. Neurobiol.* 66: 285–306, 2002.

KRISHTAL, O. The ASICs: Signaling molecules? Modulators? *Trends Neurosci.* 26: 477–483, 2003.

LE BARS, D., GOZARIU, M., and CADDEN, S.W. Animal models of nociception. *Pharmacol. Rev.* 53: 597–652, 2001.

LOESER, J.D., and MELZACK, R. Pain: an overview. *Lancet* 353: 1607–1609.

MENDELL, J.R., and SAHENK, Z. Painful sensory neuropathy. *N. Eng. J. Med.* 348: 1243–1255, 2003.

SAMAD, T.A., SAPRISTEIN, A., and WOOLF, C.J. Prostanoids and pain: Unraveling mechanism and revealing therapeutic targets. *Trends Mol. Med.* 8: 390–396, 2002.

SHAH, D.W.Y., OSSIPOV, M.H., and PORRECA, F. Neurotrophic factors as novel therapeutics for neuropathic pain. *Nature Rev. Drug Disc.* 2: 460–472, 2003.

STEIN, C., SCHÄFER, M., and MACHELSKA, H. Attacking pain at its source: New perspectives on opioids. *Nature Med.* 9: 1003–1008, 2003.

VARNEY, M.A., and GERAU, R.W. IV Metabotropic glutamate receptor involvement in models of acute and persistent pain: Prospects for the development of novel analgesics. *Curr. Drug Targ. CNS Neurol. Disord.* 1: 283–296, 2002.

ZADINA, J.E. Isolation and distribution of the endomorphins in the central nervous system. *Jpn. J. Pharmacol.* 89: 203–208, 2002.

Citations

ABO-SALEM, O.M., HAYALLAH, A.M., BILKEI-GORZO, A., FILIPEK, B., ZIMMER, A., and MÜLLER, C.E. Antinociceptive effects of novel A2B adenosine receptor antagonists. *J. Pharmacol. Exp. Ther.* 308: 358–366, 2004.

ALESSANDRI-HABER, N., DINA, O.A., YEH, J.J., PARADA, C.A., REICHLING, D.B., and LEVINE, J.D. Transient receptor potential vanilloid 4 is essential in chemotherapy-induced neuropathic pain in the rat. *J. Neurosci.* 24: 4444–4452, 2004.

CATERINA, M.J., LEFFLER, A., MALMBERG, A.B., MARTIN, W.J., TRAFTON, J., PETERSEN-ZEITZ, K.R., KOLTZENBURG, M., BASBAUM, A.I., and JULIUS, D. Impaired nociception and pain sensation in mice lacking the capsaicin receptor. *Science* 288: 306–313, 2001.

CLARE, J.J., TATE, S.N., NOBBS, M., and ROMANOS, M.A. Voltage-gated sodium channels as therapeutic targets. *Drug Disc. Today* 5: 506–520, 2000.

CLAIBORNE, C.F., MCCAULEY, J.A., LIBBY, B.E., CURTIS, N.R., DIGGLE, H.J., KULAGOWSKI, J.J., MICHELSON, S.R., ANDERSON, K.D., CLAREMON, D.A., FREIDINGER, R.M., BEDNAR, R.A., MOSSER, S.D., GAUL, S.L., CONNOLLY, T.M., CONDRA, C.L., BEDNAR, B., STUMP, G.L., LYNCH, J.J., MACAULAY, A., WAFFORD, K.A., KOBLAN, K.S., and LIVERTON, N.J. Orally efficacious NR2B-selective NMDA receptor antagonists. *Bioorg. Med. Chem. Lett.* 13: 697–700, 2003.

DIRIG, D.M., and YAKSH, T.L. In vitro prostandoid release from spinal cord following peripheral inflammation: Effects of substance P, NMDA and capsaicin. *Br. J. Pharmacol.* 126: 1333–1340, 1999.

DOODS, H., HALLERMAYER, G., WU, D., ENTZEROTH, M., RUDOLF, K., ENGEL, W., and EBERLEIN, W. Pharmacological profile of BIBN4096BS, the first selective small molecule CGRP antagonist. *Br. J. Pharmacol.* 129: 420–439, 2000.

HILL, R.G. NK1 (substance P) receptor antagonists—Why are they not analgesic in humans? *Trends Pharmacol. Sci.* 21: 244–246, 2000.

JARVIS, M.F., BURGARD, E.C., MCGARAUGHTY, S., HONORE, P., LYNCH, K., BRENNAN, T.J., SUBIETA, A., VAN BIESEN, T., CARTMELL, J., BIANCHI, B., NIFORATOS, W., KAGE, K., YU, H., MIKUSA, J., WISMER, C.T., ZHU, C.Z., CHU, K., LEE, C.H., STEWART, A.O., POLAKOWSKI, J., COX, B.F., KOWALUK, E., WILLIAMS, M., SULLIVAN, J., and FALTYNEK, C. A-317419, a novel potent and selective non-nucleotide antagonist of P2X3 and P2X2/3 receptors, reduces chronic inflammatory and neuropathic pain in the rat. *Proc. Natl. Acad. Sci. USA* 99: 17179–17184, 2002.

JI, R.R., SAMAD, T.A., JIN, S.X., SCHMOLL, R., and WOOLF, C.J. p38 MAPK activation by NGF in primary neurons after inflammation increases TRPV1 levels and maintains heat hyperalgesia. *Neuron* 36: 57–68, 2002.

JORDT, S.E., BAUTISTA, D.M., CHUANG, H., MCKEMY, D.D., ZYGMUNT, P.M., HÖGESTÄTT, E.D., MENG, I.D., and JULIUS, D. Mustard oils and cannabinoids excite sensory nerve fibers through the TRP channel ANKTM1. *Nature* 427: 260–265, 2004.

LAIRD, J.M.A., SOUSLOVA, V., WOOD, J.N., and CERVERO, F. Deficits in visceral pain and referred hyperalgesia in Nav1.8 (SNS/PN3)-null mice. *J. Neurosci.* 22: 8352–8356, 2002.

LUGER, N.M., SABINO, M.N., SCHWEI, M.J., MACH, D.B., POMONIS, J.D., KEYSER, K.P., RATHBURN, M., CLOHISY, D.R., HONORE, P., YAKSH, T.L., and MANTYH, P.W. Efficacy of morphine suggests a fundamental difference in the mechanisms that generate bone cancer vs. inflammatory pain. *Pain* 99: 397–406, 2002.

MASON, G.S., CUMBERBATCH, M.J., HILL, R.G., and RUPNIAK, N.M. The bradykinin B1 receptor antagonist B9858 inhibits a nociceptive spinal reflex in rabbits. *Can. J. Physiol. Pharmacol.* 80: 264–268, 2002.

MCMAHON, S.B., BENNETT, D.L., PRIESTLEY, J.V., and SHELTON, D.L. The biological effects of endogenous nerve growth factor on adult sensory neurons revealed by a trkA-IgG fusion molecule. *Nature Med.* 1: 774–780, 1995.

MOORE, P.K., and MARSHALL, M. Nitric oxide releasing acetaminophen (nitroacetaminophen). *Dig. Liver Dis.* (suppl. 2) 35: S49–60, 2003.

OH, S.B., TRAN, P.B., GILLARD, S.E., HURLEY, R.W., HAMMOND, D.L., and MILLER, R.J. Chemokines and glycoprotein 120 produce pain hypersensitivity by directly exciting primary nociceptive neurons. *J. Neurosci.* 21: 5027–5035, 2001.

POMONIS, J.D., HARRISON, J.E., MARK, L., BRISTOL, D.R., VALENZANO, K.J., and WALKER, K. N-(4-tertiarybutyl-phenyl)-4-(3-cholorphyridin-2-yl)tetrahydropyrazine-1(2H)-carbox-amine (BCTC), a novel, orally effective vanilloid receptor 1 antagonist with analgesic properties: II. In vivo characterization in rat models of inflammatory and neuropathic pain. *J. Pharmacol. Exp. Ther.* 306: 387–393, 2003.

PUNTAMBEKAR, P., VAN BUREN, J., RAISINGHANI, M., PREMKUMAR, L.S., and RAMKUMAR, V. Direct interaction of adenosine with the TRPV1 channel protein. *J. Neurosci.* 24: 3663–3671, 2004.

SAEGUSA, H., KURIHARA, T., ZONG, S., KAZUNO, A., MATSUDA, Y., NONAKA, T., HAN, W., TORIYAMA, H., and TANABE, T. Suppression of inflammatory and neuropathic pain symptoms in mice lacking the N-type Ca^{2+} channel. *EMBO J.* 20: 2349–2356, 2001.

SHIN, J., CHO, H., HWANG, S.W., JUNG, J., SHIN, C.Y., LEE, S.Y., KIM, S.H., LEE, M.G., CHOI, Y.H., KIM, J., HABER, N.A., REICHLING, D.B., KHASAR, S., LEVINE, J.D., and OH, U. Bradykinin-12-lipoxygenase-VR1 signaling pathway for inflammatory hyperalgesia. *Proc. Natl. Acad. Sci. USA* 99: 10150–10155, 2002.

STAATS, P.S., YEARWOOD, T., CHARAPATA, S.G., PRESLEY, R.W., WALLACE, M.S., BYAS-SMITH, M., FISHER, R., BRYCE, D.A., MANGIERI, E.A., LUTHER, R.R., MAYO, M.,

McGUIRE, D., and ELLIS, D. Intrathecal ziconotide in the treatment of refractory pain in patients with cancer or AIDS. *J. Am. Med. Assoc.* 291: 63–70, 2004.

STORY, G.M., PEIER, A.M., REEVE, A.J., EID, S.R., MOSBACHER, J., HRICIK, T.R., EARLE, T.J., HERGARDEN, A.C., ANDERSSON, D.A., HWANG, S.W., McINTYRE, P., JEGLA, T., BEVAN, S., and PATAPOUTIAN, A. ANKTM1, a TRP-like channel expressed in nociceptive neurons is activated by cold temperatures. *Cell* 112: 819–829, 2003.

TAGUCHI, A., SHARMA, N., SALEEM, R.M., SESSLER, D.I., CARPENTER, R.L., SEYEDSADR, M., and KURZ, A. Selective postoperative inhibition of gastrointestinal opioid receptors. *N. Engl. J. Med.* 345: 935–940, 2001.

TSUDA, M., MIZOKOSHI, A., SHIGEMOTO-MOGAMI, Y., KOIZUMI, S., and INOUE, K. Activation of p38 mitogen-activated protein kinase in spinal hyperactive microglia contributes to pain hypersensitivity following peripheral nerve injury. *Glia* 45: 89–95, 2004.

VAN DEN MAAGDENBERG, A.M.J.M., PIETROBON, D., PIZZORUSSO, T., KAJA, S., BROOS, L.A.M., CESETTI, T.,

VAN DE VEN, R.C.G., TOTTENE, A., VAN DER KAA, J., PLOMP, J.J., FRANTS, R.R., and FERRARI, M.D. A Cacna1a knockin migraine mouse model with increased susceptibility to cortical spreading depression. *Neuron* 41: 701–710, 2004.

WILLIAMSON, D.J., SHEPHEARD, S.L., HILL, R.G., and HARGREAVES, R.J. The novel anti-migraine agent rizatriptan inhibits neurogenic dural vasodilatation and extravasation. *Eur. J. Pharmacol.* 328: 61–64, 1997.

WOLF, G., YIRMIYA, R., GOSHEN, I., IVERFELDT, K., HOLMUND, L., TAKEDA, K., and SHAVIT, Y. Impairment of interleukin-1 (IL-1) signaling reduces basal pain sensitivity in mice: Genetic, pharmacological and developmental aspects. *Pain* 104: 471–480, 2003.

ZYLKA, M.J., DONG, X., SOUTHWELL, A.L., and ANDERSON, D.J. Atypical expansion in mice of the sensory neuronspecific Mrg G-protein-coupled receptor family. *Proc. Natl. Acad. Sci. USA* 100: 10043–10048, 2003.

Index

Drug Discovery for Nervous System Diseases, by Franz F. Hefti
ISBN 0-471-46563-1   Copyright © 2005 by John Wiley & Sons, Inc.

CPSIA information can be obtained
at www.ICGtesting.com
Printed in the USA
LVOW02s0510020716

494987LV00003B/4/P